Contents

List of contributors

David W. Altchek MD *Hospital for Special Surgery, 535 East 70th Street, New York, NY 10021, USA*

Per Bastholt RPT *F-06140 Vence, France*

Michael F. Bergeron PhD, FACSM *Assistant Professor of Pediatrics, Medical College of Georgia, Georgia Prevention Institute, HS-1640, Augusta, GA 30912-3710, USA*

Howard Brody PhD *Professor, Physics Department, University of Pennsylvania, 209 S. 33rd Street, Philadelphia, PA 19104-6396, USA*

Miguel Crespo PhD *International Tennis Federation, Tennis Development Department, Bank Lane, Roehampton, London SW15 5XZ, UK*

Jurgen Dess RPT *92318 Neumarkt, Germany*

Todd S. Ellenbecker MS, PT, SCS, CSCS *Physiotherapy Associates, Scottsdale Sports Clinic, 9449 N. 90th Street, Suite 100, Scottsdale, AZ 85258, USA*

Bruce C. Elliott PhD *Professor and Head, The Department of Human Movement and Exercise Science, The University of Western Australia, Stirling Highway, Crawley 6009, Australia*

Sue Fleshman PT, ATC *Sport Sciences and Medicine Department, Sanex WTA Tour, 133 First Street NE, St Petersburg, FL 33701, USA*

Karin G.M. Gerritsen MSc, PhD *Assistant Professor in Biomechanics, Department of Exercise Science and Physical Education, Arizona State University, Box 870404, Tempe, AZ 85287-0404, USA*

Joseph Keul MD, PhD (Deceased) *Medizinische Universitätsklinik, Rehabilitative/Präventive SportMedizin, Hugstetter Strasse 55, D-79106 Freiburg, Germany*

W. Ben Kibler MD, FACSM *Medical Director, Lexington Sports Medicine Center, 1221 S. Broadway, Lexington, KY 40504, USA*

Hartmut Krahl MD *Professor, Wörthstrasse 21, 81667 Munich, Germany*

Scott A. Lynch MD *Sports Medicine Section, Department of Orthopedics, Penn State University, Hershey Medical Center, PO Box 850, Hershey, PA 17033-0850, USA*

Ulf Michaelis MD *Department of Orthopaedic Surgery and Sports Medicine, Alfried Krupp Hospital, Alfried-Krupp-Strasse 21, D-45117 Essen, Germany*

Benno M. Nigg Dr sc. nat. *Director, Human Performance Laboratory, Faculty of Kinesiology, The University of Calgary, Calgary, Alberta, Canada*

Bill Norris ATC *Boca Raton, FL 33498, USA*

Moira O'Brien MD *Professor and Head, Anatomy Department, Trinity College, University of Dublin, Dublin 2, Ireland*

Hans-Gerd Pieper MD *Department of Orthopaedic Surgery and Sports Medicine, Alfried Krupp Hospital, Alfried-Krupp-Strasse 21, D-45117 Essen, Germany*

Babette Pluim MD, PhD *Koninklijke Nederlandse Lawn Tennis Bond, Sport Medisch Centrum Papendal, Papendallaan 60, 6816 VD Arnhem, The Netherlands*

Carsten B. Radas MD *Department of Out-patient Surgery, Orthopaedic Centre, St Josef-Stift, Westtor 7, D-48324 Sendenhorst, Germany*

Machar Reid BSc *ITF Assistant Research Officer, International Tennis Federation, Tennis Development Department, Bank Lane, Roehampton, London SW15 5XZ, UK*

Handbook of

Sports Medicine

and Science

Tennis

IOC Medical Commission Sub-Commission on Publications in the Sport Sciences

Howard G. Knuttgen PhD (Co-ordinator)
Boston, Massachusetts, USA

Francesco Conconi MD
Ferrara, Italy

Harm Kuipers MD, PhD
Maastricht, The Netherlands

Per A.F.H. Renström MD, PhD
Stockholm, Sweden

Handbook of
Sports Medicine
and Science
Tennis

EDITED BY

Per A.F.H. Renström

MD, PhD
Section of Sports Medicine
Department of Surgical Sciences
Karolinska Institutet
Stockholm
Sweden

Blackwell
Science

© 2002 by Blackwell Science Ltd
a Blackwell Publishing Company
Editorial Offices:
Osney Mead, Oxford OX2 0EL, UK
  Tel: +44 (0)1865 206206
Blackwell Science, Inc., 350 Main Street, Malden, MA 02148-5018, USA
  Tel: +1 781 388 8250
Blackwell Science Asia Pty, 54 University Street, Carlton, Victoria 3053, Australia
  Tel: +61 (0)3 9347 0300
Blackwell Wissenschafts Verlag, Kurfürstendamm 57, 10707 Berlin, Germany
  Tel: +49 (0)30 32 79 060

First published 2002

Library of Congress Cataloging-in-Publication Data

Tennis: handbook of sports medicine and science / edited by Per A.F.H. Renström.
        p. ; cm — (Handbook of sports medicine and science)
    Includes bibliographical references and index.
    ISBN 0-632-05034-9
    1. Tennis injuries—Handbooks, manuals, etc.   2. Tennis—Physiological
aspects—Handbooks, manuals, etc.   I. Renström, Per.   II. Series.
    [DNLM: 1. Tennis.   2. Athletic Injuries.   3. Sports Medicine. QT 260.5.T3 T311 2002]
    RC1220. T4 T46 2002
    617.1′027′08879634—dc21

                                                          2001052783

ISBN 0-632-05034-9

A catalogue record for this title is available from the British Library

Set in Melior by Graphicraft Limited, Hong Kong
Printed and bound in Great Britain at the Alden Press Ltd, Oxford and Northampton

For further information of Blackwell Science, visit our website:
www.blackwell-science.com

Per A.F.H. Renström MD, PhD *Professor, Section of Sports Medicine, Department of Surgical Sciences, Karolinska Institutet, SE-171 76, Stockholm, Sweden*

Arthur C. Rettig MD *Orthopedic Surgeon, Methodist Sports Medicine Center, Thomas A. Brady Clinic, Department of Education and Research, 1815 N. Capitol Avenue, Suite 560, Indianapolis, IN 46202, USA*

E. Paul Roetert PhD *Director of Administration, USA Tennis High Performance Program, 7310 Crandon Boulevard, Key Biscayne, FL 33149, USA*

Paul Settles *Director of Player Services, ATP Tennis International Headquarters, 201 ATP Tour Boulevard, Ponte Vedra Beach, FL 32082, USA*

Doug Spreen ATC *Terrace Park, OH 45174, USA*

Alex Stober RPT *90459 Nuremberg, Germany*

Kathleen A. Stroia MS, PT, ATC *Associate Vice President, Sport Sciences and Medicine Department, Sanex WTA Tour, 133 First Steet NE, St Petersburg, FL 33701, USA*

Robert S. Weinberg PhD *Professor and Chair, Department of Physical Education, Health and Sport Studies, 109 Phillips Hall, Miami University, Oxford, OH 45056-1675, USA*

Gary Windler MD *Sports Medicine Services, 321 Middleton Boulevard, Summerville, SC 29485-8027, USA*

Ian C. Wright MSc *Human Performance Laboratory, Faculty of Kinesiology, The University of Calgary, Calgary, Alberta, Canada*

Forewords by the IOC

The sport of tennis was one of the nine sports included for men participating in the Games of the I Olympiad as held in Athens in 1896. Men's tennis appeared in each of the following Olympic Games until the year 1924. Women's tennis competition in the Olympic Games was introduced in 1900 in Paris and continued until 1924, with the exception of 1904 in St Louis. Because of controversies related to the participation of amateur versus professional athletes, tennis disappeared from the Olympic programme for over 60 years until its reintroduction in 1988 in Seoul with a completely open competition.

Despite the extended hiatus, tennis must be recognized as having an important history within the Olympic programme. It is, therefore, entirely appropriate that this Handbook on the sport of tennis takes its rightful place among the other sports that have already appeared in the IOC Medical Commission series of Handbooks of Sports Medicine and Science.

My sincere appreciation goes to the Chairman of the IOC Medical Commission, Prince Alexandre de Merode, and to the IOC Medical Commission's Sub-commission on Publications in the Sport Sciences.

Dr Jacques Rogge
IOC President

Tracing its beginnings from games played some hundreds of years ago, the sport of tennis underwent major changes during the latter part of the 19th century. During the 20th century, the sport spread internationally and it is currently practised in virtually every country of the world.

Success in tennis requires a tremendous amount of physiological variables. These variables are further supplemented by the needs for proper nutrition, hydration, strategy, and being psychologically prepared. Developments in both sports medicine and sports science during the last 50 years have resulted in stronger, faster, better skilled tennis players who are utilizing the most efficient and effective equipment that the engineers and biomechanists can design. With the enhanced challenges and stresses to the human body, injury prevention and injury rehabilitation have become important issues for sports medicine physicians, health personnel, and coaches.

Our thanks go to Professor Per Renström and the contributing authors for this Handbook on Tennis who have collaborated to produce an up-to-date and complete coverage for all of the biomechanical, biological and clinical aspects of tennis play. This publication will prove to be an invaluable reference for everyone involved with the game of tennis.

Prince Alexandre de Merode
Chairman, IOC Medical Commission

Forewords by the ITF, ATP, WTA and STMS

Foreword by the International Tennis Federation

Tennis is a sport for all ages and requires speed, dexterity and endurance, especially at the professional level. Tennis is also an intellectual sport that requires court sense and strategic thinking. At the highest level, the professional tennis player competes nearly every week of the year, requiring fitness levels that are very high and an ability to play with consistency on a variety of surfaces at locations around the world.

The International Tennis Federation (ITF) takes pride in its leadership of the Joint Tennis Anti-Doping Programme in conjunction with the ATP and the WTA Tour. The ITF's Sports Medical Commission is pro-active in studying all areas that pertain to the overall health of tennis players. These areas include physiology, nutrition, bio-mechanics, the effect of the evolution of equipment on players, mental preparation and other specific issues such as jet lag, altitude, heat and humidity and the effects of playing tennis at a very young age.

The ITF, the world governing body of tennis, welcomes the *Handbook on Tennis*. This book, with contributions from international scientists and experts, will prove to be a very useful tool, a comprehensive guide to sports medicine as it pertains to tennis.

Francesco Ricci Bitti
President, ITF

Foreword by the Association of Tennis Professionals

One doesn't immediately think of professional tennis when considering the most physically demanding sports. Until, that is, one considers that the professional tennis season spans eleven months and is played on six continents in over 50 countries on a variety of playing surfaces—from carpet to hard courts to grass and clay. Until one considers that the average match lasts 1 1/2 to 2 hours and may last as long as four; that players may have to compete as many as 5 days in a row, sometimes with two matches a day, before getting a day off. Take a look at the teeming activity that is the training room on day one of an ATP tournament and you will have a sense for how physically demanding professional tennis can be.

Those of us on the ATP Medical Services Committee are increasingly aware of the physical demands placed on professional tennis players and the importance of providing the highest standards of medical care for them on a tournament-by-tournament basis. Whether you are a player, coach, athletic trainer, physiotherapist, or physician, we hope that this handbook will provide some insight into the most common tennis medical problems of professional tennis players, as well as the preferred treatment protocols recommended by ATP Medical Services personnel.

Paul Settles
Director of Player Services

Foreword by the Women's Tennis Association

Tennis presents unique challenges with one-on-one competition, typified by its demand for total athleticism, and necessitating the mental and physical strength to sustain an eleven month season that spans the globe.

In order to remain in the game and at a high level of competition, professional tennis players must utilize and incorporate the latest trends in sports medicine. The IOC *Handbook on Tennis* identifies and outlines the steps every elite tennis player must take in order to excel, a daunting but invaluable undertaking. A resource has been created that allows the tennis community (coaches, players, physiotherapists, physicians, certified athletic trainers, etc.) to access and apply the principles of tennis medicine in the creation and advancement of a successful professional tennis player.

On behalf of the Sanex WTA Tour and its group of sports sciences and medicine experts, it is my honor to be able to share our pleasure associated with the publication of this book and we look forward to the positive repercussions it will have in the game of tennis; truly a sport for a lifetime.

Kathleen A. Stroia
Director of Sports Sciences and Medicine, WTA

Foreword by the Society for Tennis Medicine and Science

The STMS was founded in 1990 to promote, educate and disseminate information about medicine and science in tennis. The STMS has initiated a newsletter which is now distributed worldwide as a joint newsletter with the ITF, ATP and Sanex WTA. The STMS also organizes courses regularly every year in the field of medicine and science in tennis, including management of injuries and medical problems in tennis.

There is a great demand in tennis for this kind of handbook. Because of increasing pressures and intensity, there is a heightened risk of injury and other medical problems. Therefore, the STMS feels that this handbook is essential reading and congratulates the IOC for its initiative in producing this publication.

Per A.F.H. Renström
President, STMS

Preface

Tennis is a truly international sport enjoyed by millions of people of all ages around the world. The players experience tennis as an exhilarating game resulting not only in stimulating competition but also in conditioning, general health benefits and camaraderie. For spectators, tennis is one of the most exciting and popular sports, not the least because of its ingenious scoring system. Because of this, a tennis match can be very dramatic and ever changing like a theatrical production by Shakespeare. A player can at some point seem to have lost a match but, in the end, emerge as the winner after three to five intensive sets.

At the top competitive levels, tennis can be a very demanding sport, both physically and mentally. Regular participation in the sport provides excellent cardiovascular exercise, improves the body's general functional capacity, and promotes both coordination and balance. This is of special importance for older tennis players. Tennis is definitely a sport for all ages, from 3 to 103 years old.

The sport of tennis provides an all-round game with quick starts and stops, repetitive overhead motions, and involvement of all the muscles of the body. During the last 10 to 20 years, the game of tennis has developed enormously as facilitated by the new designs for rackets and other equipment and new playing techniques, with special reference to serving. Training methods have also improved. The players at the top level are now stronger and faster than ever before. The rackets are larger, wider and stiffer, allowing for serve velocities of greater than 200 kilometres per hour (130 miles per hour). The players are playing much more from the back court with an open stance that permits the generation of greater forces. The game is much more intense and demanding as compared to 10 years ago.

A major concern for the sport is the extended length of the season for top-level tennis players. Tournaments are offered during 10 months of the year and this allows little time for recovery and basic training. Few other sports have such a lengthy season. Another risk factor may be the conduct of tournaments on different surfaces, including hard court, clay and grass. The shift from one surface to another may very well be the cause of a number of injury problems, especially when changing from a clay surface to a hard court with high friction.

The increasing intensity of the game and the associated physical demands also involve an increased risk of injury and other medical problems. The ATP, Sanex WTA and ITF provide excellent medical services by assigning well-educated and specialized physiotherapists and/or athletic trainers to all major tournaments around the world. Well-qualified medical doctors are also available at all the tournaments for top players. The medical services provided in tennis on a worldwide basis are probably the best any international sport can offer. The ITF has founded a medical and science committee that reviews and coordinates the medical and scientific concerns in tennis. The Society for Tennis Medicine and Science (STMS) provides education and disseminates information through newsletters and conferences in cooperation with the other international organizations. Top-level tennis players are presently offered excellent medical services but, as always, further improvement is possible, especially for the players below top level and for recreational players.

This IOC Handbook on the medicine and science of tennis should constitute a valuable reference in the effort to improve the information available to tennis players at all levels of competition. The aim of this publication is to provide all tennis players, their coaches and the associated health care personnel with an authoritative reference in which basic information is described in a clear format concerning common injuries and medical problems that can be sustained during tennis play. The available information in this book can then aid them in considering what kind of immediate, short-term or long-term treatment is available, leading to the decision as to the necessity of consulting a medical doctor.

The contributors to this book have been chosen from the outstanding experts in the field of tennis medicine and science. They are all experienced in participating in the many sports medicine/sports science conferences and meetings organized by the STMS, ATP, Sanex WTA and ITF. The Handbook leads off with a description of the biomechanics in tennis and an evaluation of the different strokes in tennis as contributed by an internationally recognized expert in this area, Bruce Elliott from Australia. Different aspects of the racket and the ball are then discussed by Howard Brody, the ITF's recognized expert in this field, who has completed extensive research in this area. An evaluation of shoes and their relation to the playing surface is discussed by Karin Gerritsen.

Michael Bergeron discusses current research information regarding the physiological and nutritional demands of tennis as well as the risks involved with playing in the heat. Babette Pluim, editor of the STMS Newsletter and a leading tennis physician, has written about the medical concerns in tennis. Moira O'Brien presents her views on the problems experienced during international travel.

Physical conditioning for tennis becomes more and more important each year. Paul Roetert and Todd Ellenbecker, who have worked for many years with the United States Tennis Association (USTA), present their views on strength and flexibility training, conditioning and physiological preparation. Younger players experience increasing injury problems and their specific problems are discussed by Ben Kibler, who is former president of the STMS and current member of USTA's medical committee. He includes a discussion of the background (pathophysiology) for tennis injuries and the rehabilitation principles after injuries have occurred with the aim of returning players to competitive play as quickly as possible following an injury.

The various injury problems are described by persons with extensive experience in the field.

David Altchek, who is ATP medical director and the US Davis Cup physician, has described current management of shoulder injuries which has become an increasing problem in tennis. Hartmut Krahl, a former medical director of the ATP and his coworkers from the ATP tournament in Essen, have discussed how to manage back problems. Arthur Rettig, the medical doctor for the Indianapolis ATP Tournament, has presented his views on the management of hand and wrist problems. The undersigned has, in cooperation with Scott Lynch, discussed knee, lower leg, ankle and foot problems as well as elbow problems in tennis. Tennis is very much a sport where a strong mind is very important. The psychological aspects of tennis competition have, therefore, been discussed by Robert Weinberg.

As mentioned above, the medical services offered to the top-level tennis players by the ATP, Sanex WTA and ITF at every tournement are of the highest quality and rather unique in international sports. In two chapters, these organizations describe their activities in the field.

It is an honour to have been invited by the IOC to coordinate this project. We are very grateful that so many of the leading experts in tennis medicine and science have been willing to share their expertise and advice with us. I would also like to thank Sue Mattingley, Julie Elliott and Nick Morgan of Blackwell Publishing for their administrative help, editorial assistance and patience throughout the time-consuming work in the production of this book. Many thanks also to Professor Howard G. Knuttgen for his strong support along the way.

It is our sincere hope that this book will be of value to all persons involved with the sport of tennis and, especially, to the players of all ages and at all levels of competition around the world.

Per A.F.H. Renström, MD, PhD
Stockholm 2001

Chapter 1

Biomechanics of tennis

Introduction

As the term suggests, biomechanics involves a study of the structure and function of the human body using mechanics. Biomechanics of tennis therefore deals with the mechanical basis of tennis, with particular emphasis on the techniques used in stroke production. The criterion measure in tennis, that is successful performance in an injury-free environment, makes it imperative that coaches and medical/paramedical personnel have an understanding of biomechanics.

The primary objective of a coach should be to develop 'good technique'. The coach who has an understanding of biomechanics can integrate the personal characteristics of the player with sound stroke mechanics to develop skills that suit the individual. Sports science and sports medicine personnel use these individual player characteristics to structure appropriate training and rehabilitation programmes.

The individualized mechanical model for performance must be developed with consideration of four broad areas.

1 *Past experiences of the coach.* Years of coaching or experiences as a player may have led a coach for example to the conclusion that a semi-western or western forehand grip should be adopted in preference to a continental grip when hitting a topspin forehand drive.

2 *The individual characteristics of the player.* The physical characteristics (e.g. lack of strength) or flair of a player may dictate that a particular technique be considered when deciding what should be learned (e.g. double-handed backhand).

3 *The current techniques used by champion players.* High-speed forehand drives that clear the net with a margin for error are an accepted example of modern technique. Coaches must therefore decide when they should teach the multisegment topspin forehand, used by a majority of leading professionals. In the multisegment forehand, the individual segments of the upper limb move relative to each other in a coordinated manner to produce a high racket speed. The alternative to this stroke is the forehand where the whole arm swings forward predominantly as a single unit.

4 *The biomechanical basis of stroke production.* The time of contact between the ball and the strings, a biomechanical consideration in stroke production, varies minimally (5 ms) irrespective of string tension. The movement of the racket and ball together with a vertical racket face at impact are therefore the key mechanical determinants of a successful topspin groundstroke.

This chapter will be divided into three sections. The first, reviews a number of general biomechanical factors that influence stroke production, while the second section deals with research specific to each of the strokes. The third section is on the analysis of technique, a key factor in the successful modification of stroke production. Chapter 2 deals with biomechanical considerations of equipment design and tennis.

General mechanical factors

The following mechanical factors are common to all tennis strokes and as such should be treated separately to a discussion of individual stroke production.

Time of ball contact

The time of contact between the ball and the strings varies minimally from 3 to 6 ms (Plagenhoef 1979; Brody 1987). No other fact has had more influence on the game, as it is not possible (within the laws of the game) to significantly alter this time. The racket must therefore be in the desired position at impact, so that the relative path and speed of both the racket and ball determine the type and amount of spin imparted, rather than any sudden movement that is attempted while the ball is in contact with the strings. (Speed is used interchangeably with velocity for ease of reading.)

Grip firmness

Tennis coaches believe that grip firmness at impact is generally critical to success in stroke production. Studies featuring *central* impacts, using a number of different experimental designs (propelling or dropping balls at freestanding or clamped stationary or swinging rackets) show that rebound ball speed is *not* significantly affected by the level of grip pressure (Elliott 1982; Grabiner *et al.* 1983; Missavage *et al.* 1984; Knudson 1989). Theoretical support for this result is provided by Liu (1983), whose model predicted that the rebound coefficient (ball speed postimpact/ball speed preimpact) is principally a function of the elastic nature of the impact between the ball and strings, which is practically independent of the condition of grip firmness.

A *decrease* in rebound coefficient was generally reported for *off-centre* impacts. Hatze (1976) reported that theoretically, an off-centre impact would be accompanied by an increase in racket recoil, which decreased postimpact ball speed. Plagenhoef (1979) using photography and an instrumented racket reported that the further away an impact occurred perpendicular to the long axis (from the centre), the lower was the rebound coefficient (2.5 cm, 15% reduction; 5.0 cm, 40% reduction). Postimpact ball speeds were less affected by off-centre impacts along the long axis, where reductions of only 10% were reported for impacts near the end of the racket compared to speeds for central impacts. These reductions in rebound speed were accompanied by increases in the forces transmitted to the hand (Plagenhoef 1979; Elliott 1982).

Higher off-centre rebound coefficients were associated with an increase in grip pressure (Elliott 1982). An approximate 20% increase in rebound coefficient was reported (approx. 0.47–0.57) for a change from a 'light to tight' grip for off-centre impacts, whereas central impacts increased to a lesser degree (0.64–0.69) (Elliott 1982). Grabiner *et al.* (1983) also investigated the relationship between resistance to rotation (about the long axis) and postimpact ball speed following off-centre impacts. They reported no significant differences between postimpact ball speed for two extreme conditions of grip firmness (maximal pressure clamped and free standing). However, they suggested that this result may have been influenced by the closing speed of both ball and racket (addition of speed of the ball and racket irrespective of direction) rather than the influence of grip firmness. Significant increases in rebound coefficients for an increase in grip pressure, particularly for off-centre impacts, were reported for closing speeds more closely related to match conditions (30 m·s^{-1}, Elliott 1982; 38 m·s^{-1}, Plagenhoef 1979) whereas at a lower closing speed (10.6 m·s^{-1}, Grabiner *et al.* 1983) no significant increase was reported.

The generation of racket speed

Coaches are continually posed the question of how to enable their pupils to develop more power in their stroke production, that is hit the ball with a higher forward speed, while still maintaining an acceptable level of control. Recent changes in stroke technique (e.g. service, Elliott *et al.* 1995; forehand, Elliott *et al.* 1989a) have further caused them to ponder if/when selected aspects of stroke production should be taught to young players. This section provides a framework for coaches to assess changes in technique associated with the development of high-speed stroke production.

The use of elastic energy

'Prepare early' is a phrase commonly used by coaches. The logic behind such a statement is that for the ball to be hit at the appropriate time and not 'late' requires this early preparation. The question then arises as to whether performance is in fact hindered by this early preparation, as elastic energy stored during the 'stretch cycle' of the movement may not be of benefit during the 'shorten cycle' of the activity. This stretch–shorten cycle is observed in tennis as a counter-movement during the racket backswing or movement preparation phase (i.e. bending of the legs during the split step in a volley) that precedes the actual forwardswing of the racket (external followed by internal rotation of the upper arm) or movement to the ball (the shortening phase).

The theory underlying the use of elastic energy in stretch–shorten cycle activities is a relatively simple process. During the stretch phase (eccentric contraction) the muscles, tendons and associated tissue are actually stretched and store elastic energy.

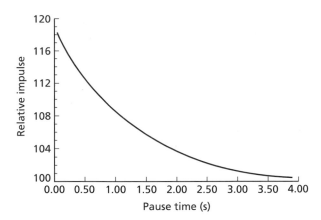

Fig. 1.1 Loss of elastic energy with increase in pause time. (Modified from Wilson *et al.* 1991.)

On movement reversal, during the shortening phase, the stretched muscles (which are in a better position to produce force) and tendons recoil back to their original shape and in so doing a portion of the stored energy is recovered and assists the movement. Research has shown that the use of elastic energy is reduced if a delay occurs between the stretch and shorten cycles of an upper limb movement (Wilson *et al.* 1991) (see Fig. 1.1). In the upper limb, after a period of approximately 1 s, 55% of the stored energy is lost; after 2 s, 80% of the stored energy is lost; and after a 4-s delay all stored energy is lost.

The recovery of this stored energy tends to occur relatively quickly and is thus of major benefit early in the forwardswing phase of the stroke or in the movement to the ball (Wilson *et al.* 1991). This is of major benefit to young children, who need the assistance of this energy source, to overcome the inertia (swing weight) of the racket during the early section of the forwardswing of for instance the forehand or serve.

Speed of movement around the court is also related to the ability to 'use elastic energy'. Groppel (1984) wrote: 'regardless of the position a skilled player assumes while awaiting the opponent's shot, upon or just prior to impact by the opponent, the player will unweight'. As the player flexes at the knees (accelerates downward) the reaction force from the court is lowered (unweighted). This unweighting is an integral part of tennis movement, whether it be before a return of serve, moving to position

for a groundstroke or as part of the split step in serve–volley and approach shot–volley play. The rapid flexion of the knees must obviously be controlled, otherwise the body would drop into a full squat position. This stopping of the downward movement has been shown to apply stretch to the muscles and other tissues of the lower limbs, which results in the storage of energy. This stored energy may then at least partially, if the movement of knee flexion is quickly followed by knee extension, be used to assist the lower limb drive in moving a player to the ball. Knee extension and the acceleration of the body upward increases the reaction force from the court and therefore allows the players to drive in the direction of the next stroke.

The distance over which racket speed can be developed

One of the main reasons of having a backswing is to increase the distance over which racket speed can be developed during the forwardswing to the ball. In a *straight backswing* (often taught to beginners), the racket is taken back in a relatively straight line, before stopping in the backswing position, prior to swinging forward to the ball. This type of backswing, which is easy to learn, is very good in developing ball *control*. It may even use some of the elastic energy stored during the stretch cycle. However, the distance the racket moves forward to the ball is often not sufficient to allow the development of a high racket speed at impact.

The *looped backswing* was introduced in ground-strokes (it has always been used in the serve) to increase the distance over which racket speed could be developed during the forwardswing to the ball. In the service action, the racket is kept away from the body when 'looped' behind the back (Fig. 1.2), which effectively increases the distance over which the player can develop racket speed when swinging up to the ball.

The *looped backswing* requires more coordination than the straight backswing and therefore control may suffer initially. However, once correctly developed this form of backswing allows for the production of greater racket speed and therefore more power in stroke production as compared to the straight back-swing. If a pause is required between backswing and

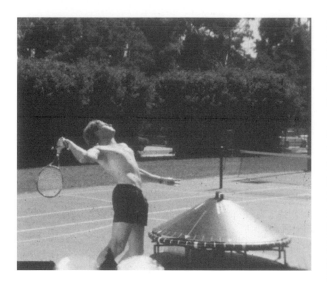

Fig. 1.2 The backswing position in the service action.

forwardswing phases of the groundstroke then the racket should stop near the top of the loop to increase the distance over which racket speed can be generated for impact. Research has shown that 2.7 m·s^{-1} of extra speed was generated with an increase of only 30 cm of racket drop during a looped forwardswing.

The use of coordinated movements

In tennis, where a high racket speed is generally required, a number of body segments must be coordinated if success is to occur. The motion of segments in high-speed tennis strokes is generally sequenced in a proximal-to-distal fashion. One of the most popular principles underlying the description of this sequencing is the 'summation of speed' principle. This concept suggests that the speed of the distal end of a linked sequence (the racket) is built up by summing the individual speeds of all segments participating in this sequence, although the principle does not provide a mechanical explanation of how this is achieved. It is generally believed that joint rotational speed data provide the clearest description of proximal-to-distal sequencing. Furthermore, these data enable coaches to visualize a movement, as motion is generally characterized as a series of coordinated segment rotations. Figure 1.3 shows how these joint rotations influence segment end

points during the forehand drive. The only joint movement that has been shown to occur very late in the forwardswing (and therefore not in proximal-to-distal sequencing) for the service (Elliott *et al.* 1995) and forehand strokes (Elliott *et al.* 1997) is internal rotation of the upper arm.

Recent developments in forehand and backhand stroke production have created some concern among coaches. The need for greater trunk rotation and the use of individual segments of the upper limb (arm, forearm and hand) in an attempt to generate a higher racket speed has created a need for changes in coaching methodologies. The extension at the elbow joint during the forwardswing of a backhand drive (note flexed elbow in Fig. 1.4) increases the racket speed at impact. Rotation of the trunk and shoulders in the backhand not only increases the distance over which the racket can generate speed but also adds another segment to the total movement (the trunk) that if coordinated with upper limb movements can assist in building racket speed.

In the serve, a 'leg drive' and 'body rotation', just to name two segments, are essential features of stroke technique. Most coaching texts include a section that deals with the flow or summation effect in the service action (as shown below), which leads to optimal racket speed at impact.

Leg drive + Trunk rotation + Upper arm elevation + Forearm extension + Upper arm internal rotation, forearm pronation and hand flexion

The role of muscle strength and endurance

The relationship between selected physical capacities such as muscle strength and performance is relatively easy to assess in sports such as weightlifting. However, such a relationship is very difficult to quantify in tennis. Varied relationships have been found between muscle strength and serving speed (Ellenbecker 1989), although more recently Kleinöder (1990) showed that a specifically designed exercise programme can improve racket speed. A prospective study by Elliott *et al.* (1990) was not able to predict with any certainty those physiological (fitness) or kinanthropometric (physical capacities) variables that would allow superior tennis performance to be identified for 11-, 13- and 15-years-olds. Players must obviously

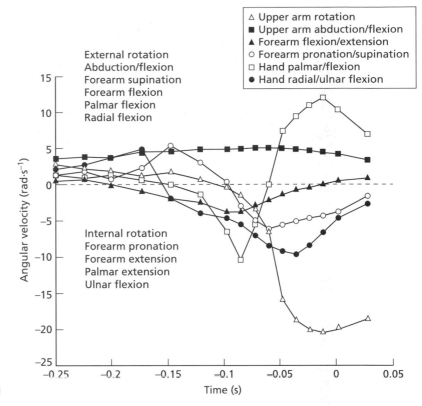

External rotation
Abduction/flexion
Forearm supination
Forearm flexion
Palmar flexion
Radial flexion

Internal rotation
Forearm pronation
Forearm extension
Palmar extension
Ulnar flexion

Legend:
△ Upper arm rotation
■ Upper arm abduction/flexion
▲ Forearm flexion/extension
○ Forearm pronation/supination
□ Hand palmar/flexion
● Hand radial/ulnar flexion

Fig. 1.3 Summation of segment velocities (speed) in the tennis forehand. (From Takahashi *et al.* 1996.)

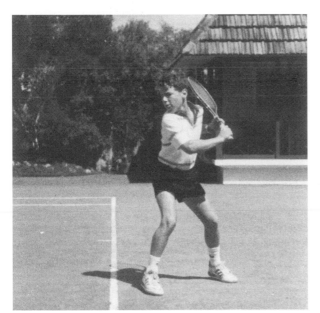

Fig. 1.4 The backswing position in the backhand drive.

develop sufficient muscle strength and endurance to perform effectively in a long match. An increase in muscle strength means that a lesser percentage of total strength is needed for each movement, which may assist in the ability to repeat the performance and protect the body from injury. Strength development is certainly needed for instance in the shoulder region, not only to produce the high upper arm rotational values for stroke production but also to protect the region from injury.

The role of equipment design

Readers are referred to the chapter on the tennis racket to further appreciate how changes in design and string tension may alter postimpact ball speed.

Margin for error and rally speed

An understanding of the concept of 'margins of error' is essential for any coach attempting to develop

Table 1.1 Error margins for a groundstroke hit with different levels of spin and speed. (Modified from Brody 1987.)

	80 km·h⁻¹ (50 mph)	108 km·h⁻¹ (67 mph)	120 km·h⁻¹ (75 mph)
No spin	9.0°	3.4°	2.0°
Backspin	5.0°	1.2°	0.0°
Topspin	10.5°	5.8°	4.0°

Approximate values for waist-height impacts.

Table 1.2 Error margins for a service hit at varying heights and speeds. (Modified from Brody 1987.)

Height	108 km·h⁻¹ (67 mph)	145 km·h⁻¹ (90 mph)	180 km·h⁻¹ (112 mph)
2.03 m (80 inches)	1.9	0.6	0.0
2.54 m (100 inches)	2.6	1.4	0.8
3.05 m (120 inches)	3.5	2.1	1.6

Approximate values for a flat service technique.

high-performance players. Brody (1987) provides a very comprehensive coverage of this and other tennis topics.

Spin and rally speed

Many players who are capable of rallying at a given level often experience a loss of control when attempting to hit the ball harder or when required to rally with a better player. The vertical error margin (the difference in the angle the ball leaves the racket for a shot that will just clear the net to the one that clears the net easily and lands on the baseline) is reduced as ball speed increases (Table 1.1) (Brody 1987). Backspin also reduces this margin for error, particularly if a player hits the ball with 'power', while topspin increases the margin for error. The relative importance of topspin increases for an increase in ball speed.

Success as a function of height in the serve

It is evident from Table 1.2 that if a player wishes to develop a high-speed service, it is also necessary to impact the ball as high as possible from the court. A near fully extended body and a good 'leg drive' such that the body is off the ground at impact will obviously enhance service technique. For instance a ball hit 2.03 m from the court's surface has no chance of success if hit at 180 km·h⁻¹. Brody (1987) also demonstrated through computer simulation that success rate improved if the ball was hit with some forward rotation (usually a combination of topspin and sidespin).

Horizontal errors and ball speed in groundstrokes

Although many coaches emphasize stance as a key determinant in postimpact ball direction, the real factors that must be considered are: the angle of the racket face and direction of the racket speed. Stance of course may affect both these factors. The poorer a player's timing the larger the angular error. If a ball leaves the strings at an angle of 6.5° from its aimed direction, it will end up approximately 2.75 m horizontally (at the baseline) away from the point at which it was aimed (Brody 1987). Table 1.3 clearly shows that the effect of horizontal angular error (error in racket angle compared to aiming point) decreases as a function of racket speed. However, it is important for coaches to also understand that the differences at high speeds are not as large as those in the lower range. Therefore, if blocking a return of service (close to 0 m·s⁻¹ racket speed), aim more for the central

Table 1.3 Horizontal angular error as a function of racket speed. (Modified from Brody 1987.)

Racket speed (m·s⁻¹)	Angle of deviation (°)
0 (0 ft·s⁻¹)	20.0
9 (30 ft·s⁻¹)	8.0
18 (60 ft·s⁻¹)	5.8
27 (90 ft·s⁻¹)	4.0

Approximate values for a preimpact ball angle of 20° to the racket direction at a speed of 18 m s⁻¹ (40 mph).

region of the court, and if attempting a passing shot always swing at the speed 'grooved during practice'. A lower speed (often mistakenly adopted to improve accuracy) will increase the effect of any error in the angle the ball leaves the racket and often leads to the ball landing out of court.

Stroke production

This section reviews the scientific literature with reference to the key mechanical factors in effective stroke production. The need to present general mechanical principles to beginners (in an appropriate manner) and certainly to college-age students or above, has been shown to be beneficial to learning. For a comprehensive understanding of stroke technique this section must be read in conjunction with the coaching literature. Specific conclusions will be drawn from the literature where this is possible; however, coaching theory based on subjective opinion will not be included.

The serve

The service action is not only the most studied stroke in tennis but is also the most strenuous, and as such a sound biomechanical basis is critical to performance. Coaches must pay specific attention to the physical characteristics of the player, along with the key mechanical features needed to develop a rhythmic action. Because of the complexity of the shot, the key mechanical factors in the service action will be presented under separate headings.

The ball toss

The height the ball should be 'pushed' using the 'straight forwards and up' or the 'rotary style' is the first service skill to be mastered. An analysis of players at the Atlanta Olympics showed that the toss was positioned such that it was in front and marginally to the left of the front foot at impact (Chow et al. 1999). High-speed photography has been used to show that many elite performers impact the ball after it has begun to drop (2.5–20.0 cm). It has been calculated that when impact occurs at the top of its flight, a player has eight times the amount of time to contact the ball (stationary ball) than when the ball is hit after

falling 1.2 m. In this situation the player has to contact a target moving at approximately 5 m·s^{-1}.

The swing to impact

Although coaching books provide guidance, weight distribution, along with the initial positioning of the feet, tends to be modified by personal preference. During the backswing the body weight initially moves back, then forwards such that at contact the vertical line from the centre of gravity (the hips) is approximately 25 cm and 40 cm forwards of the front toe in the flat and slice serves, respectively.

What movements then drive the hitting shoulder forwards and upwards for impact? Different serving techniques, with reference to movement of the feet, produce different mechanical characteristics (Elliott & Wood 1983).
• The foot-up style: this technique produces greater vertical forces over time, which results in a higher impact position and a better up-and-out racket trajectory when compared to the foot-back style.
• The foot-back style: this technique produces larger horizontal forces during the drive phase than the foot-up style and may therefore be more conducive to rapid movement to the net, following the serve.

Players may choose either style and then concentrate on eliminating weaknesses and enhancing strengths of each technique. An efficient service action was characterized by negligible side-to-side forces, and small forward forces during the preparatory phase (van Gheluwe & Hebbelinck 1986). Vertical forces should be such that the body is 'driven off the ground' for impact (Elliott & Wood 1983; van Gheluwe & Hebbelinck 1986). This lower limb drive, together with trunk rotation (Fig. 1.5a–d), then produce a forward speed of the shoulder that represents approximately 10–20% of the racket speed at impact for high-performance players (Elliott et al. 1986, 1995; van Gheluwe & Hebbelinck 1986). As the lower limb action also drives the racket 'down behind the back' this movement together with trunk rotation (to drive the racket away from the body) are key mechanical characteristics of the service action.

Research has very recently supported a commonly held view by coaches on the role of trunk rotation in the serve (Bahamonde 2000). Trunk rotations in the three planes are observed in the period prior to impact.

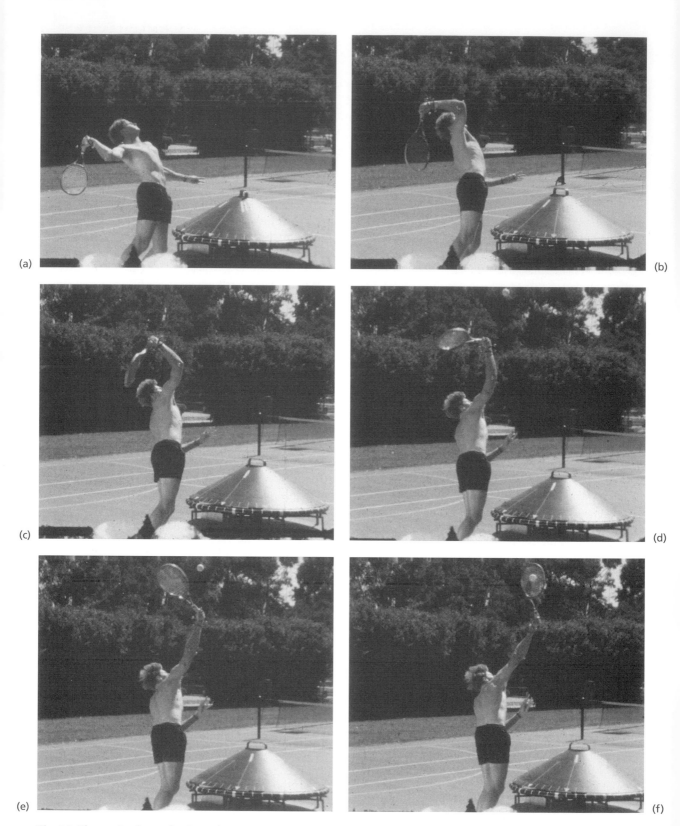

Fig. 1.5 The service forwardswing to impact.

• Minor levels of rotation about the long axis of the body help drive the racket backwards.

• Shoulder-over-shoulder rotation (cartwheel action) produces momentum that drives the racket away from the body and prepares it for impact.

• Forward rotation (somersault action) allows the player to produce angular momentum which is shifted from the trunk, to the arm, and finally to the racket.

The rotations of the upper arm, forearm and hand account for the remaining 80–90% of racket-head speed at impact. Forwards and upwards movement of the upper arm (Fig. 1.5a–c) produce approximately 15% of forward impact racket speed.

Internal rotation of the upper arm, which occurs very late in the forwardswing (Fig. 1.5c–e) accounts for approximately 40–50% of the impact speed of the racket (van Gheluwe et al. 1987; Elliott et al. 1995). Bahamonde (1997) and Noffal and Elliott (1998) showed in the flat and slice serves that the internal rotator muscles stretched eccentrically (to store elastic energy) prior to contracting to cause the vigorous internal rotation of the upper arm. A number of papers have previously shown that muscle activity was evident in the upper arm internal rotator musculature prior to impact (Miyashita et al. 1979; van Gheluwe & Hebbelinck 1986). Chandler et al. (1992), in testing muscle strength and power in a simulated tennis service action, reported 25% higher values for the internal rotator muscles of the upper arm for the preferred compared to the non-preferred upper limbs. Upper arm internal rotation is therefore a key mechanical factor in the service action and both on- and off-court training must pay particular attention to this movement.

As the upper trunk (shoulders) vigorously rotates in the early part of the serve, the upper limb trails, such that the internal rotators (as previously discussed) and elbow muscles and tissue are 'put on stretch'. While this may enhance performance, it also creates a high level of valgus (outward) stress at the elbow (Bahamonde 1997; Noffal & Elliott 1998). Care must be taken in this aspect of the service action or injury may occur.

Forearm pronation and extension (Fig. 1.5b–e), both important features of the service action, then position the racket for impact rather than assist in the generation of racket speed. While elbow extension is relatively high prior to impact, upper arm internal rotation causes elbow extension to move the racket sideways rather than forwards at impact. Any conscious action to vigorously extend the elbow near impact is therefore wasted effort.

Hand palmar (forward) flexion and ulnar flexion (side) are the last movements in the service action (Fig. 1.5d–f). Together they produce approximately 30% of the forward speed of the racket, a factor that has previously been identified by Deporte et al. (1990). The importance of wrist movement has been supported by electromyographic studies of forearm and hand musculature immediately prior to and at impact. Action about the wrist joint is therefore an important aspect of service mechanics.

At impact (Fig. 1.5f) the body should be almost fully extended to increase the height of impact. The racket should be marginally angled to the court, as it does not form a vertical line with the wrist (impact occurs with the ball in line with the front foot requiring the shoulders to be angled to the court). In baseball pitching, Matsuo et al. (2000) showed that maximum velocity and minimum stress at the shoulder and elbow joints occurred when the upper arm–trunk angle was approximately 100°. To achieve this angle in the serve requires a lateral tilt of the trunk at impact. Remember a good 'leg drive' will normally mean that impact occurs in the air.

Racket trajectory immediately prior to and following impact

Research has shown that a high-speed service is seldom hit with no forward rotation, because the height of impact for players of average stature is too low to produce a successful outcome (Elliott 1983; Brody 1987). Braden and Bruns (1977) stated that to hit a high-speed serve horizontally, impact must occur approximately 3 m above the court. Gravity, air resistance and forward rotation all affect the ball in flight. The influence of air resistance on forward speed is demonstrated by the fact that a service speed of 185 km·h^{-1} will be reduced to approximately 150 km·h^{-1} just prior to impacting the court (Plagenhoef 1979). Research generally shows that a flat service may be hit marginally downwards (0–5°) if hit approximately 2.8 m from the court with a speed of 160 km·h^{-1}. However, while forward rotation will

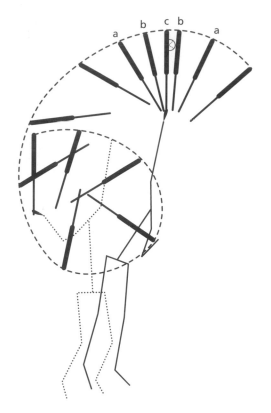

Fig. 1.6 Path of the racket from the beginning of lower limb extension to impact in a tennis serve (a = 2 frames pre-, postimpact; b = 1 frame pre-, postimpact; c = impact).

provide an extra margin for error at the net, it also requires a higher ball flight path. An up-and-out hitting action is therefore a key feature of a mature service action.

Elliott (1983) showed that high-performance players all hit a 'fast power serve' with an up-and-out action immediately preceding and through impact, which imparted forward rotation to the ball. The highest level of forward ball rotation resulted from a 5° upward racket movement immediately prior to impact, followed by a further 2° upward trajectory immediately following impact (Fig. 1.6). A group of 15-year-old high-performance players either moved their racket straight through the ball or upwards at 1° immediately prior to impact. No significant ball rotation resulted from an impact where the racket moved in a straight line both one frame prior to and following impact, a characteristic of a group of high-performance 12-year-olds.

Follow-through

Internal rotation of the upper arm and pronation of the forearm are key features of the early follow-through, such that the racket often moves away from the body prior to generally moving across the line of the body to complete the stroke.

The return of serve

The very short interval between service impact and the return obliges the player to adopt a preparatory sequence having regard to the uncertainty as to the ball's trajectory. There is a paucity of research information that assists a coach to better prepare an athlete for this stroke.

In a study that assessed the movements of the server and receiver over 230 individual trials, it was shown that a superior level performer commenced preparation prior to service impact (Hennemann & Keller 1983). As soon as the server initiates the movement, which culminates in throwing the ball into the air, the superior level receiver prepares a response. Cuing is therefore a skill that must be practised if a successful return is to follow.

Groppel (1992) revealed a common sequence that elite performers follow in initiating movement during a return of serve:
• early preparation (based largely on personal preference);
• unweights (stores elastic energy for use in movement);
• unit turn;
• movement of feet.

Lamond *et al.* (1996), through video analysis of high-performance matches, identified four common methods of foot movement:
• cross-over step;
• slide step;
• jab cross-over step (initial quick movement of foot closer to the ball, followed by cross-over step);
• gravity step (unit turn on unweighting, followed by a cross-over step).

Mean movement and total response times in both the forehand and backhand direction indicated the slide step to be significantly slower than each of the other three techniques. Coaches must be careful in interpreting these data, as quickness to the ball may not necessarily be the most important aspect for the

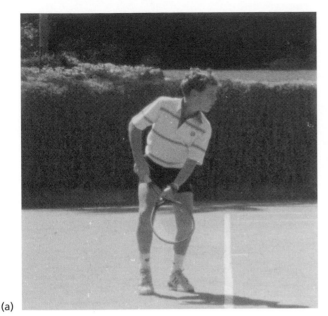
(a)

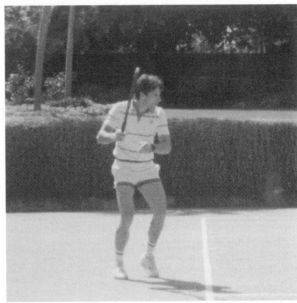
(b)

Fig. 1.7 Forehand backswing techniques.

return of serve. Of the four foot techniques listed above, the slide step is the only one that clearly results in an 'open-hitting' stance so often used in a forehand return of service.

The forehand

Modern tactics dictate that the forehand be hit with varying amounts of forward rotation (topspin). The multisegment stroke was compared to the single unit forehand by Elliott *et al.* (1989a). However, the biomechanical base to this stroke, with particular reference to the topspin forehand, is provided by Takahashi *et al.* (1996) and Elliott *et al.* (1997). Other papers will be used to provide a clearer understanding of the key mechanical features of this stroke where appropriate.

The backswing

This phase of the stroke commences with flexion of the lower limbs so that the body is moved towards the court. Deceleration then applies stretch to the quadriceps muscles, which results in the storage of elastic energy. This energy may then, at least partially, assist a player to move quickly to the ball.

The backswing may follow a number of different patterns. In the modern multisegment or 'western style' forehand a pivot of the back foot is followed by backward movement of the elbow in synchrony with the shoulder turn, so that the racket remains almost pointed at the oncoming ball (Fig. 1.7a). The racket face is then closed, while the elbow is raised and the forearm/racket then pivots about the elbow and shoulder (Elliott *et al.* 1989a). This technique contrasts with the technique where the racket is taken back in synchrony with the shoulder turn and the whole racket/arm unit rotates more about the shoulder joint (Fig. 1.7b).

The backswing, irrespective of style, is characterized by a loop, which has been shown to increase impact racket speed compared to a flatter backswing, and a large rotation of the shoulders (upper trunk rotation approximately 110°) from the ready position (Fig. 1.8a; considered 90° of rotation). (The angle convention used is: (i) upper (shoulders) and lower (hips) trunk rotations are represented by angular changes in a line drawn between the two shoulder or two hip joints; (ii) shoulder joint is the angle between the trunk and the hitting arm; (iii) elbow joint is the anterior (front) angle between the upper arm and forearm; (iv) wrist joint is the posterior (back) angle between the hand and forearm.)

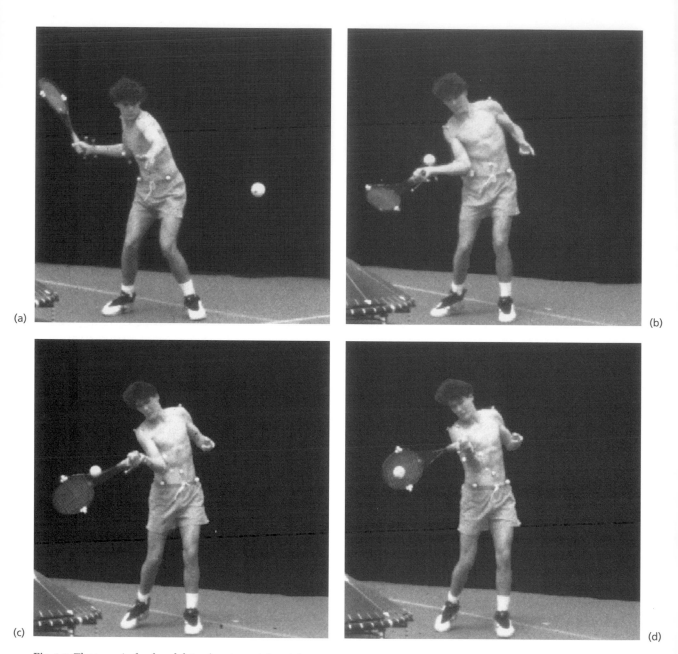

(a)

(b)

(c)

(d)

Fig. 1.8 The topspin forehand drive (western-style grip).

Similar levels of trunk twist (shoulder rotation subtract hip rotation or shoulders rotated more than hips) of approximately 30° were observed for flat, topspin and topspin lob strokes at the completion of the backswing (Takahashi *et al.* 1996). Elbow and wrist angles of approximately 110° and 140°, respectively, show that the arm is not fully extended and the hand is hyperextended in preparation for the forwardswing. The racket is not pointed at the back fence as often stated in the literature, but rotated past this orientation by approximately 45°.

Forwardswing to impact

Trunk rotation and extension of the lower limbs initiate the forward movement of the racket and are responsible for the upward and forward movement of the hitting shoulder for impact. Fujisawa *et al.* (1997) clearly showed the importance of a vigorous trunk rotation in the forehand. It was this action that created a lag in the hitting arm movement (storage of elastic energy) in the early forwardswing. The trunk continues rotating forward such that by impact the shoulders are almost parallel with the baseline (10° behind, to in-line) and the level of trunk twist is approximately 10° (shoulders forward of hips) (Fig. 1.8d). Similar forward shoulder speeds of approximately 2 m·s^{-1} at impact are observed for flat, topspin or topspin lob strokes, although the forward and upward speeds vary across strokes. Shoulder speed has been shown to contribute between 15% and 25% of the forward and upward impact speed of the racket. van Gheluwe and Hebbelinck (1986) had shown that court reaction forces were quite low in driving the body forward and therefore trunk rotation was responsible for the majority of this shoulder speed.

The rotations of the upper arm, forearm and hand then account for the remaining racket movement at impact. Elliott *et al.* (1997) clearly showed that segment contributions are influenced by the method of holding the racket (eastern vs. western grip) and level of ball rotation (flat vs. topspin vs. topspin lob strokes).

Forward movement of the upper arm (Fig. 1.8a,b) is a key feature of forehand mechanics producing 20–30% forward and approximately 20% upward speed depending on the grip being used. The elbow angle remains relatively constant (approx. 100°) throughout the forwardswing and thus is not a key feature in the development of racket speed for impact. Those players who use a western grip are certainly able to keep the elbow closer to the trunk (Fig. 1.8d) during the forwardswing to impact than those using an eastern method of holding the racket.

The upper arm, from an externally (outward) rotated position at the completion of the backswing, rotates internally in the period immediately before and after impact (Fig. 1.8b–d). This movement, which was identified in the forehand of an elite player

(Deporte *et al.* 1990), was shown by Elliott *et al.* (1997) to be an integral feature in the generation of impact racket speed (approx. 30–40%). van Gheluwe and Hebbelinck (1986) had previously shown that muscles responsible for internal rotation of the upper arm were strongly active prior to and at impact, although some variations were also evident.

The hand through forward (palmar) and upward (radial/ulnar) flexion, depending on the method of holding the racket, also plays an important role in the generation of forward and upward racket speed. The wrist joint should be hyperextended at impact by an angle of approximately 130°. Players using a western grip (Fig. 1.8c,d) are able to derive a greater proportion of upward racket speed (approx. 20%) from hand movements compared to those who use a eastern grip (approx. 5%). The ability to produce upward racket speed, an integral part of topspin stroke production, is therefore a distinct advantage for players using 'western-type' grips. All players, irrespective of grip, use the hand to generate forward speed of the racket. This should not, however, be thought of as a 'wrist flick'.

Racket trajectory, angle and speed are all key mechanical features that must be addressed in good stroke production. While the racket-face angle is perpendicular to the court or closed by up to 10° for all forehand strokes, the racket trajectory (movement of tip of racket to the court) pre- to postimpact varies (Elliott *et al.* 1997):

	Preimpact	*Postimpact*
Flat drive	20°	35°
Topspin drive	35° (Fig. 1.8b–d)	50°
Topspin lob	50°	70°

That is a steeper approach to the ball preimpact and in the early follow-through occurs for topspin compared to a flat stroke. Alternatively, racket speed reduces in the forward direction and increases in the upward direction for these strokes at impact (Elliott *et al.* 1997).

	Forward speed (m·s^{-1})	*Upward speed* (m·s^{-1})
Flat drive	17	8
Topspin drive	14	11
Topspin lob	9	12

Follow-through

During the period after impact, the upper limb segments gradually slow, while a recovery step brings the player into a position ready to move to the next shot. The high levels of upper arm internal rotation just before and after impact often means that the follow-through is across the line of the body.

The backhand

Biomechanical papers on the flat, topspin, backspin and one- vs. two-handed backhands will be reviewed to provide coaches with an understanding of the key mechanical features of these strokes. These will be presented under separate headings for ease of understanding.

The flat and topspin strokes

While a number of papers have been published on the backhand groundstroke, the most comprehensive study on the topspin drive (running, down-the-line, across-court) using three-dimensional cinemato-graphy was by Elliott *et al.* (1989b). This paper will therefore be used as the basis for the key mechanical features of this stroke, with other published material added where appropriate.

BACKSWING
Shoulder turn and back foot pivot (unit turn) must be synchronized as recommended in the coaching literature. Rotation of the shoulders by approximately 125° (Fig. 1.9a) from a position parallel to the net shows the importance of upper trunk rotation in backhand preparation. A shoulder angle (between trunk and upper arm) of approximately 50° and elbow angle of approximately 120° also show that the upper limb should be relatively close to the trunk and flexed at the completion of the backswing.

FORWARDSWING TO IMPACT
A stable front knee and minor extension of the rear knee (approx. 5°) during this period suggest that a lifting action via lower limb movement is not a mechanical factor in effective stroke production. However, hip joint extension of 10°, over the same period helps to raise the hitting shoulder and racket.

Trunk rotation (the shoulder alignment rotated approximately 65°) is primarily responsible for the forward movement of the hitting shoulder (Fig. 1.9a–c). While the upper arm remains relatively close to the trunk, the elbow joint extends approximately 40° from the backswing position to impact as a means of generating racket speed. However, the elbow joint should be both marginally flexed (approx. 15°) and stable (not extending) at impact.

Wrist extension is also a feature of the one-handed backhand stroke of advanced players. Knudson (1991) reported that advanced players produced higher and more consistent preimpact grip forces (region of the thumb) than intermediate players. This firm grip had previously been shown to be a desirable characteristic of advanced stroke production. A variation in wrist joint technique between advanced and beginner players was reported by Blackwell and Cole (1994). They reported that increased extensor muscle activity was associated with hand extension at impact for high-performance players, whereas beginners actually flexed the wrist joint following impact. Knudson and Blackwell (1997) verified these findings when they reported differences in wrist rotations following impact for professional (4 rad·s^{-1}: hand extension) and intermediate players with tennis elbow (0.4 rad·s^{-1}: hand flexion). Eccentric action following impact was theoretically supported by Riek *et al.* (1999) using computer modelling and data from novice players. This eccentric contraction of the wrist extensor musculature during hand flexion is a feature that has been associated with 'tennis elbow'.

The speed of the racket at impact is derived from a sequencing of: trunk rotation; upper arm forward movement and outward rotation; forearm extension/supination and hand extension. Racket speed reduces marginally at impact, from a peak value to achieve optimal control of the racket (this feature should *not* be coached—it will occur naturally). Ariel and Braden (1979) identified this factor in the backhand drives of the international players Ilie Nastase (one-handed) and Chris Evert (two-handed).

Mechanics for down-the-line and across-court strokes varied with respect to the position of impact. Running and stationary down-the-line strokes were impacted 15–20 cm forward of the hitting shoulder, while across-court impacts must be hit further forward (approx. 30 cm).

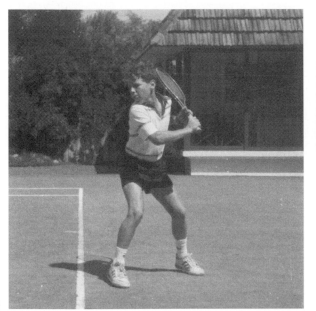

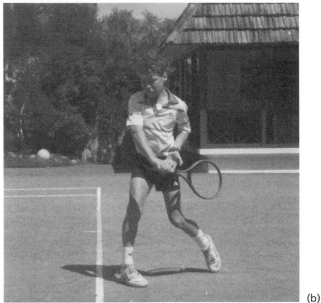

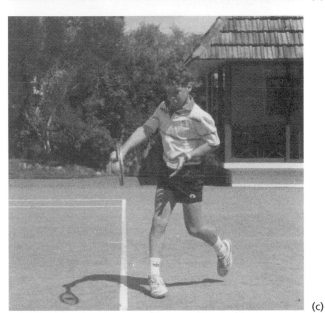

Fig. 1.9 The topspin backhand drive.

Topspin is a result of initially aligning the racket to the ball with a low-to-high trajectory (approx. 20°) prior to impact. Once impact is assured an increase in trajectory to approximately 45° just before and after impact is needed to apply spin to the ball. These values therefore supported 17° low-to-high trajectory reported by Braden and Bruns (1977) and the 45–55° angle suggested by Groppel *et al.*

(1983) if different stages of the forwardswing are assessed.

The backspin backhand drive

Modern tactics dictate that a player must be able to hit a backhand drive with topspin or backspin depending on the height of bounce of the ball or the tactical requirement of a particular rally. The mechanical basis of this stroke, as compared to the topspin stroke, with particular references to variations caused by hitting height was reported by Elliott and Christmass (1995).

Groppel (1984), in an investigation of professional players, indicated that backspin was imparted by 'brushing the back of the ball' in a downward manner with the racket face slightly open. Computer simulation was used by Brody (1987) to demonstrate that for a high-to-low racket trajectory the racket-face should be bevelled back (>90° to court), the exact angle being a function of the direction of movement

of the racket and incoming ball and the speed of the racket. A racket with a linear speed of 18 m·s^{-1} and a downward trajectory angle of 30° required a backward tilt of approximately 10° to produce the appropriate ball trajectory/speed. Results from Elliott and Christmass in Table 1.4 clearly support these data. While the racket speed remains relatively constant irrespective of the height of impact, racket trajectory with reference to the court and angle at impact alters in response to the height of impact. The racket must move 'through the impact zone' to achieve a high-speed backspin stroke (Fig. 1.10a–c).

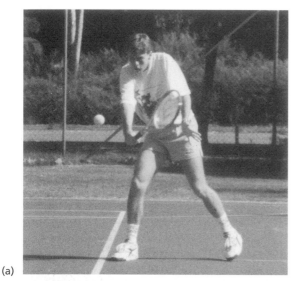

(a)

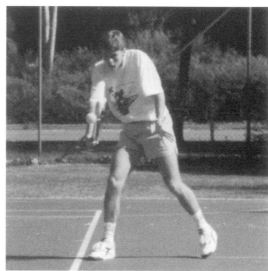

(b)

(c)

Fig. 1.10 Racket movement through the ball in a hip-height backspin backhand.

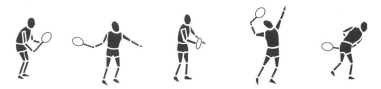

Table 1.4 Racket speed and trajectory together with ball speed in the backspin backhand. (Modified from Elliott and Christmass 1995.)

	Impact height	
	5 cm below hip (approx. hip height)	42 cm above hip (approx. shoulder height)
Preimpact		
Racket speed (m·s⁻¹)	21*	19
Racket trajectory (°)	−25	−15
Racket-face angle (°)	100	95
Postimpact		
Ball speed (m·s⁻¹)	25	25
Racket trajectory (°)	40	35

* All trajectories and angles are referenced to the court.

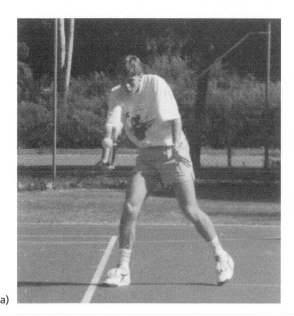

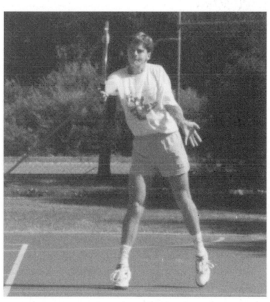

(a) (b)

Fig. 1.11 Impact position in (a) the low and (b) the high backspin backhands.

Impact in the backspin strokes occurs closer to the front foot (approx. 10 cm) than for a topspin drive (approx. 20 cm; Elliott *et al.* 1989b) (Fig. 1.11a,b). The greater control of racket speed, racket-face angle and trajectory needed in the backspin stroke (lesser margins for error) requires that the ball be hit closer to the body.

The trunk, which is angled forward in the topspin stroke (approx. 80° to the court; Elliott *et al.* 1989b), should be angled further forward at impact in high (approx. 70°) and low (approx. 60°) backspin drives. The 155° and 175° front knee angles for the low and high backspin impacts, respectively, are both larger than the 125° angle recorded in the topspin drive. The

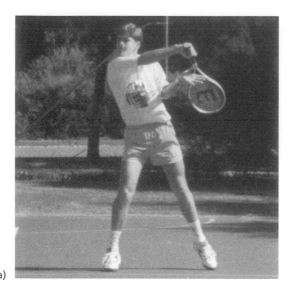
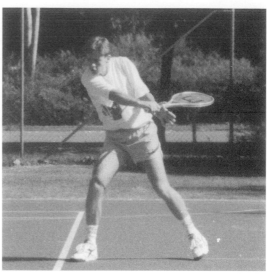

(a)   (b)

Fig. 1.12 Comparison of preparatory position for (a) high and (b) low backspin strokes.

front knee joint angle therefore plays an important role in positioning the body for impact by modifying the height of the hitting shoulder.

The upper arm was positioned a similar angle from the trunk for the low backspin backhand and a topspin drive (approx. 50°). However, this angle increased to approximately 65° for the shoulder-height backspin impact. The elbow joint angle at impact (approx. 165°), which does not change with hitting height, is similar to that used in the topspin stroke. The mean wrist angle at impact of approximately 160° was also not influenced by impact height.

At impact, the racket shoulder was moving towards the net (caused by trunk rotation and forward body movement) at a lesser level for backspin strokes (hip height approx. 0.6 m·s⁻¹; shoulder height approx. 0.4 m·s⁻¹) when compared to a topspin stroke (approx. 1.0 m·s⁻¹). Greater shoulder stability is therefore a mechanical characteristic of backspin stroke production and this factor is particularly important for higher impacts.

One major difference in the movement of the racket during the development of racket-head speed in the high and low backspin is the outward rotation of the upper arm and forearm (supination) in the high backspin stroke. A comparison of Fig. 1.12(a) and (b) clearly shows the difference in racket orientation

during the early part of the forwardswing for high and low bouncing balls.

The one- vs. two-handed backhand

A review of the coaching techniques of these strokes can be found in Groppel and Ward (1979), Reid and Elliott (2001) and in the popular tennis literature. This brief review summarizes the scientific literature in a way that provides a coach with a background to the strengths and weaknesses of each stroke. The *speed* of the racket at impact is derived from the *radius of rotation* (distance from impact location to shoulder) and the *rotational speed of the upper limb(s) and racket* plus any *forward speed of the body*. All else being equal, an increase in this radius (more extended hitting limb) will produce a higher forward impact speed, a factor that theoretically favours the one-handed technique. The reduced moment of inertia (swing weight) of the upper limb system (racket closer to hitting shoulder) and possible increase in strength (both upper limbs) with the two-handed stroke may assist the player in attaining a higher rotational speed of the racket–limb system, thus countering the effect of a reduced hitting radius. Does the increased reach of the one-handed stroke influence the reach of a player during a normal stroke? It has been shown that there is no difference in the distance between the impact location and the body (hitting radius) between the two strokes (Reid & Elliott 2001) provided the player was not required to run or stretch for the ball.

Does the increased difficulty in coordinating the five-segment single-handed stroke (hips, trunk, upper arm, forearm and hand) affect the ability to learn this skill, compared to the simpler three segment double-handed stroke (hips, trunk/upper limbs and hands)? Equally, does the increased strength requirement for the one-handed stroke further complicate this issue? Remember, advanced level two-handed strokes often are characterized by the upper limbs acting as multiple segments. No difference between the accuracy of the one-handed and two-handed strokes for beginners was reported in the literature, and college-age students demonstrated similar improvements in both strokes after 8 weeks of coaching. Reid and Elliott (2001) did show that players using two hands were better able to disguise stroke technique needed to direct the ball to different areas of the court (topspin vs. topspin lob). Research, as brief as it is, would therefore suggest that students should be allowed their own preference in backhand development unless the coach can see obvious benefits in one stroke on consideration of the playing style, flair and physical characteristics of the player.

Giangarra *et al.* (1993) demonstrated that higher upper limb muscle activity (in selected muscles) was recorded in the double-handed technique when compared to that recorded in the single-handed stroke. Any changes in the incidence of 'tennis elbow' for players using this technique are not therefore related to a reduced activity in the extensor muscles, but rather by factors associated with flawed stroke mechanics (or other factors) particularly in the single-handed stroke.

The volley

Three-dimensional cinematographic analyses of 12 highly skilled players (Elliott *et al.* 1988) and a national level performer (Deporte *et al.* 1990) are the primary sources for the key mechanical characteristics of the volley. Data that provide coaches with a better understanding of the volley are presented under separate headings for a right-handed player.

The split step

Effective volleyers need to execute a split step in preparation for both forehand and backhand volleys at the service line and at the net (Elliott *et al.* 1988). A forward lean from the vertical is also needed for the two volley strokes during this preparatory movement.

Backswing

Increased shoulder rotation is associated with the backhand volley (approx. 85°) compared with the forehand volley (approx. 60°), as the racket has to move to the opposite side of the body. At the completion of the backswing, the racket is behind the line of the shoulders for all volleys from the service line (Fig. 1.13a). This racket displacement for service-line volleys permits higher racket speeds to be generated than are required when impact occurs closer to the net.

Forwardswing to impact

The racket should move forward and down from the backswing position to impact (Fig. 1.13a,b) for forehand and backhand volleys (Elliott *et al.* 1988; Deporte *et al.* 1990). This high-to-low movement of the racket with respect to the ball produces backspin on the ball, which enhances control.

During the forward movement of the racket, the left foot (forehand volley) or right foot (backhand volley) steps towards the incoming ball. Much of the power for a volley comes from this forward step and rotation of the trunk. The relatively small upper trunk rotation of 10°, between the backswing position and impact for the forehand volley and the minimal change for the backhand volley, show the importance of general forward movement. A forward shoulder speed of 2 m·s^{-1} reported for a high-level forehand volley (Deporte *et al.* 1990), when compared to the racket speeds of approximately 11 m·s^{-1} at impact reported by Elliott *et al.* (1988), show that approximately 20% of the forward racket speed is derived from the forward movement. Coaches must also pay attention to the level of shoulder alignment at impact, which is angled further forward for across-court compared to down-the-line volleys.

Upper limb movements that reach their peak levels at similar times, a characteristic of accuracy-based activities, are, however, responsible for the development

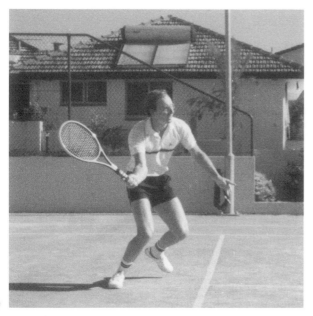

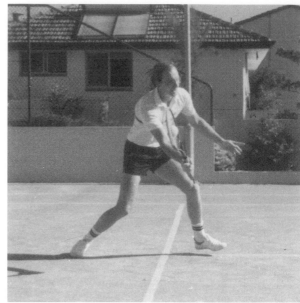

(a)

(b)

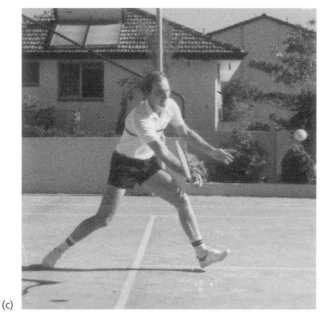

(c)

Fig. 1.13 Forwardswing in a forehand volley, hit at the service line.

of the majority of racket speed at impact. The small changes in shoulder joint angle, from the position in the backswing to impact, suggest that this joint was more involved with the orientation of the racket than with speed generation. The elbow joint angle increases (approx. 10°) from the backswing position to impact for both forehand and backhand volleys irrespective of court location (Elliott *et al.* 1988). The role of elbow

extension in the generation of impact racket speed was also reported for the forehand volley of a national level performer (Deporte *et al.* 1990). However, only small extension speeds were recorded at impact, which stresses the need for stability at the elbow joint.

Coaching literature has often stressed the importance of a 'fixed wrist joint' at impact. Elliott *et al.* (1988) and Deporte *et al.* (1990) have clearly refuted this myth and shown the importance of this movement in the generation of racket speed at impact. In the forehand volley there is an initial decrease in the posterior wrist angle due to the forward movement of the arm followed by an increase to produce a maximum rotational speed. This opening then reduces so that a relatively stable joint is a mechanical feature of impact. The wrist joint should still be hyperextended at impact (approx. 145°; Fig. 1.13b), a key feature in the forehand volley. A similar set of data was recorded for the backhand volley, although the racket was more 'in line with' the hand at impact.

Although all 12 subjects in the study by Elliott *et al.* (1988) had achieved a high level of skill, they were ranked on their ability to hit a forehand and backhand volley by three professional coaches. The four best and the four lowest ranked volleyers then formed two groups. The better group achieved higher peak speeds at all segment end points irrespective of volley and the racket top reached its peak value closer to impact compared with the lower group. Further, at impact, the higher skilled group maintained higher mean racket speed.

Follow-through

As the racket does not move as fast through impact compared to groundstrokes, it does not require as much time or distance to slow down in order to avoid injury. During the period after impact, the segments gradually decelerate prior to the racket resuming a ready position for the next volley or smash. Two clear movement patterns have been identified: (i) the racket tip moves forward and down (Fig. 1.13b–c); or (ii) movement took the form of a 'dishing action' where the racket-face opened and moved backwards and down. The better volleyers tended to move the racket by the former method, while some of the less effective volleyers mentioned above 'dished' the racket after impact.

The approach shot

The biomechanical base to the approach shot is provided by a single paper published by Elliott and Marsh (1989). This publication compared the topspin and backspin forehand approach shots hit by seven high-performance players. Only the major differences between the strokes will be reported to assist coaches to better understand their mechanics.

Preparation

All players used a grip similar to the semi-western method of holding the racket for both topspin and backspin forehand strokes. Modifications to the positioning of the wrist permitted the angle of the racket to be changed at impact for the two strokes.

The backswing

The upper arm is positioned further from the trunk at the completion of the backswing in the backspin stroke (approx. 60°) than in the topspin technique (approx. 45°) (Figs 1.14a and 1.15a). The greater hip and trunk rotation required in the topspin stroke is the major reason for the racket being positioned approximately 25° (total rotation of 205°) past a line drawn perpendicular to the back fence for this stroke, while it is only rotates 50° (total rotation of 140°) from a position parallel to the net for the backspin stroke. In the coaching literature it has been reported that a reduced backswing is needed in an approach shot when compared to that used for a groundstroke, as the distance to the opponent's baseline was reduced. This compact backswing was certainly evident in the backspin stroke, and although the racket is taken back past the perpendicular to the back fence for a topspin approach shot, it is not taken back as far as in the topspin groundstroke (Elliott *et al.* 1989a).

Forwardswing to impact

Forward movement of the body and upper limb produced a significantly higher racket speed at impact for the topspin stroke (approx. 24 m·s^{-1}) than is required for the backspin shot (approx. 16 m·s^{-1}). As the forward speed of the shoulder is only approximately 2–3 m·s^{-1} for the two strokes, it can be generalized that racket speed in the topspin stroke is created from movement of the upper arm, forearm and wrist segments (multisegment approach), whereas in the backspin stroke the upper limb moves forward more as a single unit.

A mean upward trajectory for the racket tip of approximately 25° (low-to-high path) is needed in the topspin stroke (Fig. 1.14a–c), while in the backspin stroke a high-to-low trajectory of approximately 20° is required (Fig. 1.15a–c).

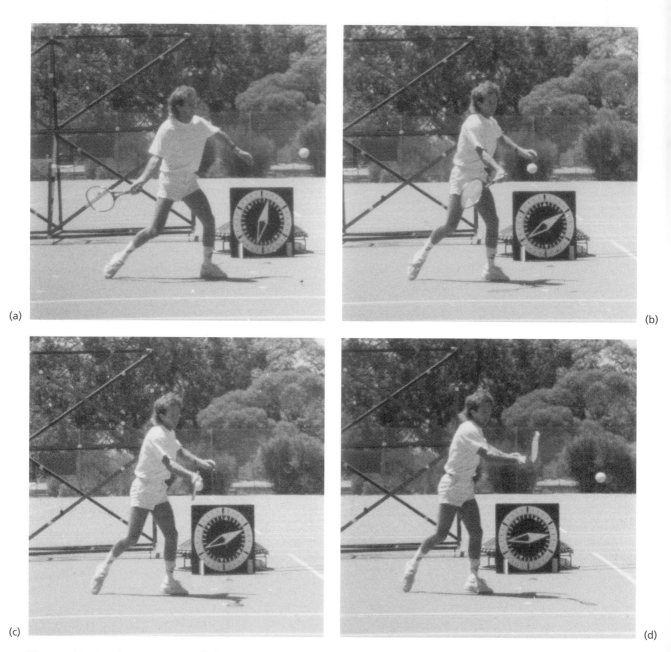

(a)

(b)

(c)

(d)

Fig. 1.14 Forehand topspin approach shot.

At impact, the hitting limb lowers in the backspin shot (knee and hip joints were flexing: Fig. 1.15c), while it raises in the topspin stroke (extension at knee and hip joints: Fig. 1.14c). The lower limb movements therefore assist the racket in its high-to-low (backspin) and low-to-high trajectories (topspin).

Forward trunk lean and shoulder angle (approx. 70° and 55°, respectively) at impact are similar for the two strokes. However, minor variations are evident in elbow and wrist angles. The elbow joint does not change during impact for the backspin stroke (approx. 150°) reinforcing the concept of the need for a stable joint at

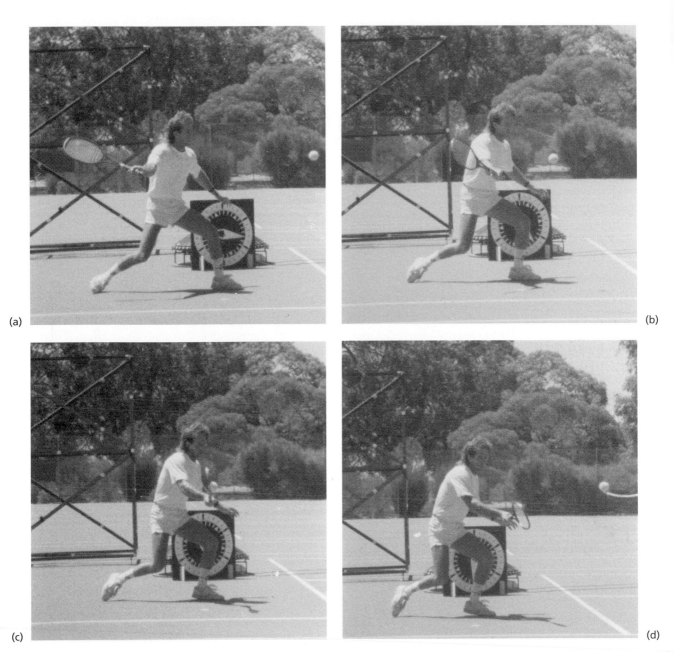

(a)

(b)

(c)

(d)

Fig. 1.15 Forehand backspin approach shot.

impact. Some elbow flexion occurs in the topspin shot about impact; however, a similar angle of approximately 150° was recorded showing that the hitting limb is relatively extended for both strokes (Figs 1.14 and 1.15c). The wrist joint is hyperextended for both shots (topspin approx. 120°; backspin approx. 115°) at

impact. Rotations of the wrist joint about impact are of insufficient magnitude to be termed a 'wrist flick'.

Clear differences are needed in the orientation of the racket face from the vertical at impact. The racket inclines backwards by approximately 5° for the backspin shot and forwards by a similar amount for the topspin stroke. These angles, together with the racket trajectories and the speed of the racket produce the various rotations of the ball.

Follow-through

The preimpact trajectory of the racket for the backspin stroke continues in the follow-through, with the racket continuing downwards at an angle of approximately 30° before moving upwards to the completion of the stroke (Figs 1.14 and 1.15c,d). Similarly the preimpact upward trajectory in the topspin stroke continues after impact at an angle of approximately 40° during the early follow-through.

The smash

There is a paucity of research data that provide the coach with objective evidence on the mechanics of the smash. It generally has been assumed that much of what has been learned about service technique can be transferred such that it also provides the scientific basis of this stroke. This belief has certainly not been tested. Tokuda *et al.* (1995) in using three-dimensional cinematography to analyse the technique of an elite male player showed:
- the elbow joint is flexed during the backswing to reduce the moment of inertia (swing weight) of the upper limb and improve movement efficiency;
- the general movement sequence is proximal to distal as in the service action (rotation about the upper arm was not examined);
- the player who impacts the ball in the vicinity of the service line must swing up to the ball (approx. 4°) and hit the ball with the racket angled backwards from the vertical (approx. 10°).

The analysis of stroke production

Effective analysis skills are an essential ingredient in developing 'good technique' in stroke production and determining the possible cause(s) of injury. Analysis methods in tennis may be classified under three general areas; namely *subjective*, *objective* and *predictive*.

Most coaches and medical/paramedical professionals use a variety of subjective evaluation techniques during their normal interaction with players or patients. They watch the service action with an eye to identifying flaws in technique that may lead to injury. Objective techniques refer to the collection, measurement and evaluation of data from the stroke of interest. A coach may measure the speed or angle of a racket from video in an endeavour to increase postimpact ball speed and spin. Predictive techniques attempt to answer the 'what if . . . ?' question. For example, what effect would increasing the length of the racket or the level of upper arm internal rotation in the serve have on impact speed?

Subjective analysis methods

Subjective analysis, a 'natural' ability of good coaches, is a skill that can be learned and improved through practice. The importance of the development of this skill in coaches is often understated, although it is the most common analysis technique employed by them. A book by Knudson and Morrison (1997) discusses the varied subjective analysis techniques that may be used by coaches. Further work to refine the techniques and structure of qualitative analysis (McPherson 1996) has produced systems that help clarify this previously 'intuitive' approach (Fig. 1.16). A mechanical model of each stroke (e.g. Fig. 1.17: the tennis serve) must therefore be developed if such an analysis system is to be used. Not all sections of each model are of the same importance and therefore *key* variables must be identified.

Coaches, having established the mechanical features for each stroke, must then decide what parts are critical to performance (e.g. coordinated forwardswing) and those parts that may be optional (e.g. selected grips or position of feet in a 'foot-up' or 'foot-back' service action). Objective data reported in applied sports science research studies usually provide the ranges of acceptability for each of the variables in the model as set out in Fig. 1.17. That is, in evaluating the extent of upper arm internal rotation (a key movement in the generation of racket speed at impact in the serve) a coach may do the following:
- Look at upper arm range of movement (flexibility) in external rotation.
- Look to see if internal rotation is a vigorous/very rapid rotation immediately prior to and through impact.
- Ensure that strength/power training of the shoulder region includes rotator cuff and major

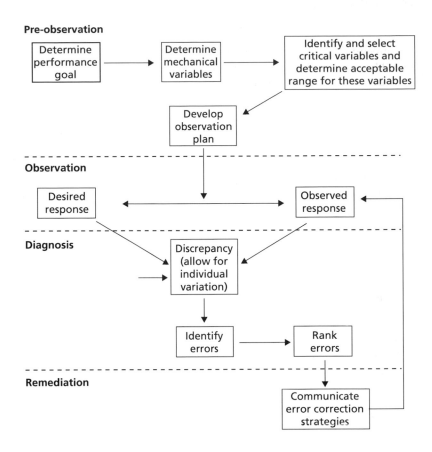

Fig. 1.16 An approach to subjective skill analysis. (Modified from McPherson 1996.)

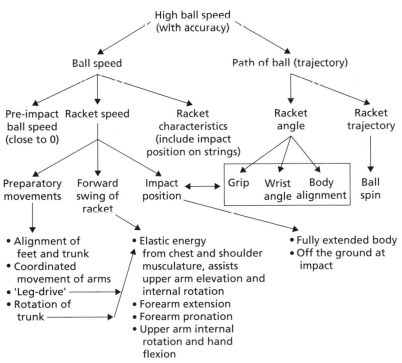

Fig. 1.17 A mechanical model of the tennis serve.

rotator musculature (latissimus dorsi, pectoralis and anterior deltoid). This must also include eccentric muscle activity as the internal rotators eccentrically contract to slow external rotation prior to contracting concentrically to 'drive' the internal rotation of the upper arm.

The next phase in this subjective evaluation is the observation of the movement, and a comparison between the response and the previously determined desired response. This is followed by the determination of primary errors, from which error correction strategies are communicated to the player. The aim of this is to determine the *cause* of a technique fault, as opposed to correcting *effects*, which emanate from the original cause, and to determine the best way to correct each fault. A tennis serve, where there is insufficient time to complete the preparatory racket movement 'behind the back' is often rectified by pushing the ball higher into the air (an effect). The appropriate correction strategy may have been to coordinate the movement of both arms. A high ball toss may only lead to further technique errors.

Objective analysis methods

Objective evaluation, which generally requires the assistance of a biomechanist, is associated with a permanent record for a number of trials, so that each can be viewed and/or analysed. In general terms objective analysis performed with assistance from a biomechanist may involve:
- dynamometry—the recording of force against the court during selected stroke production (e.g. Elliott & Wood 1983; van Gheluwe & Hebbelinck 1986);
- electromyography—the recording of muscle activity during each stroke (e.g. van Gheluwe & Hebbelinck 1986; Kibler 1995);
- cinematography—the high-speed recording of segment motion during stroke production (e.g. Elliott *et al.* 1989a; Elliott *et al.* 1995).

The coach will normally use video photography as a subjective research tool, although objective data may eventually be derived from video.

Predictive analysis methods

The general aim of this analysis method is to use a computer model to predict changes that would occur in a movement as a consequence of alterations to input values. That is, one aims to answer the question, 'What would happen to the speed of the racket if the level of wrist flexion during the service action changes from 10 rad·s^{-1} to 15 rad·s^{-1}?'. Legnani and Marshall (1993) have used analyses of experimental data and simulations to predict joint forces during the tennis serve. These authors modified joint motions, extracted from experimental data, as input to examine their effects on racket motion and joint forces. Preliminary results indicated that increasing the linear speed or range of motion of the trunk (a consequence of altered leg drive) or the timing and therefore the speed of upper arm internal rotation both contributed to increased racket-head speed. From an injury perspective it was evident that changes in the extent of elbow extension and rate of upper arm internal rotation influence forces at the elbow. The complexity of the 'real-world' system has been a major stumbling block for this type of research, but improvements in computer models of performance over coming years should see this approach providing better answers for the coach and player.

References

Ariel, G. & Braden, V. (1979) Biomechanical analysis of ballistic vs tracking movements in tennis skills. In: Groppel, J., ed. *Proceedings of a National Symposium on the Racquet Sports*, pp. 105–124. University of Illinois Press, Champaign, IL, USA.

Bahamonde, R. (1997) Joint power production during flat and slice tennis serves. In: Wilkerson, J., Zimmermann, W. & Ludwig, K., eds. *Proceedings of the XVth Symposium on Biomechanics in Sports*, p. 92. Texas Woman's University, TX, USA.

Bahamonde, R. (2000) Angular momentum changes during the tennis serve. *Journal of Sports Science* **18**, 579–592.

Blackwell, J.R. & Cole, K.J. (1994) Wrist kinematics differ in expert and novice tennis players performing the backhand stroke: implications for tennis elbow. *Journal of Biomechanics* **27** (5), 509–516.

Braden, V. & Bruns, C. (1977) *Vic Braden's Tennis for the Future*. Little, Brown, Boston, MA, USA.

Brody, H. (1987) *Tennis Science for Tennis Players*. University of Pennsylvania Press, Philadelphia, PA, USA.

Chandler, J., Kibler, B., Stracener, E., Ziegler, A. & Pace, B. (1992) Shoulder strength, power and endurance in college tennis players. *American Journal of Sports Medicine* **20**, 455–459.

Chow, J., Carlton, L., Chae, W., Lim, Y. & Shim, J. (1999) Pre- and post-impact ball and racket characteristics during tennis serves performed by elite male and female players. In: Sanders, R. & Gibson, B., eds. *Proceedings of the XVIIth International Symposium on Biomechanics in Sports*, pp. 45–48. Edith Cowan University, Perth, Australia.

Deporte, E., van Gheluwe, B. & Hebbelinck, M. (1990) A three-dimensional cinematographical analysis of arm and racket at impact in tennis. In: Berme, N. & Cappozzo, A., eds. *Biomechanics of Human Movement: Applications in Rehabilitation, Sport and Ergonomics*, pp. 460–467. Bertec Corporation, Worthington, USA.

Ellenbecker, T. (1989) Total arm strength isokinetic profile of highly skilled tennis players and its relation to functional performance measurement. In: Gregor, R., Zernicke, R. & Whiting, W., eds. *Congress Proceedings of the XIIth International Congress of Biomechanics*, p. 141. University of California, Los Angeles, USA.

Elliott, B.C. (1982) Tennis: the influence of grip tightness on reaction impulse and rebound speed. *Medicine and Science in Sport and Exercise* **14** (5), 348–352.

Elliott, B.C. (1983) Spin and the power serve in tennis. *Journal of Human Movement Studies* **9** (2), 97–104.

Elliott, B. & Christmass, M. (1995) A comparison of the high and low backspin backhand drives in tennis using different grips. *Journal of Sports Sciences* **13**, 141–151.

Elliott, B. & Marsh, T. (1989) A biomechanical comparison of the topspin and backspin forehand approach shots in tennis. *Journal of Sports Sciences* **7** (4), 215–227.

Elliott, B.C. & Wood, G.A. (1983) The biomechanics of the foot-up and foot-back tennis service techniques. *Australian Journal of Sports Science* **3** (2), 3–6.

Elliott, B., Marsh, T. & Blanksby, B. (1986) A three-dimensional cinematographic analysis of the tennis serve. *International Journal of Sports Biomechanics* **2** (4), 260–271.

Elliott, B.C., Overheu, P. & Marsh, P. (1988) The service line and net volleys in tennis: a cinematographic analysis. *Australian Journal of Science and Medicine in Sport* **20** (2), 10–18.

Elliott, B., Marsh, T. & Overheu, P. (1989a) A biomechanical comparison of the multisegment and single unit topspin forehand drives in tennis. *International Journal of Sport Biomechanics* **5** (3), 350–364.

Elliott, B., Marsh, T. & Overheu, P. (1989b) The topspin backhand drive in tennis. *Journal of Human Movement Studies* **16** (1), 1–16.

Elliott, B.C., Ackland, T., Blanksby, B. & Bloomfield, J. (1990) A prospective study of physiologic and kinanthropometric indicators of junior tennis performance. *Australian Journal of Science and Medicine in Sport* **22** (4), 87–92.

Elliott, B.C., Marshall, R.N. & Noffal, G. (1995) Contributions of upper limb segment rotations during the power serve in tennis. *Journal of Applied Biomechanics* **11**, 433–442.

Elliott, B., Takahashi, K. & Noffal, G. (1997) The influence of grip position on upper limb contributions to racket-head speed in the tennis forehand. *Journal of Applied Biomechanics* **13** (2), 182–196.

Fujisawa, T., Fuchimoto, T. & Kaneko, M. (1997) Joint moments during tennis forehand drive: an analysis of rotational movements on a horizontal plane. In: *Book of Abstracts from the XVIth ISB Tokyo Congress*, p. 354. International Society of Biomechanics, Tokyo, Japan.

van Gheluwe, B. & Hebbelinck, M. (1986) Muscle action and ground reaction forces in tennis. *International Journal of Sports Biomechanics* **2** (2), 88–99.

van Gheluwe, B., De Ruysscher, I. & Craenhals, J. (1987) Pronation and endorotation of the racket arm in a tennis serve. In: Jonsson, B., ed. *Biomechanics X-B*, pp. 666–672. Human Kinetics, Champaign, IL, USA.

Giangarra, C.E., Conroy, B., Jobe, F., Pink, M. & Perry, J. (1993) Electromyographic and cinematographic analysis of elbow function in tennis players using single- and double-handed backhand strokes. *American Journal of Sports Medicine* **21** (3), 394–399.

Grabiner, M., Groppel, J. & Campbell, K. (1983) Resultant tennis ball speed as a function of off centre impacts and grip firmness. *Medicine and Science in Sport and Exercise* **15** (6), 542–544.

Groppel, J. (1984) *Tennis for Advanced Players and Those Who Would Like to Be.* Human Kinetics, Champaign, IL, USA.

Groppel, J. (1992) *High Tech Tennis*, 2nd edn. Leisure Press, Champaign, IL, USA.

Groppel, J. & Ward, T. (1979) Coaching implications of the tennis one-handed and two-handed backhand drives. In: Terauds, J., ed. *Science in Racquet Sports*, pp. 81–87. Academic Publishers, Del Mar, CA, USA.

Groppel, J., Dillman, C. & Lardner, T. (1983) Derivation and validation of equations of motion to predict ball spin upon impact in tennis. *Journal of Sports Science* **1**, 111–120.

Hatze, H. (1976) Forces and duration of impact and grip tightness during the tennis stroke. *Medicine and Science in Sports and Exercise* **8**, 88–95.

Hennemann, M. & Keller, D. (1983) Preparatory behaviour in the execution of a sport-related movement. The return of serve in tennis. *International Journal of Sport Psychology* **14**, 149–161.

Kibler, W.B. (1995) Biomechanical analysis of the shoulder during tennis activities. *Clinics in Sports Medicine* **14** (1), 79–85.

Kleinöder, H.K. (1990) *The effect of tennis specific power-training towards an increase of service speed and speed of leg movements.* PhD Thesis, The German Sports University, Cologne, Germany (unpublished).

Knudson, D. (1989) Hand forces and impact effectiveness in the tennis forehand. *Journal of Human Movement Studies* **17** (1), 1–7.

Knudson, D. (1991) Forces on the hand in the tennis one-handed backhand. *International Journal of Sports Biomechanics* **7** (3), 282–292.

Knudson, D. & Blackwell, J. (1997) Upper extremity angular kinematics of the one-handed backhand drive in tennis players with and without tennis elbow. *International Journal of Sports Medicine* **18**, 79–82.

Knudson, D. & Morrison, C. (1997) *Qualitative Analysis of Human Movement*. Human Kinetics, Champaign, IL, USA.

Lamond, F., Lowdon, B. & Davis, K. (1996) Determination of the quickest footwork for teaching return of the tennis serve. *ACHPER Healthy Lifestyles Journal* **43**, 5–8.

Legnani, G. & Marshall, R. (1993) Evaluation of the joint torques during a tennis service: analysis of experimental data and simulations. In: Landjerit, B., ed. *Proceedings of the IVth International Symposium on Computer Simulation in Biomechanics*, pp. 8–11. International Society of Biomechanics, Paris, France.

Liu, U.K. (1983) Mechanical analysis of racket and ball during impact. *Medicine and Science in Sports and Exercise* **15** (5), 388–392.

McPherson, M.N. (1996) Qualitative and quantitative analysis in sports. *American Journal of Sports Medicine* **24** (6), 85–88.

Matsuo, T., Matsumoto, T., Takada, Y. & Mochizuki, Y. (2000) Influence of lateral trunk tilt on throwing arm kinetics during baseball pitching. In: Hong, Y. & Johns, D., eds. *Proceedings of the XVIIIth International Symposium on Biomechanics in Sports*, pp. 882–886. Chinese University of Hong Kong, HK, China.

Missavage, R.J., Baker, J.A. & Putnam, C. (1984) Theoretical modeling of grip firmness during ball–racket impact. *Research Quarterly for Exercise and Sports* **55**, 254–260.

Miyashita, M., Tsunoda, T., Sakurai, S., Nishizono, H. & Mizuno, T. (1979) The tennis serve as compared with overhand throwing. In: Groppel, J., ed. *Proceedings of a National Symposium on the Racquet Sports*, pp. 125–140. University of Illinois Press, Champaign, IL, USA.

Noffal, G. & Elliott, B. (1998) Three-dimensional kinetics of the shoulder and elbow joints in the high performance tennis serve: Implications for injury. In: *Proceedings of the 4th International Conference of Sports Medicine and Science in Tennis*. Society for Tennis Medicine and Science, Coral Gables, FL, USA.

Plagenhoef, S. (1979) Tennis racket testing related to 'tennis elbow'. In: Groppel, J., ed. *Proceedings of a National Symposium on the Racquet Sports*, pp. 291–310. University of Illinois Press, Champaign, IL, USA.

Reid, M. & Elliott, B. (2001) The one- and two-handed backhands in tennis. *Sport Biomechanics* **1**, 47–68.

Riek, S., Chapman, A.E. & Milner, T. (1999) A simulation of muscle force and internal kinematics of extensor carpi radialis brevis during backhand tennis stroke: implications for injury. *Clinical Biomechanics* **14**, 477–483.

Takahashi, K., Elliott, B. & Noffal, G. (1996) The role of upper limb segment rotations in the development of spin in the tennis forehand. *Australian Journal of Science and Medicine in Sport* **28** (4), 106–113.

Tokuda, J., Sato, Y., Yamada, Y. & Mitsuhashi, D. (1995) A three-dimensional motion analysis of the overhead smash. In: Sasahara, H. & Tomosue, R., eds. *Proceedings of the First Asian Congress of Tennis Science*, pp. 12–13. Hiroshima University of Economics, Hiroshima, Japan.

Wilson, G.J., Elliott, B.C. & Wood, G.A. (1991) The effect on performance of imposing a delay during a stretch–shorten cycle movement. *Medicine and Science in Sports and Exercise* **23** (3), 364–370.

Chapter 2

The tennis racket

Introduction

Today, tennis rackets are quite different from the ones that were in use for most of this century (Fig. 2.1). This big change in the racket was facilitated by the introduction of composite materials and advanced manufacturing technology. When rackets were made of wood, the strength to weight ratio of that material determined many of the racket parameters. To have a racket frame with sufficient stiffness to produce the desired playing characteristics and also be able to withstand the forces due to high string tensions and the repeated pounding of high-speed balls, the racket had to be fairly heavy. The length of the racket and the size and shape of the head were limited by the necessity to keep the racket weight within the bounds that an average player could easily handle.

With the introduction of metal rackets and almost immediately afterwards the introduction of composite materials, many of the structural limitations set by wood were eliminated. Racket designers were given almost a free licence to use their imagination and apply the dynamic laws of physics, rather than have the strength of materials as the determinant of the design criteria. Today we find longer frames with longer and wider heads, head shapes that deviate from oval, much stiffer rackets, and considerably more durable frames, all weighing up to 30% less than the traditional, classic wooden frames.

With these new rackets available, many players have modified both their strokes and their style of play to take advantage of them. On the faster surfaces that tennis is played, such as grass, the serve has become more dominant. It is also possible for players to occasionally hit clean winners from the baseline, even on some of the slower court surfaces. With this new equipment in the hands of the bigger, stronger, better conditioned athletes that play tennis today, both the men's and the women's games now put more emphasis on power and speed. The modern tennis racket has helped today's player hit the ball harder and go for 'big' shots more often.

The frame

The tennis racket designer attempts to provide rackets that have predictability (a uniformity of response), comfort (minimum shock and vibration) and power (high rebound ball speed with less player effort). The term 'sweet spot' is used to indicate the area on the racket where the ball impact results in those desired characteristics. A racket with a large sweet spot will allow players to hit the ball over a large region of the strings, and still have the desired results.

There are classically three sweet spots (Brody 1987) on a tennis racket, each having a preferred reason why the player wants to hit the ball at that location. They are:

1 the centre of percussion (located where the resulting shock or jar to the hand is a minimum);

2 the node (located where the resulting vibrations are a minimum);

3 the maximum of the coefficient of restitution (the region where the rebounding ball speed is a maximum).

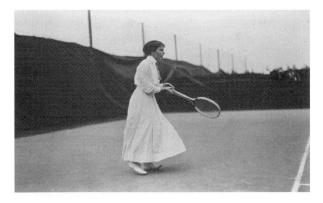

Fig. 2.1 Typical wooden racket in use during the first half of the 20th century. Photo © IOC/Olympic Museum Collections.

The centre of percussion

In the frame of reference of the tennis racket, if a ball strikes the racket at the racket centre of mass (the CM or balance point) and then rebounds, the racket will recoil in order to conserve linear momentum. Because the CM is usually near the throat of the racket, this is not a likely or desirable place for a ball to strike. If the ball strikes the racket near the centre of the head (more likely), the racket still recoils to conserve linear momentum, but now it also will twist or rotate about the CM in order to conserve angular momentum. The motion of the racket due to linear momentum conservation and the motion of the racket handle or grip due to angular momentum conservation are in opposite directions as is shown in Fig. 2.2. Therefore, it is possible, at a particular ball impact location, for the two motions to cancel exactly at the point where the hand holds the racket. If this were to happen, then the shock or jar that the hand experiences due to the ball–racket interaction would be minimized. That particular ball impact location where the two motions cancel at the hand is called the centre of percussion (COP). It depends upon the mass distribution of the racket as well as where the hand is located on the handle.

The location of the COP can be determined by turning the racket into a pendulum, with a pivot at the point on the grip where the hand is located. The period (time for a complete swing of the racket-pendulum) is obtained, and the distance between the pivot point and the COP location (in centimetres) is given by $25\ T^2$ where T is the period (in seconds).

Assuming a pivot point about 7–9 cm from the butt end of the racket, the COP for a typical old classical wooden racket came out near the throat of the frame, and not near the centre of the head, where players tend to hit the ball. With the introduction of the oversize head, the COP point is close to the centre of the head. This was not because the COP is a different distance from the hand, but because the centre of the enlarged head has been moved down towards the racket handle.

The node

The tennis racket, even when made with the most advanced composite material, is not a rigid body.

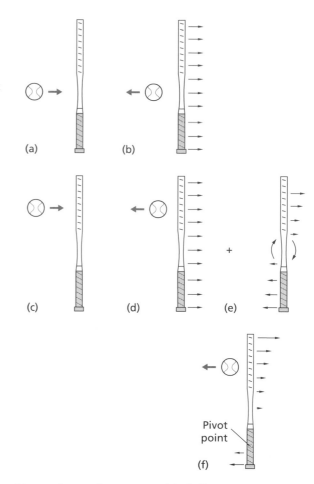

Fig. 2.2 Centre of percussion. If the ball is incident on racket centre of mass (a), the racket recoils (b) to conserve linear momentum. If the ball is incident near centre of head (c), the racket recoils (d) to conserve linear momentum and it twists (e) to conserve angular momentum. Combining the two previous motions (f) leads to a cancellation of motion at the handle of racket (the pivot point).

When the racket interacts with a ball, the frame can vibrate. If the racket handle is rigidly clamped in place, the lowest two modes of transverse vibrations are shown in Fig. 2.3(a,b). If the racket is essentially completely free, the lowest mode of vibration is shown in Fig. 2.3(c). If the racket is struck at some location other than the node (located as shown in the figure), then the frame will vibrate in one or more of these modes, depending on how the handle is held. Each of these modes of vibration has a unique frequency associated with it, and that identifies

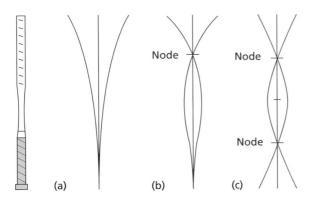

Fig. 2.3 Vibration modes of a tennis racket with its handle clamped (a,b) and with both ends free (c).

which mode it is, and therefore whether the handle is clamped or free. A hand-held racket vibrates at a frequency very close to the frequency of a free racket, and there is no sign of the clamped handle mode of oscillation (Brody 1995).

When a ball strikes the racket at the node of a particular mode of oscillation, that mode is not excited. The farther the impact is from the node, the greater is the amplitude of the vibration. This is shown in Fig. 2.4. These vibrations have a frequency in the range of 100–200 Hz, depending on the frame stiffness, frame length and the racket mass. You can determine the location of the node without electronic equipment by holding the racket between two fingers at the approximate location of the node in the handle and striking the strings at various locations with the other hand. You will be able to feel which impact locations cause vibrations and which location does not cause the frame to vibrate.

Much design effort has gone into both reducing vibrations and damping out vibrations. A racket that is stiffer will have a smaller amplitude of vibration for the same off-node ball impact. Various methods have been tried to damp out those vibrations that do occur, and the best one seems to be the human hand. In fact, the tighter the racket handle is gripped, the quicker the vibrations damp out (with the energy of the racket vibration going into the hand and arm).

The small, soft objects that are placed in the string bed close to the throat with the hope of reducing or eliminating vibrations, do essentially nothing to prevent, reduce or damp out vibrations of the frame

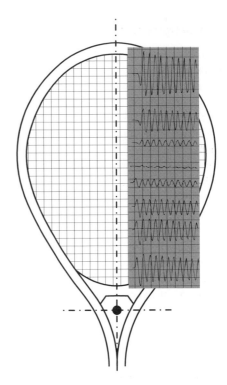

Fig. 2.4 Oscilloscope traces of vibrations of a free racket for various locations of ball impact. The node is located close to the centre of the head, and the vibrations increase in amplitude as the impact point moves away from the centre.

of the racket. However, they do quickly kill off the 500–600 Hz string vibrations. The energy contained in string vibrations is quite small compared to the energy in frame vibrations, because the frame has about 20 times the mass of the strings.

It is obviously very desirable to hit the ball at the node, or close to it, because this eliminates or minimizes the subsequent annoying vibrations of the frame. With the old, small-headed, wooden rackets, the node location tended to be near the throat of the frame. When racket heads were enlarged by extending them down toward the handle, the centre of the head was moved closer to the node. It is also possible to move the location of the node by changing the stiffness or mass distribution of the frame.

While vibrations are annoying and bothersome, there is no clinical evidence that vibrations of either the frame or the strings can cause any type of hand, wrist, arm or elbow damage.

The power of the tennis racket

The term power, as used in tennis, refers to the speed of the outgoing ball relative to the effort the player has exerted in swinging the racket. This is to be distinguished from the definition of power used in physics and engineering where the term means the rate at which work is done or energy transformed.

As important as the power of a racket is, the variation of the power with respect to ball impact location may be more important. If the ball strikes the strings at a small distance from the desired location and the result is a very different ball rebound, then the power sweet spot is considered to be very small and the racket will be difficult to play with. If, on the other hand, some miss-hits still lead to acceptable ball trajectories, the racket is said to have a large sweet spot, be 'forgiving' and enjoyable to play with.

If the ball strikes the racket at the CM of the frame, the amount of power (rebound ball speed) would be determined primarily by the strings and the mass of the racket, assuming a fairly rigid frame. The recoiling racket would have translational kinetic energy, but no rotational kinetic energy. As it is rare that a ball is struck at the CM (it is usually located outside of the strung region of the head), the mass moments of inertia about the principal axes and the distance of the ball impact from these axes come into play. The moment of inertia of an object about a particular axis is that property of the object that determines how much the object's rotational motion changes when struck off-axis. The larger the moment, the less an object's rotational motion changes for a given angular impulse. Moment of inertia is usually denoted by the symbol I, and it is equal to the sum of all the mass in the object multiplied by the square of the distance of that mass from the axis of rotation. The farther from the axis a ball strikes, the greater is the transfer of rotational momentum to the racket, and the larger is the racket's rotational kinetic energy. The more kinetic energy the racket ends up with, the less energy the rebounding ball ends up with. Increasing the moment of inertia about an axis will reduce the amount of rotational kinetic energy the recoiling racket takes away. This means the ball will end up with an increase in its energy.

Polar or roll moment of inertia

As an example, the magnitude of the moment of inertia about the long axis of the racket (the axis running along the handle, called the polar or roll moment) is determined primarily by the head width squared and the racket weight. If a racket head is increased in width from 20 cm to 25 cm (a 25% increase), the polar moment increases by 50%, because it goes as the square of the distance of the frame from the axis.

If a ball strikes the racket away from the long axis, the racket will twist around that axis. The farther the impact is from the axis and the higher the ball speed, the more the racket will twist. A simple calculation of the impulsive torques involved and the force that the hand can generate shows that for impacts that miss the axis by a few centimetres or more, the hand cannot prevent the racket from twisting. The more the racket twists, the more rotational kinetic energy it acquires, and therefore, the less rebound energy the ball ends up with. Since the moment of inertia of a racket about the long axis is very small, the effective power of the racket degrades quickly as the impact location moves further off-axis. In addition, since the racket is twisting, the angle at which the ball rebounds depends on exactly where, relative to the axis, the ball strikes.

The way to reduce this degradation of power and erroneous angle of rebound is to increase the moment of inertia of the racket about the long axis (the polar moment or the roll moment). This is one of the reasons why the oversize racket with a 25% wider head (and a 50% greater moment) gained immediate acceptance by the tennis-playing public when it was introduced. It would then seem logical that players should adopt a racket with the widest head allowed by the International Tennis Federation (31.75 cm). However, along with these benefits that the wider head provides, there is also a drawback. As the moment of inertia increases, the racket becomes somewhat less manoeuvrable. For a baseline player who does not twist and turn the racket a great deal in the course of stroking the ball, this may not be a serious detriment. For the aggressive serve and volley player, or a player whose strokes involve much arm rotation and pronation, a large polar moment can be a problem. This type of player usually selects a racket with a mid-size rather than oversize head as a compromise solution.

The polar moment of any racket can be increased by placing additional weight (lead tape) at the 3 o'clock and 9 o'clock position of the head. About 5 g on each side of the head will add about 10% to the polar moment, adding stability and power on off-axis impacts.

Longitudinal power distribution

As the ball impact position moves away from the CM toward the racket tip, the power (rebound ball speed) decreases, if the racket is at rest (which is how most rackets are tested). The fall-off in power is not as great in this direction as the fall-off for impacts away from the long axis, because the moment of inertia in this case is about eight times greater than the polar or roll moment (the racket is much longer than it is wide). Racket designers and manufacturers have attempted to move the maximum power point away from the throat area and up towards the centre of the strung area, where players tend to hit the ball. This also places it closer to the other two sweet spots. They have produced rackets that are head heavy (actually handle light) to move the CM up higher on the head, adjusted the string pattern to provide greater string plane deformation higher in the head, and made the head much stiffer.

It is also possible to move the power up higher on the head of the racket by adding weight (usually in the form of lead tape) to the tip of the racket. This will both move the CM up higher in the racket and increase the moment of inertia about the axis through the CM. Both of these effects will increase the speed of the rebounding ball when the impact is near the centre of the head. Adding weight to the tip has its disadvantages as well. If 10 g are added to the tip of a 300-g racket, the swingweight of that racket increases by more than 10%. Swingweight (moment of inertia about the butt end) is a measure of how difficult it is to swing the racket. An increase in swingweight means that the player will have to exert more effort (torque) to get the racket up to speed.

Racket weight and balance

Because a 300-g tennis racket is so much more massive than a 58-g tennis ball, the rebound speed of the ball is surprisingly insensitive to the exact racket weight. As the collision of the ball and the racket lasts

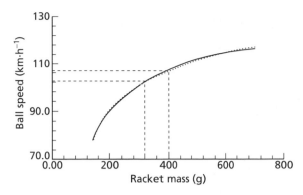

Fig. 2.5 Struck ball speed vs. mass of racket for a groundstroke. Both incident ball and racket head speed are 50 km·h^{-1}. A change in racket mass from 320 g to 400 g (a 25% increase) will only increase the ball speed from 102.5 km·h^{-1} to 107 km·h^{-1} (a 4% increase), assuming the racket head speed does not change.

only about 4 ms, the hand and arm do not add much momentum to the racket during the actual impact. Therefore, the collision can be considered to conserve momentum (the vector momentum of the ball and racket before the collision will equal the vector momentum of the ball and racket after the collision). Making use of this fact, and keeping the incident ball and racket speed fixed, it is possible to calculate the outgoing ball speed for various racket masses. This is shown in Fig. 2.5. Note that a large change in racket mass results in very little change in outgoing ball speed. All of this is assuming that the initial racket speed does not change when the racket is made heavier or lighter.

If the racket head speed changes there is a large change in ball speed. Therefore, if changing the racket weight results in a change in racket head speed, there also will be a change in ball speed. However, as smaller racket weight should lead to higher head speed, decreasing the racket weight can often lead to higher ball speed. If, on the other hand, the player does not change racket head speed when the racket weight is changed, there will be a very slight effect in the other direction.

The strings

It is interesting that most of the major advances in tennis technology have concerned the racket frame and not the strings that go into the frame. Yet it is the strings that contact the ball, and not the frame. There have been improvements in the various synthetic strings that are used in tennis, but the preferred material by the top professional tennis players is still gut (animal intestines), as it was half a century ago.

Strings are used in tennis rackets instead of an elastic membrane because of the reduced air resistance that an array of very thin strings (about 1–1.5 mm diam.) has compared to a membrane. One needs only to place a piece of paper over the strings and swing the racket to feel the effect of air resistance. In addition, strings tend to bite into the ball, where a membrane will not.

The purpose of the strings is to transfer some of the kinetic energy or momentum that the racket frame has to the ball as efficiently as possible. By the official rules of tennis, the ball must dissipate almost half the energy it brings into a collision with a hard surface. There are no rules concerning the energy return of strings. Good-quality strings will return to the ball about 95% of the energy that they absorb when they deform. When the ball hits the strings, both deform and both store energy in the process. It is clear where you want most of the energy stored. Because the strings only dissipate 5% of the energy they absorb, while the ball dissipates a considerably larger percentage of the energy it absorbs, to get maximum rebound ball speed, one wants the strings to absorb as much of the initial kinetic energy of the ball as is possible. Reducing the tension in the strings allows this to happen more readily, and results in higher rebound ball velocities for the same racket head speed.

It is generally accepted among many tennis players and coaches that tighter strings provide better control over the ball. However, this result is based mainly on anecdotal evidence. There is no scientifically valid data in the literature either to substantiate or refute this conjecture.

Even though most players and racket manufacturers specify the string tension (in pounds, Newtons or kilopods), it is actually the string plane stiffness or deformation that determines how the strings behave and respond in the racket. String plane deformation is a measure of the excursion of the strings from their equilibrium position, in a direction perpendicular to the string plane, as a function of applied force. In this respect, the string plane is acting like a simple spring,

deforming and storing energy. Lower string tension, lower string density (fewer strings per centimetre), more elastic strings and longer string lengths (due to a larger racket head) all contribute to a larger string plane deformation for a given external force. The larger the string plane deformation, the longer the ball will remain in contact with the strings (dwell time or contact time) and the greater the recoiling ball speed will be. As the dwell or contact time increases, the peak magnitude of the forces transmitted to a player's hand and arm are reduced. Longer contact time gives the racket a softer, more comfortable feel at impact.

There are several ways to measure string plane stiffness, including a direct measurement using a Babolat Racket Diagnostic Center. This device applies a force perpendicular to the string plane and measures the plane deformation. There are also various small electronic instruments that sense the frequency of the vibration of the entire string plane with the instrument clamped to the strings, and get string-plane stiffness from this measurement. Knowing the head size and the string spacing, it is possible to convert from string-plane deformation (or stiffness) to average string tension. The small electronic instruments do this automatically, by requesting that the head size and string spacing be entered. Because most players and racket stringers talk about tension, and not string-plane deformation or stiffness, this chapter will continue to use the term 'tension'. Players often try to determine the string tension in their racket by plucking, strumming or striking the strings, and listening to the pitch of the resulting sound. This is at best only a relative measurement. The frequency (pitch) of the vibrating string plane depends on the average length of strings, gauge (thickness) of the strings, and density of the material the strings are made of, in addition to the tension. If you have two rackets with identical head sizes, identical stringing patterns, and using the same type of strings, then the pitch of the ping of the strings is a good indication of their relative tensions. When you compare rackets with different head sizes, different gauge (thickness) of string, or different types of string, your ear may detect a difference in the pitch, but it may not be due to a difference in string tension.

The tension in the strings decreases with time and with use. To get around this problem, some of the top players insist that every racket they use be freshly strung on the day of a match. For many recreational players, the strings are not replaced until one breaks. Other players replace their strings when the racket is not responding the way they think it should. There are some guidelines on how often to restring a racket, but none of the suggestions is based on anything but anecdotal information. There are no objective tests or measures that will tell a player that it is time to get fresh strings in the racket. As the strings age, they probably lose some of their elasticity. However, looser strings tend to produce higher ball speeds, so the two effects may tend to cancel each other out. If it is true that tighter strings give better control, then there is good reason to replace the strings as they age and soften.

When the ball hits the strings, they deform and then snap back, propelling the ball off the strings. The strings then overshoot their equilibrium position and oscillate for a short time at about 400–600 Hz or vibrations per second. (This is the same frequency that you get when you strum or pluck the strings.) This vibration feeds into the frame of the racket and may annoy some players. It is possible to damp out the string vibration by placing a small commercially available absorber in the string bed, close to the periphery of the head. This absorber also changes the sound that is made by the ball string interaction from a 'ping' to a 'thud'. It is very unlikely that the vibrations of the strings can cause any damage to the hand, arm or elbow of the player. This is because the strings have a mass of about 15 g, so the energy involved in their oscillation is very small compared to the other energy terms in the ball–racket interaction. These vibration dampers are very successful in reducing string plane oscillations. They do essentially nothing to reduce or damp out vibrations of the frame of the racket.

If the racket head is firmly clamped so that it cannot move and tennis balls are fired towards it, the rebound ball speed as a function of impact location can be determined. (The ratio of rebound to incident ball speed is called the coefficient of restitution or COR for short.) It is usually found that the COR is a maximum near the centre of the head (where the string plane deformation is a maximum) and the COR falls off slightly as the impact location approaches the frame, where the string plane is stiffer. This pattern can be modified somewhat by adjusting either the string

tension in individual strings or changing the spacing between adjacent strings. A fan or diverging pattern of strings (as opposed to a uniform rectangular grid) will have a higher COR where the strings are further apart compared to the same location on a rectangular grid with small spacing.

Thinner strings (of the same material and construction) should be more elastic and might bite into the ball somewhat better. Since the elasticity of a string is inversely proportional to the string's cross-sectional area, a 10% reduction in string diameter should lead to a 20% change in elasticity. There is some evidence that as the tension increases, some elasticity is 'pulled' out of synthetic strings and they become stiffer and somewhat 'boardy'. Gut strings, on the other hand, seem to retain more of their elastic nature until they reach their tensile limit.

The modern racket

Tennis rackets are tested both for static and dynamic properties such as weight, size, balance, stiffness and moments about the principal axes, and for their interaction properties, such as COR. The stiffness of a racket frame can be measured by applying forces at various locations and measuring the deformations. The stiffness also can be obtained by determining the racket's resonant frequency and knowing that the stiffness goes approximately as the frequency squared divided by both the racket mass and the cube of its length. The moments of inertia are usually measured by suspending the racket from a calibrated wire (torsion pendulum) and measuring the period of the oscillation (Brody 1985).

The interaction properties (COR) are measured by firing tennis balls at the racket and measuring the ratio of rebound to incident ball speed for various locations on the racket head. Years ago, this was done with the racket handle firmly clamped in place, but now it is done with either a free racket or one that has some minimal constraints on the handle. This change came about because it has been shown that a hand-held racket is not well represented by a racket with its handle clamped in place. With a free racket, the ratio of rebound ball speed to incident ball speed is called the apparent coefficient of restitution (ACOR) (Hatze 1994). (It is not the coefficient of restitution because the recoil of the racket is neglected.) For most rackets, the ACOR is a maximum near the CM, falls off quickly as the impact point moves away from the long axis, and falls off slowly as the impact point moves from the CM towards the tip along the main axis of the racket. However, this testing will give you the power distribution for various ball impact locations on the head only for a static racket. If the racket is being translated with a speed V (racket), then the speed of the struck ball is given by:

$$v \text{ (struck)} = (\text{ACOR} \times v \text{ (incident)}) + ((1 + \text{ACOR}) \times V \text{ (racket)}) \qquad (1)$$

where v (incident) is the speed of the incident ball. This equation would give the correct answer for the maximum power point if the racket were being translated only, but on the court it is being swung, not translated. The term V (racket) in the formula is the racket head velocity at the point of ball impact, and for a swung racket, this varies with position on the head. The tip of the racket is moving much faster than the throat, which means that the impact location of maximum struck ball speed is considerably higher on the head of the racket than the ACOR map of the head at rest would indicate. For a modern head-heavy frame being swung with an effective pivot point near the butt end of the racket, the maximum power point (maximum ball rebound speed) can come out close to the centre of the racket head for a groundstroke. For a serve, where the first term of eqn 1 is zero (no initial ball speed), the maximum power point comes out well above the centre of the head of the racket.

Errors and the racket

Errors are those shots that go wide of the sidelines, hit the net or sail over the baseline. The acceptance window for hitting a shot that lands in the court is usually much greater in the horizontal direction ($\pm 9°$) than it is in the vertical direction, where it is primarily determined by how hard the ball is hit. The higher the ball speed, the less time gravity has to pull the ball into the court, and the more difficult it is to have the shot land good. Yet, the modern game is played with what seems to be much more pace on the ball, and not the corresponding increase in errors that the previous argument would predict. The improvement in the players, the changes in strokes and the improvement in the racket are responsible for this.

On the serve, the improvement in rackets (lighter, more power near the tip) has allowed more high-speed serves to go in. Because the rackets are much lighter, the player can whip them around faster on the serve, yielding higher racket head speed. This in turn leads to higher ball speeds, as eqn 1 shows. By the logic of the previous paragraph, if the ball speed increases, the first serve percentages should go down. However, the modern racket allows the player to maximize the serve speed while striking the ball close to the racket tip, which increases the height at which the ball is struck. Add to this the change in the foot fault rule, which allows a player to be off of the ground when striking the ball, and even more height is available. This combination of additional heights increases the service acceptance window that the higher ball speed had decreased. The result is the serve has become a much more formidable weapon, particularly on fast courts.

The groundstrokes also are being hit harder, even though in theory this also will reduce the window or margin for error in the shot. The new rackets, coupled with the newer style of groundstroke has produced an interesting error reducing effect that allows this higher ball speed to be used.

When balls are hit with topspin, the Magnus Effect produces a downward force in addition to gravity. This extra downward force means that a ball can be hit very hard, spend very little time in its flight, yet still end up landing within the court. This would not be the case for a flat or backspin shot.

At the increased ball speed, the acceptance window can be so small that slight variations in impact location of the ball on the racket head may lead to balls hitting the net or sailing long. With the classic tennis stroke and the classic wooden racket, the power peaked near the racket throat and decreased as the impact location moved toward the tip. Most players aim to strike the ball near the centre of the racket head, so slight errors in impact location (which are very common) would lead to less rebound ball speed or more rebound ball speed, depending on exactly where the ball was struck. If the player aimed central impacts on the head so that the ball would land deep in the court ('getting good depth'), impacts that were closer to the throat would come off with greater speed and go long. To avoid this common error, players would either aim somewhat shorter in the court, or hit the ball somewhat softer to increase their margin of error.

With the modern racket and groundstroke, the peak power is near the centre of the head, which is usually the preferred impact location. If the player attempts to hit shots near the centre of the head and aims those shots quite deep in the court, any ball missing the centre of the head will come off with less speed and land somewhat shorter. Slight miss-hits then cannot go long, and errors of that type are avoided. This allows the player to swing out and hit the ball hard, confident that the shot will land in the court.

Side-to-side errors can be much less important because the court is so wide, unless you are aiming for the corner or trying to pass someone at net. If you aim for the centre of the court, you have ±9° margin of error. When you aim for the corner or try to go down the line, you determine your own margin of error by how close to the edge you aim your shot. There is also another safe play. If you attempt to return a ball to the location it is coming from, you will tend to make fewer errors in the horizontal direction. If you return a cross-court shot cross-court or if you return a down-the-line shot down the line, you will have more control over the ball direction. In each of these cases, the ball approaches and leaves the racket perpendicular (normal) to the string plane. If the racket is aimed correctly at impact, the ball will go in the direction you want it to. This is not the case when you change the ball direction. Then the ball is not impacting perpendicular to the racket face, and the angle at which the ball emerges not only depends on the racket head angle, but also on how hard the racket is being swung. The harder the ball is hit, the closer will the ball's trajectory follow the racket's direction. The softer the shot, the larger will be the angle between the normal to the racket face and the ball trajectory. This effect is caused by the fact that the rebounding component of ball velocity parallel to the racket face does not depend on the ball or racket head speed, while the normal component of the rebounding ball velocity depends on ball and racket speed as is given in eqn 1. When you are returning shots coming at you cross-court by hitting them hard down the line, and they are going in, if you ease up

on your stroke (possibly to play cautiously), the ball may land in the alley.

The speed of the game

Every year there is a cry by some tennis fans, players and the media to slow the game down, particularly the serve on grass courts. One of the principal suggestions is to modify the racket design specifications, possibly returning to wooden rackets. If eqn 1 is examined, for a serve, the speed of the outgoing ball is

$$v\,(\text{struck}) = (1 + \text{ACOR}) \times V\,(\text{racket}).$$

Assume a player is capable of hitting a serve at 210 km·h^{-1} (130 mph) when the ACOR of the racket is 0.30 at a particular ball impact location on the racket. If the racket or ball specifications are changed so as to reduce the ACOR by 1/3 (the new ACOR would be 0.20, which corresponds to a very dead racket or ball), the corresponding speed of the serve would only be reduced to 194 km·h^{-1} (120 mph). Since the ACOR of a typical old wooden racket was considerably greater than 0.20, changing the racket power or even taking some of the air out of the ball is not the solution to this problem.

New size of tennis ball

What seems to be the best idea to slow the game down is to make the ball slightly larger (Haake *et al.* 2000). This is the solution adopted by the International Tennis Federation (ITF) and it is called the Type 3 ball. It is approximately 6% larger (in diameter) than a standard ball (Type 2), but is essentially identical to the standard ball in every other property.

A ball that is 6% larger will have a cross-sectional area that is over 12% larger than a standard ball. This means that in its flight through the air it will run into many more air molecules than a standard ball would. Each of these collisions with an air molecule slows the ball down just a little, and if there are more collisions, the ball will slow down more. Elaborate wind tunnel and computer modelling studies have been done, as well as video analysis of the actual ball trajectories, to verify this hypothesis. Players using this larger ball are in general agreement that the game is slowed down.

For a typical groundstroke, a standard ball reached the other baseline moving at 50% of its original speed. The same shot, hit with the larger ball, will reach the opposite baseline moving at 47% of its original speed.

Several unpublished studies of on-court testing of the larger ball against the standard ball by the ITF and by the United States Tennis Association (USTA) show that the number of strokes per rally increases, since the players have more time to get to and prepare for shots. On the basis of preliminary data, there seem to be no deleterious health problems associated with the enlarged ball.

References

Brody, H. (1985) The moment of inertia of a tennis racket. *Physics Teacher* **23**, 213.

Brody, H. (1987) *Tennis Science for Tennis Players.* University of Pennsylvania Press, Philadelphia, PA, USA.

Brody, H. (1995) How would a physicist design a tennis racket? *Physics Today* **48** (3), 29.

Haake, S.J., Chadwick, S.G., Dignall, R.J., Goodwill, S. & Rose, P. (2000) Engineering tennis—slowing the game down. *Sports Engineering* **3**, 131–144.

Hatze, H. (1994) The relationship between the coefficient of restitution and energy losses in tennis rackets. *Journal of Applied Biomechanics* **9**, 124.

Chapter 3

Shoes and surfaces in tennis: injury and performance aspects

Introduction

Tennis is an exciting game, and an excellent way to develop cardiovascular endurance and muscular strength for both upper and lower extremities. Unfortunately, injuries in tennis are very common, not only amongst athletes at the professional level but also amongst athletes at the recreational level. A retrospective study showed that 32% of recreational tennis players, who played on average 1–2 h per week, suffered at least one tennis-related injury during a regular season (Nigg & Denoth 1980). The incidence of injuries increased with playing time up to 49% amongst people who played tennis on average more than 9 h per week. Several factors will determine if one sustains an injury. Amongst these factors are physical conditioning level, technique, shoes and playing surface. Tennis is a very interesting sport in that there are substantial differences in the surfaces that are played on. This is expressed in the four Grand Slam tournaments, which are played on hard courts (Australian Open and US Open), on clay (Roland Garros) and on grass (Wimbledon). This chapter will examine the effects of shoes and playing surfaces on lower extremity injury rates, investigating the potential of shoes and surfaces to decrease lower extremity injuries in tennis.

In addition to influencing injury rates, shoes and playing surfaces also affect physical performance in tennis. Tennis involves a variety of physical movements including running, sprinting, cutting, twisting, starting and stopping movements, and jumping. The overall performance in tennis will to some extent depend on the ability to execute these movements well. Shoes and playing surface are important determinants of whether a movement can be executed well. Therefore, this chapter will also examine possible

effects of shoes and playing surfaces on tennis performance, investigating the potential of shoes and surfaces to increase performance in tennis.

It is the purpose of this chapter to summarize the current knowledge on the role of shoes and playing surfaces related to both injury and performance aspects of tennis. Firstly, data on the incidence and prevalence of lower extremity injuries in tennis are summarized, and a closer look at the biomechanical environment that a tennis player may experience is provided by presenting experimental kinetic and kinematic data for a side-shuffle movement. The possible effects of such biomechanical loading on the musculoskeletal system are examined in light of the lower extremity injury statistics to explore potential injury mechanisms. Secondly, the role of shoes and surfaces with respect to performance aspects of tennis is described. Finally, possible modifications to both shoes and tennis surfaces that may help to either decrease lower extremity injury rates or increase performance are explored.

Injury aspects

Lower extremity injuries in tennis

Injuries can be divided into two groups according to how they occur, namely as either acute (i.e. traumatic) or chronic (i.e. overuse) injuries. It is very important to study the incidence and prevalence of lower extremity injuries to identify possible risk factors. This section first presents a general picture of the kind of acute and chronic lower extremity injuries that occur during tennis. Subsequently, findings of several studies that have combined data on lower extremity injuries with data on specific shoes or playing surfaces are described.

Acute injuries

An injury surveillance amongst young elite male tennis athletes ($n = 1440$) showed that 21.1% of this population sustained new (10.1%) or recurrent injuries that required medical attention (Hutchinson *et al.* 1995) during the US National Championships for juniors (under 18 years of age), which were held on a hard-court surface similar to the one used at the US Open Grand Slam tournament. In these athletes,

48.8% of all injuries were lower extremity injuries, which occurred almost twice as frequently as upper extremity (26.5%) or central injuries (24.7%). Sprains (55%) and strains (17.1%) were most commonly observed amongst all injuries while fractures and dislocations were very rare (1.3%). The majority of sprain-type injuries occurred in the lower extremity. These data are consistent with data that were reported on another group of elite young tennis players at the Australian Institute of Sport (Reece *et al.* 1986). Over a 4-year period, the tennis athletes reported on average between two and three injuries each. This study also reported a dominance of lower extremity injuries (59%) vs. upper extremity (20%) and trunk (21%) injuries. The most commonly observed intrinsic injury was a sprained ankle. Calf and quadriceps strains were next in order. All courts at the Australian Institute of Sport are non-slip Plexipave surfaces. Most of the knee injuries (70%) that occur in tennis are of an acute, traumatic nature (Renstrom 1995). Knee injuries comprise a total of 19% of all tennis injuries. The medial collateral and the anterior cruciate ligament are the most commonly injured knee ligaments in tennis.

Chronic injuries

Thirty per cent of all knee injuries are overuse injuries (Renstrom 1995). Patellofemoral pain is quite common amongst young tennis players. Amongst players under 14 years of age, 7% (boys) to 11% (girls) report anterior knee pain. Most meniscus injuries occur in the middle-aged and elderly tennis players. Degenerative cartilage problems, either on the femoral condyles or on the posterior surface of the patella, are commonly observed in elderly tennis players.

Surfaces and shoes

Several studies have shown that the playing surface has an influence on lower extremity injury rates in tennis. Senior tennis players have fewer knee problems when they have spent most of their tennis careers on clay courts (Kulund *et al.* 1979). A small sample (*n* = 15) of elite tennis athletes reported back pain and lower extremity pain when playing on hard courts, but did not complain of pain when playing on clay courts (von Salis-Soglio 1979). Knee overuse

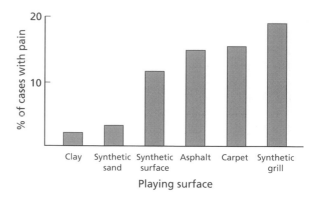

Fig. 3.1 Percentage of pain and injuries on different playing surfaces (*n* – 1003 tennis players). (Data from Nigg and Denoth 1980.)

injuries and knee ligament sprains occur more commonly on concrete surfaces than on clay surfaces (Renstrom 1995). Significantly fewer injuries were observed (*n* = 1003) on clay courts or synthetic surfaces with a loose granular topping (2–3% of all injuries) when compared to hard courts (up to 18% of all injuries) (Fig. 3.1) (Nigg & Yeadon 1987). In other words, subjects experienced significantly less pain when playing on surfaces that allow a controlled sliding movement. The cushioning properties of the playing surfaces appeared to be less important than the sliding characteristics. Surfaces with very similar stiffness characteristics, namely the 'synthetic sand' and the 'synthetic surface', show a significant difference in the number of players reporting pain while playing on these surfaces (Fig. 3.1). Therefore, it was speculated that the differences in injury frequency are directly related to the differences in frictional properties of the surface (Nigg & Segesser 1988). It was also investigated whether shoe properties affect tennis injury rates. In an experimental study, 33% of the subjects that were using a soft and flexible tennis shoe reported pain, discomfort or injuries. Many more subjects (49%) reported pain, discomfort or injuries amongst a group of subjects that were using a harder and stiffer tennis shoe (Luethi *et al.* 1986).

Summary

A variety of acute and chronic lower extremity injuries are commonly observed amongst tennis players of all ages. Young tennis players appear to experience mostly acute injuries, such as ligament and muscle sprains, whereas older tennis players experience mostly chronic injuries, such as degenerative cartilage problems. The frictional characteristics of the tennis shoe–surface interface is a very important risk factor for lower extremity injuries in tennis. Specifically, shoe–surface interfaces that do not allow a player to execute controlled sliding movements are associated with a much higher risk of injury.

Biomechanical environment

The physical demands on the lower extremity during tennis can be great. Tennis involves a variety of movements including running and shuffling from side to side. The magnitude of the net ground reaction force vector averaged over 10 subjects during heel–toe running at 4.0 m·s^{-1} exceeds two times bodyweight (Fig. 3.2). During a maximum-effort side-shuffle movement (moving to the right, planting the right foot, and pushing off again moving now to the left as rapidly as possible), the magnitudes of the peak external forces are not as great as during running, but the time over which the force is acting on the musculoskeletal system is much longer.

The forces in the muscles and joints of the leg can be much greater than the externally measured ground reaction forces. In both running and in the side-shuffle movement, the ground reaction force rises rapidly to a peak shortly as a result of the collision of the leg with the ground. These impact forces are associated with large decelerations of the lower extremity. Active forces, which are caused by actively contracting muscles (either eccentrically to break the movement or concentrically to generate push-off), can result in very high internal forces.

The range through which the joints move during tennis can be greater than during other movements such as running. Figure 3.3 (top) shows the position of the leg at the time of maximum knee flexion during a running trial, while Fig. 3.3 (bottom) shows the position of the leg at the time of maximum knee flexion during a side-shuffle movement (same $n = 10$ from Fig. 3.2). Both the hip and the knee joints are flexed more during the side-shuffle movement than during running. Also, the ankle joint reaches a much more inverted position, that is the sole of the foot is rotated more inwards during the side-shuffle movement than during running. Large joint flexion and inversion angles effectively increase the moment arm of the ground reaction force about the joint, increasing the joint moments and consequently increasing the required muscle forces. As a result of the higher muscle forces, there will be higher forces between the joint surfaces.

Summary

During a tennis game the human body experiences large forces (both impact and active) on the lower extremity. Areas where high loading, large muscle forces and extreme ankle joint positions occur are visually presented in Fig. 3.3. The external load on the lower extremities during a side-shuffle movement is created largely by friction generated between the tennis shoe and the playing surface.

Injury mechanisms

This section will examine the possible effects of the biomechanical environment (impact and active forces, extreme joint positions) on the musculoskeletal system (bones, cartilage, muscles, tendons, and ligaments).

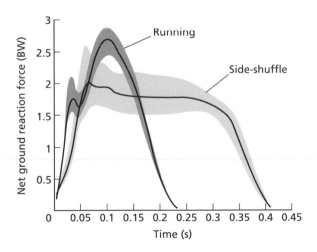

Fig. 3.2 Mean ($n = 10$) and standard deviation (grey area) of the net ground reaction force profiles (normalized to bodyweight (BW) and expressed as N force/N bodyweight) during running and during a side-shuffle movement.

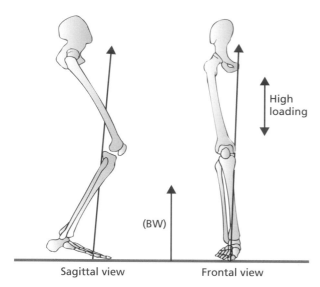

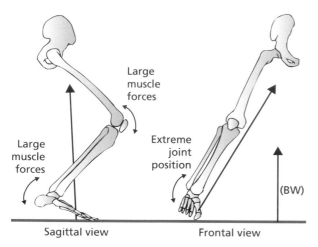

Fig. 3.3 Mean ($n = 10$) maximum knee flexion during running (top) and during a side-shuffle movement (bottom). Corresponding net ground reaction force vectors are also shown. BW, Bodyweight.

loading may be highly osteogenic, that is it induces formation of bone. However, excessive repetitive loads may also cause stress fractures in bone and repeated exposure to impact forces may cause microdamage in cartilage as has been observed in animal models. Nevertheless, a relationship between impact forces and running injuries has yet to be shown in epidemiology studies. Degenerative cartilage problems, which are generally observed in the elderly tennis population, may be caused by the cumulative effect of repeated trauma from excessive external loading (see Figs 3.2 and 3.3) during many years of tennis.

The landing movements during tennis cause eccentric muscular actions. Eccentric muscle forces are required to break the side-shuffle movement shown in Fig. 3.3. This breaking action is followed by concentric muscle action to generate the push-off. Eccentric contractions have been associated with injuries to the musculotendon complex. Eccentric muscular contractions can result in damage to muscle fibres. Particularly, the strain during active lengthening appears to be an important determinant for muscle damage. Nevertheless, this process is reversible. Muscle fibres have the ability to return to their normal conditions, and may even adapt, such that future bouts of exercise will cause less injury to the muscle. The tendon, on the other hand, is not as richly vascularized as the muscle belly, and therefore it has no similar regenerative capabilities to help return it to normal. Tendon injuries can become chronic injuries (tendinitis) as repetitive mechanical strains can cause injuries to all soft tissues. This occurs when the microdamage caused by the repetitive motion exceeds the normal remodelling capacity of the tissue. When the loading on the tendon exceeds its failure load, the tendon ruptures.

Impact and active forces

High loading environments have been shown to have beneficial effects on the human body, especially on bones. Values for bone mineral content (BMC) and bone mineral density (BMD) of the dominant arm in young professional tennis players were significantly higher than for the non-dominant arm (Pirnay *et al.* 1987), indicating a higher quality extracellular bone matrix. This finding demonstrates that dynamic

Extreme joint positions

When joints approach the limits of their range of motion, ligaments are at risk. Forcing a joint to extremes rapidly increases the loading of the ligaments, which may result in ligament sprains. Ligament injuries are often acute injuries, and are often quite severe in nature. Ligaments have only limited regeneration capabilities. Once a ligament has ruptured it does not appear to be able to return to a 'normal' ligament. During a purely lateral side-shuffle movement (see Fig. 3.3, bottom) the ankle joint is at risk. Excessive inversion may result in an ankle sprain. In addition to purely lateral movements, tennis also involves a lot of twisting and turning motions. Excessive varus/valgus or internal/external rotation may result in a knee sprain, in particular the anterior cruciate ligament and the medial collateral ligament of the knee joint may be sprained.

Summary

The effect of impact and active forces, eccentric loading and extreme joint positions acting on the musculoskeletal system may be beneficial. However, there is a delicate balance between benefits and disadvantages. A biomechanical overload may easily result in injuries to structures in the lower extremity, including articular cartilage, muscles and tendons, and ligaments. These types of injuries are consistent with the tennis-related lower extremity injuries described above. The high loads on a variety of different structures in the lower extremity are primarily caused by friction between the lower extremity and the playing surface. Lower frictional forces would reduce the load in these structures, and are likely to result in fewer injuries.

Performance aspects

Performance in tennis is not as clearly defined as in the 100-m sprint or in the high-jump event. Overall performance in tennis depends on many factors. Elite coaches attribute success in tennis to mental and tactical skills, technique and physical performance. Performance in tennis is also very surface specific. Some players prefer one surface to another, because as the surface affects the character of the game, their specific qualities are more effective on that particular surface. In addition to strength and conditioning level, sporting performance is also affected by the tennis shoe and the playing surface. The influence of shoes and surfaces on sporting performance in tennis may be quantified by looking at specific subsets of performance one at a time. The following quantities might be measured to assess specific performance using various shoes and surfaces:

- time on running circuits;
- jump height; and
- oxygen consumption to estimate energetic cost.

Frictional forces are required for propulsion. The sliding that may occur in cases where there is low friction can be considered a loss of energy. Higher coefficients of friction between shoe or surface are likely to result in a better specific performance on various performance tests, in particular those including sprinting and turning movements.

To summarize, overall performance in tennis depends on many factors, including physical performance. The influence of shoes and surfaces on sporting performance can be assessed by measuring performance-related variables on very specific subsets of sporting performance.

Modifications to shoe and surface

The next step is to combine the (potential) injury mechanisms with the performance aspects, and to determine whether there are conflicts of interest. Higher coefficients of friction are associated with a higher specific performance; however, higher friction coefficients are also associated with a higher risk of injury. People playing tennis on surfaces with high friction characteristics experience significantly more injuries than people playing tennis on surfaces with low friction characteristics (see Fig. 3.1). Lower frictional forces decrease the ground reaction force vector (Fig. 3.3) and will therefore substantially decrease the muscle forces and the loading in the joints. It must be noted that frictional forces should not be too small either, because propulsion would be very difficult, and slipping might occur. It appears that the shoe and surface characteristics should be such that optimal friction between shoe and surface exists. As the rate of injuries on courts that permit sliding is substantially lower than on courts that do not permit sliding, it appears that clay courts in combination with today's tennis shoes approach the optimal friction much closer than any hard court in combination with any shoe that is currently on the market.

One could argue that injury avoidance should also be considered as a performance criterion. The benefits of a lower friction between shoe and surface, that is the decreased risk of an injury, may outweigh the compromises in sporting performance. Furthermore, because overall performance in tennis depends on many factors other than shoes, there is a good chance that potential injury-reducing modifications will not substantially limit overall tennis performance. It appears that the focus of shoe construction should be aimed at reducing the rate of lower extremity injuries in tennis, rather than be aimed at increasing performance aspects.

In spite of the substantial differences in characteristics of tennis playing surfaces, the tennis shoes that are currently on the market are often marketed as shoes that may be used on all different playing surfaces: 'one shoe fits all'. To achieve lower friction levels between tennis shoe and playing surface, one should therefore play tennis on surfaces that permit sliding movements. Considering the fact that the injury rates are substantially lower on such playing surfaces, it may be worthwhile investigating the possibilities to either adopt the rather expensive clay courts, or to construct low-maintenance, cost-effective artificial playing surfaces with a loose granular topping. Constructing specific tennis shoes for specific playing surfaces could reduce the rate of injuries even further.

Determining the relationships between injury mechanisms, tennis shoes, playing surfaces and performance aspects is extremely difficult. A complete understanding of the complex relationships between the external loading environment and its action on the lower extremity is still lacking. Even though footwear design criteria that aim for injury minimization have yet to be established (Barnes & Smith 1993), a well-designed shoe in combination with a well-designed playing surface has potential to assist in reducing the number of lower limb injuries arising from tennis activities. Shoes could:
• increase comfort;
• provide lateral stability by controlling the movement (inversion/eversion) using heel counters and lacing systems;
• help reduce impacts (shock absorption/cushioning);
• alter the pressure distribution; and
• provide rotational and translation friction.

Some elite players have turned to high-cut tennis shoes similar to developments in basketball, and some coaches encourage ankle bracing (Reece et al. 1986). Lateral stability of the shoe is very important in relation to ankle sprains. High-topped shoes may provide enhanced sensation of ankle position (Barnes & Smith 1993) or may mechanically stiffen the ankle joint. Whatever the mechanism, high-topped shoes have led to a decrease in ankle injuries among basketball players (Garrick & Requa 1973) and bracing has led to a fivefold decrease in recurrent ankle injuries amongst soccer players (Surve et al. 1994). It must be noted that it is very difficult to design a shoe that prevents excessive inversion while allowing eversion and full plantar flexion and dorsiflexion movements. These movements are a very important factor in, for example, sprinting performance. A restriction of the normal range of joint motion may lead to a decrease in sporting performance.

Summary

Modifications to tennis shoes and playing surfaces should be aimed at reducing the risk of lower extremity injuries during tennis. Even though there are a lot of indications to do so, it would probably go too far to ban all hard-court, high-friction surfaces. The character of the play is altered significantly when playing on a different surface. Different aspects of performance become more important and the Grand Slam tournaments often feature different champions. As long as the majority of the important tournaments is still played on hard courts, young elite tennis players will practice on these types of tennis courts. With regard to the general public, whereas many clay courts are available in Europe and South America, you will hardly find one in North America. Many more should become available for use by the general public. Artificial playing surfaces with a loose granular topping are a cost-effective way to obtain the advantages of clay courts at a much lower cost, as they require low maintenance only. If guidelines on frictional characteristics of a surface were adopted, shoe companies could focus all their attention on designing a specific shoe for these particular surfaces that would further reduce the risk of injuries. The effects of all modifications to either shoe or surface will have to be evaluated carefully by well-designed studies, to determine whether the prevalence of injuries indeed has decreased and overall tennis performance is not compromised.

Acknowledgements

The authors gratefully acknowledge the assistance of Marco Medik in the literature search.

References

Barnes, R.A. & Smith, P.D. (1993) The role of footwear in minimizing lower limb injury. *Journal of Sports Sciences* **12**, 341–353.

Garrick, J.G. & Requa, R.K. (1973) Role of external support in the prevention of ankle sprains. *Medicine and Science in Sports* **5**, 200–203.

Hutchinson, M.R., Laprade, R.F., Burnett, Q.M. II, Moss, R. & Terpstra, J. (1995) Injury surveillance at the USTA Boys' Tennis Championships: a 6-yr study. *Medicine and Science in Sports and Exercise* **27**, 826–830.

Kulund, D.N., McCue, F.C., Rockwell, D.A. & Gieck, J.H. (1979) Tennis injuries: prevention and treatment. *American Journal of Sports Medicine* **7**, 249–253.

Luethi, S.M., Frederick, E.C., Hawes, M.R. & Nigg, B.M. (1986) Influence of shoe construction on lower extremity kinematics and load during lateral movements in tennis. *International Journal of Sports Biomechanics* **2**, 166–174.

Nigg, B.M. & Denoth, J. (1980) *Sportplatzbelaege (Playing Surfaces)*. Juris Verlag, Zurich, Switzerland.

Nigg, B.M. & Segesser, B. (1988) The influence of playing surfaces on the load on the locomotor system and on football and tennis injuries. *Sports Medicine* **5**, 375–385.

Nigg, B.M. & Yeadon, M.R. (1987) Biomechanical aspects of playing surfaces. *Journal of Sports Medicine* **7**, 117–145.

Pirnay, F., Bodeux, M., Crielaard, J.M. & Franchimont, P. (1987) Bone mineral content and physical activity. *International Journal of Sports Medicine* **8**, 331–335.

Reece, L.A., Fricker, P.A. & Maguire, K.F. (1986) Injuries to elite young tennis players at the Australian Institute of Sport. *Australian Journal of Science and Medicine in Sport* **18**, 11–15.

Renstrom, P.A.F. (1995) Knee pain in tennis players. *Clinics in Sports Medicine* **14**, 163–175.

von Salis-Soglio, G. (1979) Sportverletzungen und Sportschaeden beim Tennis (Sport injuries in tennis). *Deutsche Zeitschrift für Sportmedizin* **8**, 244–247.

Surve, I., Schwellnus, M.P., Noakes, T. & Lombard, C. (1994) A fivefold reduction in the incidence of recurrent ankle sprains in soccer players using the Sport-Stirrup orthosis. *American Journal of Sports Medicine* **22**, 601–606.

Chapter 4

The physiological demands
of tennis

Introduction

The physiological demands and metabolic characteristics of tennis have not been described or understood as clearly as with some other sports or exercise activities. Consequently, tennis coaches and players have often developed and utilized diverse, and sometimes inappropriate, training strategies. Tennis is an activity characterized by intermittent exercise bouts of varying intensities and numerous recovery periods over a duration ranging from less than 60 min to over 4 h. Adding to the confusion, tennis can be played on a variety of surfaces, indoors or outdoors with myriad influential environmental factors and with contrasting styles of play. Furthermore, of course, there are singles and doubles. Each one of these variables has a measurable impact on the underlying physiological demands of a match and a player's corresponding physiological responses.

So what is meant by the 'physiological demands' in tennis, and why should a better understanding of this aspect of tennis be important to players, coaches or health professionals? Tennis physiology encompasses a wide range of biological processes relating to bodily functions and adaptations during play. Many of these processes involve the conversion of stored chemical energy to mechanical energy for running and hitting forehands, backhands and other strokes of the game, as well as the continual ongoing restoration of energy during and between points. To meet the varying physiological demands of a tennis match, a player's body must appropriately respond to extensive stop-and-go activity, short points, long points, intense play, not-so-intense play, and various environmental circumstances. This chapter primarily focuses on the requirements and physiological responses that relate to oxygen delivery

and utilization, cardiovascular function, and using and restoring energy during play, as well as some of the potential health-related physiological effects that have been observed in tennis players who play tennis regularly. Subsequent chapters cover other applied anatomical, physiological and morphological responses to tennis play and training, including suggested training and conditioning methods.

A basic understanding of the physiological principles described here should be important to coaches and players. Why? For one reason, so that the training methods presented in this book (and elsewhere) can be carefully evaluated. Moreover, a better understanding of the physiological challenges of tennis and adaptations associated with play and conditioning will help coaches and players to select and utilize the most appropriate practice and conditioning approaches to prepare their players or themselves for the sometimes-extraordinary physiological demands that are encountered on the court. Additionally, health professionals will readily recognize the cardiovascular and other conditioning effects of regular tennis and, thus, should consider tennis as a preferred alternative for many persons who are looking to enhance their fitness and well-being.

The demand for energy

A tennis player's ability to run, hit the ball and recover for the next shot is in large part determined by his or her own physiological capacity to acquire, convert and utilize energy. The longer the points and the match go on, and the more intense play becomes, the more challenging it is for a player's muscles to meet the demands for energy. Heart rate and contraction force increase, various hormones are secreted, metabolic rate goes up, breathing rate increases and there is a consequent rise in body temperature, all in response to a higher energy demand. Is this process limited or can a player respond increasingly and sufficiently to any degree of physiological demand? Of course, there are limitations. But, what physiological factors limit a tennis player's ability to continue playing at a desired level of intensity and for as long as is necessary? To answer this, it is important to understand some basic concepts.

During a tennis match, the ability to sustain play depends on the ongoing consumption and use of oxygen. As play progresses from the warm-up through the early games of the first set, the rate of oxygen consumption ($\dot{V}o_2$) increases. Although a player's maximal oxygen consumption rate ($\dot{V}o_{2max}$) is usually never required during a match, a good and efficient capacity to consume and utilize oxygen is critical to one's ability to recover during and between points. The cardiovascular system plays a key role in this. Thus, good cardiovascular fitness is not only important for a tennis player's health, it is also extremely helpful for on-court performance. But the cardiovascular system and the utilization of oxygen are not the only energy-related physiological systems important to a tennis player. There are three primary energy systems that continually function together to power and sustain on-court muscular activities—immediate, non-oxidative glycolysis and oxidative metabolism. The first two systems are not dependent on oxygen and the third one is; thus, the former are considered to be anaerobic and the latter is referred to as the aerobic energy system.

Immediate energy for play

Central to the process of energy conversion and utilization is a chemical called adenosine triphosphate (ATP). ATP is used in muscle cells as an immediate source of energy for muscle contraction. With all muscle contractions, whether they be for a serve, volley, running to a ball, recovering to regain position, or even for changing grips, the breakdown of ATP supplies the necessary chemical energy for the contractions to occur. As ATP is used, another chemical that stores cellular energy called creatine phosphate (CP) almost immediately replenishes the active muscles' ATP supply. Both of these immediate-energy processes (i.e. breakdown of ATP and the restoration of ATP from CP) are anaerobic; that is, oxygen is not required or directly involved.

There is considerably more CP stored in resting muscle (about five to six times as much) than ATP, which gives a tennis player's muscles an effective energy reserve to rapidly regenerate ATP. Some ATP is also regenerated from degraded ATP (i.e. adenosine diphosphate or ADP). But despite the effectiveness of these two phosphagen (ATP and CP) energy reserves,

sustained play (i.e. for more than several seconds or so) requires the assistance of other energy sources to support repeated muscle contractions. Moreover, other energy-providing processes are also used to restore the phosphagen energy reserves, during and between points, when the muscles are temporarily relaxed or less activated.

Other non-oxidative energy sources

Two other rapid biochemical processes for providing energy in the form of ATP are glycolysis and glycogenolysis, which, respectively, refer to the breakdown of glucose and glycogen (a readily mobilized stored form of carbohydrate made up of glucose subunits). Dietary glucose, from the ingestion of starches (e.g. rice, pasta, potatoes, etc.) and dietary sugars, enters the bloodstream and is taken up by many cells, including those of the liver and muscles. In the liver and muscles, glucose can be either used for immediate energy or stored as glycogen for later energy requirements. Glycogenolysis (in the liver or muscle cells) 'feeds' glycolysis by providing glucose via the breakdown of glycogen. Ultimately, glucose is converted to pyruvate with a net resultant increase in ATP. Pyruvate can be subsequently oxidized to carbon dioxide and water (see 'Oxidative metabolism' below) to yield even more energy or it can be reduced to lactic acid. Although glycolysis itself does not involve oxygen, when glucose is ultimately oxidized to carbon dioxide and water, this slower, extended form of glycolysis is considered to be an aerobic process, because oxygen is eventually involved. Otherwise, when pyruvate is reduced to lactic acid (without using oxygen), then glycolysis remains anaerobic, and energy is provided at a much faster rate. Importantly, lactic acid can still form in the presence of oxygen.

Selected muscles have a greater dependence on glycogen breakdown and glycolysis for energy during play when they repeatedly contract, as when a player runs hard to hit one or several successive strokes. Moreover, the proportional reliance on glycolysis and glycogenolysis for energy provision increases further with the duration and intensity of each point. Furthermore, when the demand for a rapid rate of ATP production is high, substantially more lactic acid is produced in order to keep the glycolysis process going and to provide a faster energy (ATP) yield. During these moments of play, aerobic metabolism is not providing ATP fast enough to keep up with the high-energy demand. If pyruvate is not converted to lactic acid, glycolysis cannot continue at a high rate and the rapid energy requirements will not be met. However, a large accumulation of lactic acid (or lactate—the salt form of lactic acid) in the muscles does *not* often occur during tennis. Because of the intermittent nature of play and typical irregularity of muscle recruitment, a constant or repeated high-intensity load on any one muscle or muscle group(s) does not last long or occur very often. Thus, there is an overall low reliance on lactic acid-producing glycolysis in a player's muscles (examples of measured blood lactate levels during tennis are presented later in this chapter). Although, even with a constant low level of lactate in the blood, anaerobic glycolysis can still be, at times, significantly active in selected muscles during play. Such low circulating lactate levels merely suggest that the removal and utilization of lactate for energy (primarily by oxidative metabolism) kept pace with its formation and entry into the blood. Again, the intermittent nature of play certainly permits such a scenario. But even though the immediate energy sources (ATP and CP) and non-oxidative glycolysis can effectively and rapidly provide energy for muscular activity during play, oxidative metabolism can provide substantially more energy and plays an important role throughout any tennis match.

Oxidative metabolism

Carbohydrate, fat and protein (amino acids) are all potential oxidative energy sources during a tennis match (their utilization during play and suggested dietary intake are comprehensively described in Chapter 5). Even though glycogen and glucose can be broken down and metabolized to effectively provide energy without the use of oxygen, oxidative (aerobic) metabolism of glucose along with other macronutrients (fats and protein) yields far more energy, albeit at a slower rate. Moreover, aerobic metabolism can provide energy during play, while lessening the extent of fatigue-related factors, such as rapid glycogen depletion and lactic acid accumulation. Thus, the ongoing use of oxygen is

critical in allowing one to keep playing without having to rely solely on other energy systems that would readily induce play-halting fatigue. In fact, even when the intensity of play is high and anaerobic gylcolysis *is* called upon to meet a larger proportion of the muscles' energy needs, oxidative metabolism continues. Subsequently, aerobic energy restoration readily contributes to a rapid cellular recovery during less intense portions of play and between points. This emphasizes why it is important for a tennis player to have a fairly efficient and effective aerobic capacity.

Cellular oxidation takes place in the mitochondria. These are specialized structures in muscle cells that use oxygen to link the breakdown of carbohydrate, fat and protein to the restoration of a tennis player's immediate energy sources (ATP and CP) through a process called cellular respiration. Again, because oxygen is used, this is an *aerobic* process. As play continues, and ATP and CP levels are reduced, breathing and heart rate increase so that more oxygen can be delivered to the muscles and the mitochondria can do their job.

Pyruvate (the end product of glycolysis) enters the mitochondria and is processed through a series of enzymatic steps referred to as the Krebs cycle. Carbon dioxide and several important high-energy constituents (NADH and FADH—these are reduced forms of nicotinamide adenine dinucleotide and flavine adenine dinucleotide, respectively) are formed at this stage. Intermediate products of fat and protein breakdown can also enter the Krebs cycle, as energy sources, to yield the same high-energy compounds. Next, NADH and FADH give up their hydrogen. Electrons stripped from the hydrogens move along through a process called the electron transport chain and are eventually combined with oxygen. The resultant hydrogen protons (H^+)—each stripped of an electron—ultimately provide energy for ATP production (via phosphorylation of ADP) and combine with oxygen to form water.

Aerobic or anaerobic?

Is tennis aerobic or anaerobic? The answer to this seemingly often-debated question depends, in part, on the duration of tennis activity that is under consideration. If one only considers a single (or a few successive) stroke(s) or short ballistic movement to

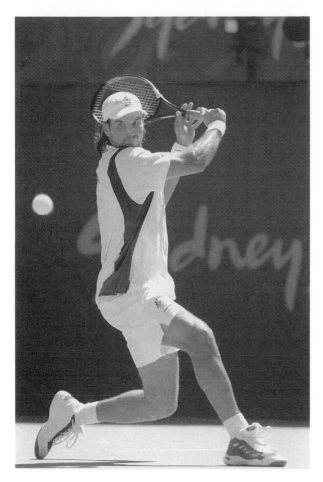

Fig. 4.1 The energy demands of tennis play are met by a combination of high-energy phosphates, anaerobic glycolysis and aerobic metabolism. Photo © Allsport/C. Brunskill.

the ball, then the predominant energy systems utilized to support such a brief individual subunit of tennis activity are not dependent on the presence and use of oxygen (Fig. 4.1). The immediate energy processes (ATP and CP metabolism), perhaps in combination with some additional production of ATP via a small contribution from non-oxidative glycolysis, are activated quickly, provide energy at a fast rate, and have the capacity to sufficiently meet those limited energy demands. Thus, anaerobic (without oxygen) metabolism would arguably appear to be capable of playing the major energy-provision role. However, many points are played over the course of a match that usually lasts more than an hour and many of the points last (sometimes considerably) more than

several seconds. Consequently, the much larger energy capacity of the oxidative energy system is essential to a tennis player, and aerobic metabolism is constantly relied upon to help resynthesize the phosphagen energy stores (ATP and CP) between and during points. Thus, oxidative phosphorylation is the major source of ATP production and energy restoration during a tennis match. So, is tennis aerobic or anaerobic? It is both! Perhaps a more accurate classification that would highlight this perspective, along with the relatively low reliance on lactic acid-producing anaerobic glycolysis, would be to say that tennis is primarily *alactic* (ATP-CP)–*aerobic*.

Physiological responses to tennis

As stated earlier, the physiological demands and metabolic characteristics of tennis have not been described as extensively or understood as clearly as with some other sports. Nevertheless, a number of researchers have evaluated certain physiological aspects of tennis play. Below is a description of some of these selected findings.

Physiological responses during play

During 2 h of singles tennis on clay courts, Ferrauti (1997) found that nationally ranked senior tennis players (men, 47.0 ± 5.4 years; women, 47.2 ± 6.6 years) had a mean oxygen uptake of 23.3 ml·kg^{-1}·min^{-1}. In addition, these players had an average heart rate of 140.1 ± 15.5 beats·min^{-1}, a respiratory exchange ratio (RER) of 0.94 ± 0.04, and a blood lactate of 1.5 ± 0.7 mmol·l^{-1}. Moreover, free fatty acid and glycerol concentrations increased significantly (+450% and +300%, respectively). Ferrauti stated that intermittent periods of high-intensity play contributed to elevated sympathetic activity (i.e. adrenaline (epinephrine) release), which appeared to contribute to a rapid and persistent breakdown and utilization of fat and glycogen for energy.

Bergeron *et al.* (1991) measured heart rate, haematocrit, haemoglobin, blood glucose and plasma concentrations of lactate, cortisol and testosterone in 10 Division I male tennis players (20.3 ± 2.5 years), during singles play. The mean heart rate during the 85 min of play was 144.6 beats·min^{-1}, which represented 61.4% of these players' maximal heart rate reserve. Plasma lactate and blood glucose concentrations did not significantly change over the duration of the match, although there was a 23% increase in blood glucose following the measured post-warm-up value. Plasma cortisol levels progressively decreased, while plasma testosterone levels went progressively up. Bergeron *et al.* (1991) concluded that the overall metabolic response during tennis resembles prolonged, moderate-intensity exercise, with ample opportunities for oxidative metabolism to predominate and anaerobic by-products to be readily cleared.

Therminarias *et al.* (1991) evaluated the effects of a 'strenuous' tennis match on heart rate and plasma lactate, free fatty acids, glucose and selected hormone levels in young (21.2 ± 1.9 years) and veteran (46.6 ± 1.3 years), regionally ranked women tennis players. During the singles matches, at times, heart rates were near or at maximum, with only moderate drops demonstrated during less intense periods of play. Notably, relatively high heart rates were maintained during phases of rest (i.e. when players changed sides), especially with the older players. In contrast, plasma lactate concentration stayed low (on average, less than 1.8 mmol·l^{-1}, at the end of play) in each of the players. Free fatty acid concentrations were higher at the end of play, although adrenaline (epinephrine) levels were not, indicating that the 'strenuous tennis matches' were not particularly stressful for these well-trained women. ·

One of the earlier investigations to evaluate the physiological responses during tennis was conducted by Seliger *et al.* (1973). In this classic study, 16 top-50 nationally ranked tennis players from Czechoslovakia were monitored during a 10-min long, indoor training 'match'. Based on expired air measurements, the oxygen uptake during play was 27.3 ± 5.5 ml·kg^{-1}·min^{-1}, which means that the subjects competed at approximately 50% of their maximal aerobic power (i.e. $\dot{V}o_{2max}$). Moreover, these players expended an estimated 10.4 ± 1.2 kcal·min^{-1} and had an average heart rate of 143.0 ± 13.9 beats·min^{-1}, during the on-court session. While it was agreed that singles tennis could be categorized as a moderate- to heavy-intensity activity, Seliger *et al.* characterized the overall energy metabolism in their tennis study as 88% aerobic and 12% anaerobic.

A number of other studies (Misner *et al.* 1980; Docherty 1982; Copley 1984; Friedman *et al.* 1984; Elliott *et al.* 1985; Morgans *et al.* 1987; Jetté *et al.* 1991) have also reported similar heart-rate and metabolic profiles as were shown in the above selected investigations. Collectively, these findings indicate that the alactic (ATP-CP) and aerobic (oxygen) energy systems, without a significant reliance on anaerobic glycolysis, can meet the variable on-court energy demands of moderate- to high-intensity tennis. Moreover, despite the intermittent nature of play, heart rate is generally maintained in a range that would indicate an overall exercise intensity (% of $\dot{V}o_{2max}$) capable of providing a beneficial cardiorespiratory conditioning effect. The heart-rate response during play can, of course, be affected by other factors such as dehydration and thermal stress, which can result in a compensatory increase in a tennis player's heart rate in order to maintain cardiac output. Psychological factors can also affect on-court heart rate responses. However, as further shown below, the cardiovascular stress of singles tennis is generally high enough to potentially yield an increase in aerobic power and myriad positive health benefits, which might improve performance and lower the risk of cardiovascular disease in players who compete regularly.

Physiological adaptations to play

Selected metabolic and cardiovascular adaptations were examined in 14 professional tennis players (7 men, 23 ± 3 years; 7 women, 18 ± 2 years) by Keul *et al.* (1991). Heart volume was 20–30% larger, compared to untrained persons, with corresponding increases in end-diastolic and end-systolic volume, left-ventricular muscle mass, and stroke volume. These changes were consistent with the phenomenon termed the 'athlete's heart' (Pluim 1998). Moreover, Keul *et al.* (1991) found that these players performed well on a treadmill test, demonstrating an anaerobic threshold that suggested further physiological adaptations, as a result of supplemental interval and endurance training.

Vodak *et al.* (1980) examined cardiorespiratory characteristics in 50 middle-aged, above-average skilled tennis players, whose participation in regular exercise was limited to only tennis. The 25 men (42 ± 6.0 years) and 25 women (39 ± 3.3 years) demonstrated a mean $\dot{V}o_{2max}$ (men, 50.2 ± 5.7 ml·kg⁻¹·min⁻¹; women, 44.2 ± 5.4 ml·kg⁻¹·min⁻¹) that was well above previously reported values for untrained, middle-aged persons, although somewhat less than the aerobic power reported for dedicated middle-aged runners, for each group. In addition, the male and female tennis players had mean resting heart rates of 54.0 ± 5.8 beats·min⁻¹ and 61.0 ± 8.4 beats·min⁻¹, respectively. Vodak *et al.* (1980) stated that these values were about 10 beats·min⁻¹ slower, compared to resting heart rates observed in more sedentary middle-aged persons. Notably, the tennis players had resting blood pressures much lower than what was found in a large group of randomly selected men and women from the same region.

Powers and Walker (1982) reported that a group of high-school girls, who were experienced tennis players engaged in regular tennis training and competition, had an average resting heart rate, blood pressure and body fat percentage. However, these female players had higher values for vital capacity and maximal voluntary ventilation (121.2 ± 3.5 l·min⁻¹) than that reported for untrained females of the same age group. Moreover, the aerobic power of these players (48.0 ± 2.1 ml·kg⁻¹·min⁻¹) was considerably higher than previously reported values for similarly aged females in the general population, and somewhat higher when compared to selected female athletes in other sports, such as basketball, field hockey and Olympic speed skating.

The long-term effects of tennis training on selected lipoprotein measures were examined by Ferrauti *et al.* (1997). In this study, 22 healthy, middle-aged recreational tennis players participated in 6 weeks of 'running intensive' tennis training (three 90-min sessions per week). Ferrauti *et al.* observed a decrease in bodyweight, an increase in anaerobic threshold, and lower average levels of total cholesterol, triglycerides and total cholesterol/high-density lipoprotein cholesterol (TC/HDL-C), as a result of the 6 weeks of training. These data suggest that tennis training, characterized by sufficient running and intensity and short rest periods, may yield several antiatherogenic adaptations, similar to those achieved via more traditional programmes of regular aerobic exercise (e.g. jogging, swimming and cycling).

Evidently, playing tennis (and training for tennis) regularly helps to develop and maintain certain aspects of cardiovascular fitness (Kulund *et al.* 1979;

Buono *et al.* 1980; Keul *et al.* 1982, 1991; Powers & Walker 1982; Friedman *et al.* 1984; Morgans *et al.* 1987; Bergeron *et al.* 1991; Therminarias *et al.* 1991). In fact, several studies have reported even higher aerobic power levels in tennis players than described above (Buti *et al.* 1984; Carlson & Cera 1984; Elliott *et al.* 1985). However, it is difficult to distinguish the effects of tennis alone on parameters such as aerobic power, for example, because many tennis players regularly participate in activities such as middle- and long-distance running and/or cycling, as part of their supplemental training programmes. Either way, whether it is the tennis or the supplemental training that is primarily responsible for establishing and maintaining good aerobic fitness in players, enhanced pulmonary function and an improved capacity for oxygen utilization are clearly beneficial to on-court endurance and performance. Importantly, today's game seemingly requires greater levels of fitness than even just two decades ago, to meet the physiological demands of successful performance. Thus, although there are limited data to compare, some of the reported physiological characteristics, responses and adaptations from earlier tennis studies might not be indicative of the fitness level and tennis-induced physiological adaptations of today's players.

Training effects that enhance performance

There is, of course, a wide array of on- and off-court training exercises to enhance a tennis player's endurance, strength, speed and power. Which of these performance factors should a coach and player emphasize during training? To a large extent this depends on the specific level of play, current needs, and goals of the player in question. However, successful competitive tennis requires all players to have a suitable degree of all four factors. Thus, any comprehensive, periodized, age-appropriate, individual-specific and long-term training programme for tennis should develop all of these attributes. (A number of suggested training methods are presented in Chapter 9.) The following is a description of some of the adaptations associated with training that affect a player's ability to meet the physiological demands of tennis described above. For the purpose of tennis conditioning, 'endurance' training includes moderate-to high-volume, interval or continuous, on- or off-court, tennis-specific movement drills (with and without hitting balls) that raise the heart rate but are generally (or effectively, *overall*) below lactate threshold intensity, as well as distance running and cycling, for example.

The cardiovascular system will adapt in many ways, in response to endurance training. For example, from a regular increased blood volume load, the heart can improve its capacity and efficiency for pumping blood, through an increase in stroke volume. Consequently, tennis players can have a lower heart rate at rest and during a given intensity of subsequent play or training. Weightlifting and other strength exercises increase the pressure load on the heart, which can cause a further increase in left-ventricle mass. High-intensity interval training can also elicit similar cardiovascular changes. However, tennis players will generally find that such training is more effective in achieving optimal endurance during play when it is combined with sufficient on- and off-court endurance exercises and drills (e.g. some distance running and high-volume hitting).

Again, an ample and efficient capacity to consume and utilize oxygen is critical to a player's ability to effectively recover during and between points. Can a tennis player improve his or her maximal oxygen consumption ($\dot{V}o_{2max}$)? Yes. How much? It depends primarily on one's current level of cardiorespiratory fitness. Generally, most active and reasonably fit tennis players should expect no more than a 20% increase in $\dot{V}o_{2max}$, as a result of intense, long-term endurance training. If initial cardiorespiratory fitness is low, however, greater increases in $\dot{V}o_{2max}$ are possible. Will an increase in $\dot{V}o_{2max}$ help on-court performance? Probably, to some degree. Importantly, many tennis players can improve on-court endurance by much more than 20%, by enhancing body composition, strength, speed, technique and other physiological attributes described in this section.

Endurance training appears to have a minimal effect on the inherently already high glycolytic activity of muscle (especially in fast-twitch muscle). However, enzyme activity associated with glucose entry from the blood into the muscle's glycolytic pathway can increase significantly with endurance training. This enhancement would be particularly beneficial to a tennis player during long matches, when blood glucose (ingested or from the liver)

is relied on to a greater degree to support ongoing energy needs. Speed and power training does not have much of an effect on the activity of enzymes associated with glycolysis either. However, any resultant muscle hypertrophy will probably increase the overall glycolytic capacity and activity of the affected muscles.

On the other hand, the effects of endurance training on components more closely related to oxidative metabolism are much more pronounced. An increase in mitochondria number and size will be associated with a proportional increase in the muscle's overall activity involving the Krebs cycle and electron transport chain. Such an increase in mitochondrial capacity should improve a player's endurance. More mitochondrial material can mean enhanced utilization of oxygen and fat (and less carbohydrate) at a given intensity of play. This can delay fatigue. Notably, resistance training generally does not enhance mitochondrial capacity. Moreover, endurance training can increase the capillary-to-muscle fibre ratio, which will enhance an active muscle's ability to extract nutrients and oxygen from the blood. This will further improve a player's oxidative capacity and muscle endurance. Such training can also affect lactate turnover in muscle—lactate production may go down in some muscle fibres, while its uptake and oxidation is enhanced elsewhere. Thus, lactate accumulation is reduced.

Again, based on findings from many of the studies cited above, the overall metabolic response to tennis indicates that oxidative energy metabolism is the *primary* (not sole) mechanism for ATP restoration through the course of an entire tennis match (between and during points). Thus, training should emphasize a variety of conditioning exercises and drills performed just below a player's 'anaerobic' (lactate) threshold; that is, not quite a high enough intensity to elicit a rapid rise in blood lactate. The adaptations associated with such training could optimize the capacity and efficiency for ongoing energy recovery during play.

Summary

The heart-rate responses, oxygen uptake, low plasma lactate levels and fatty acid mobilization observed during play indicate that tennis can induce a high metabolic demand for energy that is primarily met by phosphagen breakdown and the aerobic catabolism of carbohydrate and fat. The intermittent, short work bouts (albeit at a high intensity, at times), interspersed with numerous recovery periods, reduces the overall reliance on anaerobic glycolysis for ATP production and also provides numerous opportunities for lactate to be removed and utilized. Tennis and supplemental conditioning for tennis can improve cardiorespiratory endurance, which further enhances the aerobic-like physiological responses observed during play (e.g. lower lactate levels and increased utilization of fat). From a cardiovascular conditioning and health perspective, tennis should be considered an attractive alternative activity for many people looking to develop or maintain fitness and reduce the risk of cardiovascular disease.

References

Bergeron, M.F., Maresh, C.M., Kraemer, W.J. *et al.* (1991) Tennis: a physiological profile during match play. *International Journal of Sports Medicine* **12**, 474–479.

Buono, M.J., Constable, S.H. & Stanforth, P.R. (1980) Maximum oxygen uptake and body composition of varsity collegiate tennis players. *Arizona Journal of Health, Physical Education, Recreation and Dance* **23**, 6–7.

Buti, T., Elliott, B. & Morton, A. (1984) Physiological and anthropometric profiles of elite prepubescent tennis players. *The Physician and Sportsmedicine* **12**, 111–116.

Carlson, J.S. & Cera, M.A. (1984) Cardiorespiratory, muscular strength, and anthropometric characteristics of elite Australian junior male and female tennis players. *Australian Journal of Science and Medicine in Sport* **16**, 7–13.

Copley, B.B. (1984) Effects of competitive singles tennis playing on serum electrolyte, blood glucose and blood lactate concentrations (Abstract). *South African Journal of Science* **80**, 145.

Docherty, D. (1982) A comparison of heart rate responses in racquet games. *British Journal of Sports Medicine* **16**, 96–100.

Elliott, B., Dawson, B. & Pyke, F. (1985) The energetics of singles tennis. *Journal of Human Movement Studies* **11**, 11–20.

Ferrauti, A. (1997) Tennis versus running: substrate utilization during intermittent and continuous exercise. In: Bangsbø, J., Saltin, B., Bonde, H. *et al.*, eds. *Second Annual Congress of the European College of Sport Science Book of Abstracts II*, pp. 920–921. HO & Storm, Copenhagen.

Ferrauti, A., Weber, K. & Strüder, H.K. (1997) Effects of tennis training on lipid metabolism and lipoproteins in recreational players. *British Journal of Sports Medicine* **31**, 322–327.

Friedman, D.B., Ramo, B.W. & Gray, G.J. (1984) Tennis and cardiovascular fitness in middle-aged men. *The Physician and Sportsmedicine* **12**, 87–91.

Jetté, M., Landry, F., Tiemann, B. & Blümchen, G. (1991) Ambulatory blood pressure and holter monitoring during tennis play. *Canadian Journal of Sport Sciences* **16**, 40–44.

Keul, J., Berg, A., Huber, G. *et al.* (1982) Kardio-zirkulatorische und metabolische anpassung-svorgänge bei tennisspielern [Cardiocirculatory and metabolic adaptation of tennis players]. *Herz-Kreislauf* **7**, 373–381.

Keul, J., Stockhausen, W., Pokan, R., Huonker, M. & Berg, A. (1991) Metabolische und kardiozirkulatorische adaptation sowie leistungsverhalten professioneller tennisspieler [Metabolic and cardiovascular adaptation and perform-ance of professional tennis players]. *Deutsche Medizinische Wochenschrift* **116**, 761–767.

Kulund, D.N., Rockwell, D.A. & Brubaker, C.E. (1979) The long-term effects of playing tennis. *The Physician and Sportsmedicine* **7**, 87–92.

Misner, J.E., Boileau, R.A., Courvoisier, D., Slaughter, M.H. & Bloomfield, D.K. (1980) Cardiovascular stress associated with the recreational tennis play of middle-aged males. *American Corrective Therapy Journal* **34**, 4–8.

Morgans, L.F., Jordan, D.L., Baeyens, D.A. & Franciosa, J.A. (1987) Heart rate responses during singles and doubles tennis competition. *The Physician and Sportsmedicine* **15**, 67–74.

Pluim, B.M. (1998) *The athlete's heart: a physiological or pathological phenomenon?* Thesis, Rijksuniversiteit Leiden, Leiden, The Netherlands.

Powers, S.K. & Walker, R. (1982) Physiological and anatomical characteristics of outstanding female junior tennis players. *Research Quarterly for Exercise and Sport* **53**, 172–175.

Seliger, V., Ejem, M., Pauer, M. & Šafařík, V. (1973) Energy metabolism in tennis. *Internationale Zeitschrift fur Angewandte Physiologie* **31**, 333–340.

Therminarias, A., Dansou, P., Chirpaz-Oddou, M.-F., Gharib, C. & Quirion, A. (1991) Hormonal and metabolic changes during a strenuous tennis match. Effect of ageing. *International Journal of Sports Medicine* **12**, 10–16.

Vodak, P.A., Savin, W.M., Haskell, W.L. & Wood, P.D. (1980) Physiological profile of middle-aged male and female tennis players. *Medicine and Science in Sports and Exercise* **12**, 159–163.

Chapter 5

Nutrition in tennis

Introduction

Proper nutrition is important in any tennis player's quest to reach peak performance. At all levels of competition, whether to win a local recreational league championship or in preparation for a Grand Slam event, players look for ways to improve their performance and gain a competitive edge. Often this includes trying the latest fad in nutritional supplements, in hope of getting closer to that elusive experience of playing the best tennis possible. Nutrition for tennis, as for all sports, can be somewhat confusing. Suitable dietary strategies should be adjusted for a player's age, fitness, level of competition and intensity of play, environment, time of competition, duration of play, amount of time between matches, and many other factors. Match preparation, from a nutritional standpoint, is further challenged by the unpredictability of how long any given match will go: will it be 90 min or 4 h?

Although a healthy diet and body can clearly contribute to being a better tennis player, this chapter will not focus on general nutrition guidelines to eating for good health. Thus, following the next section on a balanced diet, the remainder of this chapter will review several basic nutrition principles, as well as other selected current nutrition issues, primarily as they relate to *tennis performance*. Unfortunately, to date, there has been very little research on nutrition and tennis. Hence, many of the following recommendations are based on established results from research on other sports and exercise activities, as well as observations and anecdotal reports from tennis. Moreover, the discussion and guidelines presented here are mostly specific to adults; while there has been extensive research on nutrition and exercise performance, such studies on children and adolescents are lacking.

Much of the following information on match preparation, play and recovery is also generally appropriate for on-court training and practice; players should therefore incorporate many of the following suggestions into their training and practice routines as well. It is important that players, parents, coaches and trainers also realize that the effectiveness of any sound nutrition game plan is greatly enhanced when integrated with proper training and adequate rest.

A balanced diet

The primary dietary concern for all tennis players should be to generally avoid the known nutritional risk factors that are associated with health problems and to follow those nutritional guidelines that will help to promote good health. A diet that includes excessive calories, saturated fat or alcohol, or chronic vitamin, mineral or caloric deficiencies should be avoided by anyone interested in good health *or* good tennis. Simple as it seems, a balanced and varied diet, which provides all the necessary nutrients (carbohydrates, fats, protein, minerals, vitamins, etc.) to sufficiently support growth and development, regulate metabolism, maintain normal menstrual status and provide adequate energy during train-ing and competition, will go a long way to help tennis players play their best tennis. These days, the widespread availability of varied and good nutrient-dense food choices gives all players ample opportunity to maintain a well-balanced diet. Unfortunately, habitual selection of only favourite food items may limit important key nutrients. By following any one of the various scientifically based food guides, such as the *United States Food Guide Pyramid*, players, coaches and parents can achieve appropriate variety, proportions and balance in their daily dietary planning, so that an adequate regular intake of all the essential nutrients is not just left to chance.

Carbohydrates

Bread, cereal, rice, pasta, fruits and vegetables are all good primary sources of carbohydrate that should be regularly included in a tennis player's diet, and today a variety of sport drinks and sport bars add to a player's dietary options for this much-needed nutrient. How much dietary carbohydrate does a tennis player need? It depends. Although it is often recommended that 55–70% of a player's daily dietary calories comes from carbohydrates, such a goal is not always appropriate or practical, particularly if the daily total caloric intake requirement is very high. A more precise guideline for a competitive tennis player would be to ingest at least 7 g of carbohydrate per kg of bodyweight each day. This is equivalent to 490 g (or 1960 calories from carbohydrates) for a 70-kg person, which would represent roughly 65% of a 3000-calorie daily diet, for example. This relative amount should provide enough dietary carbohydrate to replenish muscle and liver glycogen (the body's storage form of carbohydrate) each day. Although a small amount of carbohydrate is available as blood sugar (glucose), most of the body's carbohydrate is stored as glycogen in the muscles and, to a lesser degree, in the liver.

Before they are absorbed into the blood, dietary carbohydrates, including sucrose (table sugar), are eventually broken down by digestion to single sugar units called monosaccharides, which include glucose, fructose and/or galactose. Glucose is the body's primary fuel for energy. Fructose (the very sweet sugar of fruit and also found in soft drinks and some sport drinks) and galactose (part of lactose or milk sugar) are first converted to glucose by the liver before they can be used for energy. Foods that raise the blood sugar (glucose) level a lot and quickly are categorized as having a high glycaemic index (Foster-Powell & Brand Miller 1995), and for tennis players the glycaemic effect can be very important. For example, certain foods, such as bagels, ready-to-eat cereals (e.g. corn or rice), white bread, honey, baked potatoes, white rice (low-amylose) and some sport drinks (those whose primary carbohydrate content is derived from glucose, sucrose or glucose polymers), will raise the blood sugar quickly and thus can provide a rapid and more readily utilizable energy source. On the other hand, apples, yoghurt and fructose-predominant sport drinks, for example, will provide energy at a slower rate, because the carbohydrate will not be absorbed as readily and because it must be then converted to glucose in the liver. In addition, high consumption of fructose may also slow down fluid absorption and

may cause a feeling of gastrointestinal distress, particularly during play.

Several of the following sections discuss the importance of, and specific ways to ensure, adequate carbohydrate intake prior to play, so that the body's carbohydrate stores in the liver and muscles are maximized to prevent premature fatigue on the court. Appropriate ways to provide carbohydrate for energy during play and to restore carbohydrate after a match are also presented.

Fats

The general recommendation for dietary fat intake is 20–30% of total daily calorie intake. Further, saturated fats should account for less than 10% of each day's total calories. Not only is fat needed for many biological functions, it provides considerable energy during play. Fortunately, most tennis players have enough body fat to support their on-court energy requirement for fat, and fat intake *during* or *just prior* to play is not necessary or appropriate. A little bit of fat can be found in blood in the form of free fatty acids or triglycerides. And while a much larger portion of the body's stored fat resides as muscle triglycerides, most triglycerides are stored in fat cells. Triglycerides, of course, must be broken down to fatty acids and glycerol before they can be used for energy.

Some players' daily fat intake regularly exceeds the recommended amount. This may be for convenience or preference; but, for those involved with extensive playing or training, it is often a practical means to help maintain bodyweight without having to consume an excessive bulk of carbohydrates (especially from solid foods) each day to match a very high calorie expenditure on the court. Does this hurt a player's performance? After all, this practice is common (Chen *et al.* 1989; Grandjean 1989; Heinemann & Zerbes 1989; Faber *et al.* 1990) among other athletes and has been, in fact, promoted as being beneficial (Sears 1993). As long as the daily carbohydrate requirement is still met, and as long as the player is not adding unneeded body fat, then from a performance point of view, a periodic high-fat diet may be okay. From a long-term health perspective, the risks associated with such a diet with fit, very active tennis players have not yet been studied. Presumably, however, excessive fat intake will adversely affect the diet-related risk factors for coronary heart disease to some degree, even in a fit population.

Protein

The need for extra protein in an athlete's diet has long been a topic of considerable debate. Although the general recommendation for daily protein intake has been, for some time now, 0.8 g of protein per kg of bodyweight (about 10–15% of daily calories), tennis players do not have to look very hard to find numerous claims that, as athletes, their protein needs are supposedly much higher, and according to a growing body of research (Lemon 1991; Brouns 1993; Evans 1993), this may be true in many cases.

During and immediately after strenuous exercise, there is an increase in protein breakdown. This is followed by an increase in protein synthesis during the recovery period. Because of these activities, many people think that athletes need to consume more protein to maintain their body or to support desired increases in muscle size and muscle energy-producing components. Current recommendations (Lemon 1991; Brouns 1993; Evans 1993) for endurance athletes generally fall between 1.2 and 1.8 g of protein per kg of bodyweight per day. Given the strong endurance component and physiological demands of competitive singles tennis (see Chapter 4), players involved in extensive regular training and competition may require this much protein each day to keep up with potential high rates of protein breakdown and synthesis, as well as to offset any additional small exercise-induced protein losses through sweat and urine. Fortunately, such an increase in dietary protein is probably already met by the typically higher daily caloric intake that these athletes usually have. So unless a tennis player is inappropriately restricting calories, protein supplements are not needed.

Carbohydrate and fat: primary energy sources for tennis

Many factors contribute to the number of calories a player expends on the court, although 600–800 calories per hour would not be difficult for many adults to achieve during competitive singles. Which nutrients provide the most support for such an expenditure of energy? Carbohydrate, fat, protein, water, vitamins and minerals all play a role; however, carbohydrate and fat are the primary energy sources for tennis.

During a tennis match, the emphasis shifts to utilizing more carbohydrate and proportionately less fat, as the intensity of play and overall energy expenditure increase. This is necessary because carbohydrate can supply energy for muscle contraction at a much faster rate than fat can. However, the intermittent nature of tennis reduces the duration of a continuous high demand for energy within any specific muscle group during and between points. Consequently, even during intense singles play, fat is used to supply considerable energy throughout the course of the match.

Importantly, using fat for energy still requires a continual simultaneous breakdown of carbohydrate. Therefore, all players, regardless of the intensity of play, will eventually feel the effects of depleting carbohydrate stores if the match is long enough and carbohydrate is not consumed during play (see sections on 'Nutrition during play' and 'Nutrition and fatigue'). The availability of sufficient carbohydrate for energy can be further challenged in hot environmental conditions. As the temperature goes up, the rate of carbohydrate usage can also increase (Hargreaves *et al.* 1996); thus, fatigue can occur more rapidly without regular and adequate carbohydrate intake.

During the latter part of a tennis match, protein could become a more significant contributor in meeting a player's energy demands, especially if the prematch and during-play dietary carbohydrate intake is inadequate. Ways to reduce potential protein utilization for energy, through ensuring sufficient carbohydrate intake and availability, are addressed in subsequent sections.

Effects of training on carbohydrate, fat and protein use during play

As noted here and in Chapter 4, tennis has a significant endurance component. Playing tennis or regularly participating in other endurance-enhancing exercise or activities (such as bicycling or running) will cause specific changes in a player's body that will positively affect performance. Many of the physiological changes are described in Chapter 4 and other chapters. However, several adaptations relating to the use of nutrients for energy during play are worth noting here.

As a result of several months or so of regular endurance training, there will be an increase in the muscle enzymes that are used to break down and utilize carbohydrate, especially those that are associated with aerobic (with oxygen) metabolism. This, along with other changes that improve the delivery and use of oxygen in the muscles, permits a more efficient use of carbohydrate for producing energy. In addition, well-trained players can store more carbohydrate (as glycogen) in their muscles, which can help to maintain performance and delay fatigue. As far as the use of fat is concerned, endurance training has some positive effects here as well. Changes include improved availability of fat for energy, along with enhanced efficiency of fatty acid uptake and use by the muscles. Overall, after training, one's body will tend to use proportionately more fat for energy during exercise and recovery. This has important implications for any well-trained tennis player who consequently might not have to rely on blood glucose as much and deplete glycogen stores as readily as a lesser trained individual; again, fatigue could be delayed, even during high-intensity competition. At the same time, these changes could indirectly defer an undesirable increased reliance on protein for energy, as the length of a match is extended and when carbohydrate stores would be otherwise diminished.

Interestingly, some research (Henriksson 1991) shows that trained individuals may have an enhanced ability and tendency to use protein for energy during exercise. However, this may be an advantage only when the body's carbohydrate stores are too low and there is no supplemental energy intake during play.

Prematch nutrition

How well a tennis player eats before playing can have a significant impact on the outcome of a match. Many prematch nutritional strategies are designed to ensure adequate prematch hydration and sodium balance. These are discussed briefly here and much more extensively in Chapter 6. Appropriate fat, protein, mineral and vitamin intake are also important, but, because tennis is overall a prolonged endurance event, the other primary prematch nutritional concern

for all players is adequate carbohydrate intake. How to begin a match with carbohydrate stores replenished is therefore the focus of this section.

Before a tennis match begins, a player's carbohydrate stores (muscle and liver glycogen) should be full (remember, players involved in training and competition generally need at least 7 g of carbohydrate per kg of bodyweight each day). And the emphasis on prematch dietary carbohydrates ought to begin at least by the previous evening. This is usually not a problem for players, because, particularly during tournaments, the evening meal is typically when the majority of daily caloric intake occurs, unless a late-night match is played. Moreover, a progressive increase over several days in carbohydrate intake and a concomitant decrease in training duration and intensity, just before the start of an event, can better optimize a tennis player's internal carbohydrate stores prior to beginning a first-round match.

The prematch meal is often more of a challenge. Here, the goal is to eat a well-balanced meal with an emphasis on carbohydrate-rich foods and fluid intake. The recommended number of calories depends, in part, on when the match is scheduled to begin. As a guide, players should try to eat a moderate amount of food. However, by the time play begins, a player's stomach should be relatively empty, but without feelings of hunger. If there is time, then a variety of nutritious, easily digestible, non-distress-causing (e.g. low-fibre) solid foods can be consumed about 3–4 h prior to play. Based on a person's bodyweight, a general guideline is to consume approximately 4–5 g of carbohydrate per kg of bodyweight with the prematch meal. The recommendation, for example, for a 70-kg player would be 280–350 g of carbohydrate, which is a fairly sizeable meal. Although a little fat and protein can be included, too much can extend the digestion period for too long. Various fluids (e.g. water, juice, milk, sport drinks) can be consumed with the prematch meal, so long as alcohol and excessive caffeine are avoided.

Of course, a prematch meal, in essence, might be breakfast, lunch or something in between; it may even consist of a combination of one of these plus a snack or two. Whichever meal or combination it is, players should not completely skip other regularly scheduled meals. For example, if a match is to be played in the early or middle afternoon, a good-sized early breakfast (emphasizing carbohydrates) should be eaten, followed by a smaller prematch lunch during the late morning or midday. Alternatively, if play begins 3–4 h after a prematch breakfast or lunch, players should eat an additional small (1–1.5 g of carbohydrate per kg of body weight), easily digestible carbohydrate snack about 1–1.5 h prior to the start of the match. A combination such as 500 ml of a sport drink along with a sport bar or other solid carbohydrate food works well to 'top off' carbohydrate stores and body water.

A common problem encountered at some events arises when an early morning match is scheduled—say, for 8 or 9 a.m.; players, parents and coaches often wonder how to manage breakfast. In this case, it's usually best to have a smaller-than-usual breakfast, again with an emphasis on carbohydrates and easily digestible foods, at least 90 min before play begins. Commercial high-carbohydrate, low-fat liquid meals work well here, because they have no bulk and are easily digested and absorbed. Then, during the match, it will be important to consume a carbohydrate–electrolyte drink throughout play, because the body's stored carbohydrate levels will be initially somewhat lower at the outset, and the supplemental carbohydrate will likely have a more readily prominent role in providing energy and deferring hunger (see next section).

Whether it is because of scheduling, preference or prematch anxiety, many tennis players simply do not eat enough calories before they compete. Again, liquid carbohydrate meals work well in many of these situations. It is important to eat enough, because inadequate prematch calories and even partially depleted carbohydrate stores can set a player up for premature fatigue on the court.

Another common mistake is to neglect regular fluid and carbohydrate intake during the prematch warm-up session, which often lasts 30 min or more. Such an oversight, especially if it is compounded by a warm-up that is too long and consists of excessive hitting and running, only helps to ensure that the player will begin the match more fatigued, dehydrated and carbohydrate-depleted than is desired. Similar rates of fluid and carbohydrate intake should be followed during the prematch warm-up as are appropriate during play (see next section and Chapter 6). If carbohydrate is not consumed during the warm-up

period, a small carbohydrate snack right after could be sufficient; its content depends on how much time is available before the match begins.

Lastly, numerous 'performance-enhancing' dietary supplements are available today and are regularly used by many tennis players to prepare for a match. Several of the popular and newer ones are discussed later (see section on 'Nutritional ergogenic aids').

Nutrition during play

Carbohydrate and fat are the primary energy sources used during tennis. Yet, because a tennis player's body fat supply is not going to run out in the course of a match, carbohydrate and water are the only principal nutrients that need to be consumed while playing tennis (Fig. 5.1). In some situations, salt intake during play has a more significant role in maintaining fluid balance and preventing heat cramps (see Chapter 6); but generally, it is not an important on-court dietary concern for most players.

Even if a tennis player eats well prior to playing, after 60–90 min of intense singles, liver and muscle glycogen stores will probably be significantly decreased. Further, the ability to maintain blood glucose and meet the muscles' demand for energy may be seriously challenged (Bergeron *et al.* 1991; Ferrauti *et al.* 1997), which could lead to fatigue. Lack of carbohydrate, of course, can be prevented by periodically ingesting carbohydrate during play. How much supplemental carbohydrate does a player need? It depends on a number of factors (e.g. prematch dietary status, body weight, environment, and intensity of play), but generally, up to 60 g·h^{-1} is about the maximum rate that the body can utilize. How does a player get 60 g of carbohydrate? Because fluids should be consumed anyway, the easiest way to obtain enough carbohydrate during play is to drink about a litre of a carbohydrate–electrolyte drink over the course of each hour. More specific and complete on-court fluid replacement guidelines are covered in Chapter 6; however, the following discussion addresses several related important points regarding carbohydrate intake.

Again, the on-court nutritional priorities for all tennis players are water and carbohydrate, and today a number of commercial sport drinks are designed to rapidly deliver these two nutrients so

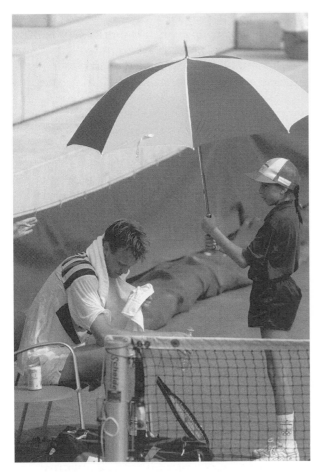

Fig. 5.1 While a balanced diet is the general recommendation for tennis players, the ingestion of both carbohydrate and water is important during the course of a match. Photo © IOC/Olympic Museum Collections/J.-J. Strahm.

that performance can be maximized. Are sport drinks better than water? Clearly, carbohydrate–electrolyte sport drinks can have several distinct advantages over water alone: (i) they provide energy in the form of carbohydrate; (ii) they have been shown to delay the onset of fatigue and perception of effort; (iii) they increase voluntary fluid intake; and (iv) they provide electrolytes which help to maintain mineral and fluid balance. Moreover, some carbohydrate–electrolyte drinks may be absorbed a little faster than water. Any of these factors can be an important contributor to maintaining performance, especially when playing in a hot environment. In fact, supplemental energy intake may be more readily beneficial during play in

the heat, because glycogen utilization tends to occur more rapidly as body temperature rises (Hargreaves *et al.* 1996). Furthermore, the positive performance effects of carbohydrate and water ingestion, during long-term exercise, are additive. In other words, appropriate carbohydrate *and* water consumption (e.g. as a sport drink), during play, is better than carbohydrate or water consumption alone. Today's sport drinks, designed for consumption during exercise, generally have a carbohydrate concentration of 5–8%. This means, for each litre consumed, a player will get 50–80 g of carbohydrate, respectively. Research shows that higher carbohydrate concentrations (i.e. >10%) delay emptying of the stomach, which, in turn, delays water and carbohydrate from getting into the bloodstream where they are needed. However, ingesting sufficient volume of a sport drink (alone or in combination with water) usually helps to maintain a better rate of gastric emptying than when too little is consumed.

During the first hour or so of a tennis match, liver and muscle glycogen often support most of the body's demand for glucose. Thus, from a standpoint of providing energy, the supplemental carbohydrate from a sport drink may not have much of an effect on performance, especially if a player's carbohydrate stores are fully replenished at the start of play. However, it may still be best to drink a carbohydrate–electrolyte drink (perhaps at a diluted concentration *at first*) from the onset of play, even though glycogen stores may not be low. This will help to maintain blood glucose levels and enhance fluid absorption. Moreover, ingesting carbohydrate throughout the first set might have a sparing effect on some of the body's carbohydrate stores, which may help to maintain performance toward the last set or for a subsequent match on the same day (see section on 'Postmatch nutrition').

Often tennis players drink more than 1 litre during each hour of play, in an attempt to offset very high rates of fluid loss from sweating. Exclusive use of a sport drink (even if the carbohydrate content is in the 5–8% range) in these situations might not be well tolerated (and may be detrimental), because of the overall excessive amount of carbohydrate that would be ingested. So as an alternative many players drink a sport drink *and* plain water at each changeover. This combination permits the desired amount of fluid replenishment without taking in too much carbohydrate. At first, the emphasis can be on water (e.g. four swallows of water and two of a sport drink during each changeover). As the match continues, players should make a progressive transition towards consuming more carbohydrate at changeovers (e.g. two swallows of water and four of a sport drink). Similarly, eating too large a snack (such as fruit or a sport bar) during play, while regularly drinking a sport drink at the same time, might also delay stomach emptying and fluid delivery, again, because of the excessive carbohydrate intake. Further, ingesting a high amount of fructose (liquid or solid) could also cause gastrointestinal distress, since fructose is absorbed more slowly from the intestine, compared to other carbohydrates in sport drinks, such as glucose, sucrose and glucose polymers. However, a small, easily digestible, high-glycaemic index snack (e.g. crackers, raisins, jelly beans, etc.) may provide additional needed energy late in the match.

All in all, sufficient hydration and appropriate carbohydrate intake, during play, can make a big difference in a player's overall performance and, as recently found (Vergauwen *et al.* 1998), stroke quality.

Postmatch nutrition

After a match, a tennis player's primary nutritional interest should be the restoration of lost fluid, electrolytes and carbohydrate. How immediate and aggressive this effort needs to be depends on how much carbohydrate was used (roughly suggested by how intense and long the match was), how much sweat was lost, and, most importantly, when the next match will begin. Once again, more specific rehydration recommendations and considerations are detailed in Chapter 6.

If the next match is scheduled to begin shortly after the completion of play (i.e. within 1–2 h), rehydration and carbohydrate intake (about 50–100 g or 1–1.5 g of carbohydrate per kg of body weight) should begin immediately (i.e. within 15 min of the end of the match). High-carbohydrate sport drinks, along with sport bars, gels and other carbohydrate-rich foods with a high glycaemic index (e.g. bagels, crackers, certain ready-to-eat cereals, white bread and jelly beans), are good choices. These will facilitate the rapid restoration of muscle glycogen more so than

high-fructose foods or meals with an emphasis on low glycaemic index carbohydrate sources (e.g. flavoured yoghurt, apples, oranges, pasta and mixed-grain bread). Notably, some research (Zawadzki *et al.* 1992) suggests that a carbohydrate and protein combination might be better than just carbohydrate for rapid glycogen resynthesis. If convenience is a priority, there are several commercial high-carbohydrate sport drinks and sport bars available that provide appropriate amounts of carbohydrate and protein for this purpose. Otherwise, certain combinations of breads, cereals and dairy products, for example, can provide similar ratios of carbohydrate and protein. Once the next match begins, regular consumption of a carbohydrate–electrolyte drink, designed for consumption during play, may be *necessary* to maintain blood glucose, provide energy and defer hunger, since the short between-match recovery period is probably not going to be long enough to adequately replenish carbohydrate stores.

When preparing for a second match that begins 4–5 h or more after the completion of the first, players should generally follow the prematch meal guidelines described earlier. But many tennis players would rather not eat a large meal between matches, even if there were plenty of time. Thus, if smaller quantities of food are preferred, 50–100 g of carbohydrate, for example, ingested immediately after play, and again every 2 h, can be an effective method for replenishing (at least partially) one's carbohydrate stores. Having more time to accomplish this task means that a player can choose from a wider variety of foods (low, medium and high glycaemic index). Although, it is always a good idea to consume some rapidly absorptive carbohydrates and fluid (i.e. high glycaemic index) right after play, so that glycogen and hydration status will be more promptly and completely restored for the next match.

If a player is not scheduled to compete again until the next day, appropriate regularly scheduled meals and snacks (according to the above guidelines) should provide enough of the necessary nutrients to nutritionally recover from the previous match and adequately prepare to play again.

Lastly, if sweat losses from the previous match were extensive, and especially if a player just experienced (or is prone to experience) heat cramps, additional salt may have to be added to the diet (see Chapter 6).

Nutrition and fatigue

From a nutritional standpoint, fatigue during tennis occurs when there is an inadequate supply of carbohydrate and/or a diminished ability to use all available sources (i.e. carbohydrate, fat and protein) to produce energy at a fast enough rate to meet the body's muscular demands. At this point, the fatigued tennis player can no longer continue playing at the desired level of intensity.

At the beginning of play, a player's blood glucose level tends to increase, in response to a variety of hormonal influences designed to mobilize carbohydrate. Without supplemental carbohydrate intake during the match, a continued high rate of glucose utilization in the muscles will eventually lead to a much greater reliance on blood glucose for energy, which will, in turn, quickly deplete liver glycogen stores. As play continues, blood glucose will progressively decrease (Bergeron *et al.* 1991). Prematch carbohydrate status, of course, plays a role in how readily this occurs. But also, high-intensity play, repeated long points, and dehydration can significantly change the way the muscles use energy, such that carbohydrate will be utilized at an even faster rate. Eventually, carbohydrate availability will be diminished to the point that performance may be severely hindered (Vergauwen *et al.* 1998). This is why regular carbohydrate and fluid intake during difficult, long matches is so important, especially in hot environmental conditions. Moreover, if carbohydrate is not consumed during an extended match, there may be a significant increase in the conversion of protein to glucose, in order to have a continued supply of available energy. This could lead to a lower concentration of the branched-chain amino acids (BCAA) in the blood, which could act as another contributory factor in a player's sense of fatigue (see section on nutritional ergogenic aids).

Once again, carbohydrate and fat are the principal sources of energy utilized during tennis, and although much has been stated here and elsewhere in this chapter regarding the importance of adequate carbohydrate intake before and during play to defer fatigue, a tennis player's diet should also regularly include sufficient protein, vitamins, minerals and water. These other important nutrients support the ongoing utilization of carbohydrate and fat for energy throughout the course of a match; a deficiency in one or more of them could readily accelerate the onset of fatigue.

Nutritional ergogenic aids

Advocates of today's growing and seemingly endless selection of nutritional ergogenic ('work-enhancing') aids promote these products with promises such as enhanced energy, increased strength, power and lean body mass, more endurance, better performance and faster recovery. Like many other athletes who are constantly in search of anything that will provide a competitive advantage, some tennis players are very susceptible to such tantalizing claims. But do the products work? Are the latest supplements just what a player needs to perform better? To date, very few nutritional 'ergogenic' supplements have lived up to their claims. More importantly, some have been found to actually *impede* optimal performance. On the other hand, as a result of well-controlled experimental studies, certain products have shown some promise as being effective ergogenic aids. Too often, however, the purported benefits of many new supplements are based on unsubstantiated claims or testimonials, poor research or research findings taken out of context, or simply just misinformation. In this section, several currently popular and well-studied nutritional ergogenic aids are discussed, with particular mention of their appropriateness for tennis.

Medium-chain tryglycerides

To take advantage of the enhanced utilization of fat during exercise as a result of training, several dietary fat supplements have been suggested for athletes. From this category, medium-chain tryglycerides (MCTs) are one of the ergogenic aids used by athletes today, because of the professed ability of MCTs to enhance energy levels, fat metabolism and endurance. Once ingested, MCTs are rapidly emptied from the stomach, quickly absorbed from the intestine, and readily made available for energy. This may lead to a greater utilization of fat, but, thus far, MCTs or other fat-loading techniques have not been shown to improve performance. Therefore, despite the need for fat in a tennis player's diet and the important role of fat in providing energy during competition, fat loading prior to play or fat supplementation during a match are not currently validated or recommended procedures for tennis.

Creatine

Creatine monohydrate has become one of the most popular 'performance-enhancing' nutritional supplements in use today, and for good reason. Supportive preliminary evidence associated with creatine supplementation includes increased one repetition maximum (1-RM) performance (i.e. how much weight a person can lift one time, such as with a bench press or squat) and peak power, as well as enhanced rowing performance and repetitive sprint performance in swimming, running and cycling. In addition, many studies have demonstrated increases in body weight.

Does such laboratory data mean that creatine supplementation will enhance performance during tennis? Will the same effects be shown with highly trained and conditioned athletes, as have been demonstrated with moderately trained or untrained individuals? Is creatine supplementation appropriate for the physiological demands of tennis? Are the observed weight gains actual gains in muscle or mostly fluid retention? What about the long-term effects and health risks associated with continued supplementation? The answers to these questions are not known at this point.

Creatine is a natural compound that is made by your own body from two amino acids (arginine and glycine). You can also get creatine from eating fish, meat and other animal products. During very brief, explosive-type exercise, your muscles' capacity to adequately meet the high demand for energy is largely dependent on the availability of creatine phosphate (CP), a high-energy compound found in your muscles. It has been thought that, by increasing the amount of creatine in the muscles, more CP will be readily available to provide energy at a faster rate during very high-intensity exercise.

Before reasoning that the above preliminary research findings and rationale sound like perfect justification for taking creatine supplements to improve one's tennis, a few things should be considered. Reports of increased muscle creatine and CP levels, enhanced performance and desirable changes in body composition have been inconsistent and remain somewhat equivocal. Regarding potential gains in muscle protein, there are proven and more effective ways to gain the necessary lean body mass required for tennis. Importantly, the long-term consequences and health risks associated with continued creatine supplementation have not yet been comprehensively examined. Concerns over potential negative effects on the kidneys, heart and liver, for example, should be carefully studied. Lastly, given the specific loading patterns and metabolic demands on individual muscle groups during tennis, the muscle creatine and CP levels are probably (without supplementation) already more than adequate in any well-conditioned player. At present, creatine supplementation for tennis does not appear to be justified.

Sodium bicarbonate

During very high-intensity exercise, there is an increasing concentration of hydrogen ions (H^+) in the muscle cells, as a result of a continuous rapid production of lactic acid. A high level of H^+ will rapidly lead to fatigue. Unless there is something to offset the growing concentration of H^+, there will soon be a decrease in muscle force output, a lower production of energy, and a resultant decrease in performance, even in the presence of adequate carbohydrate supplies. Fortunately, sodium bicarbonate, which is naturally present in the body, buffers a portion of the H^+ associated with the accumulating lactic acid during anaerobic exercise. This helps to delay fatigue. Would augmented sodium bicarbonate levels do a better job in delaying the onset of fatigue during high-intensity exercise by helping to buffer more lactic acid? Probably. Will ingested bicarbonate enhance a tennis player's overall performance during a match? Probably not.

As outlined in Chapter 4, the intermittent nature and overall moderate intensity of tennis precludes the necessity for a great reliance on anaerobic carbohydrate metabolism during play. Consequently, lactic acid production is seldom very high (Bergeron *et al.* 1991). Thus, sodium bicarbonate supplementation would not be very helpful for tennis, because a player does not need to compensate for a large accumulation of H^+, as it probably rarely occurs.

Branched-chain amino acids

When carbohydrate is in short supply, your body relies more on protein for energy. This can lead to lower blood levels of the branched-chain amino acids (BCAA). Moreover, during prolonged exercise, there is an increase in the concentration of free fatty acids in the blood, which leads to higher levels of free tryptophan (another amino acid). The resultant effect will be a higher free tryptophan : BCAA ratio. This is thought to be an important factor in the development of fatigue, especially during endurance activities. When free tryptophan enters the brain it is converted to serotonin; high amounts of this neurotransmitter may be associated with making one feel fatigued. Conceivably, tennis players could be susceptible to fatigue related to lowered BCAA levels and increased free tryptophan, particularly during lengthy matches (Strüder *et al.* 1995). Would BCAA supplementation help to alleviate this situation by maintaining higher levels of BCAA in the blood? As one might expect, some researchers have shown improved performance with BCAA supplementation and others have demonstrated no change in performance. Although BCAA might, in theory, be helpful in delaying the onset of fatigue during long matches, especially if carbohydrate stores are significantly diminished, adequate carbohydrate intake prior to and during play could achieve the same effect, by reducing the amount of free fatty acids released and by minimizing any potential increase in the free tryptophan : BCAA ratio. Furthermore, BCAA supplementation could lead to higher levels of ammonia in the blood; this would accelerate fatigue.

Vitamins and minerals

Vitamin and mineral supplements are widely used by tennis players, often in great excess, not only to 'maintain health', but also with the hope that performance will be enhanced as well.

B-complex vitamin supplements are particularly popular, probably because of their important role as coenzymes in helping carbohydrate and fat to be used for energy. Logically, it seems like B-complex supplementation would be, in theory, helpful in enhancing the utilization of these nutrients during activities such as tennis. But, despite the essential role of these and other vitamins in a variety of physiological processes, including energy metabolism, unless an athlete has a vitamin deficiency, vitamin supplementation will not enhance physical performance. In fact, excessive intake of the fat-soluble vitamins (A, D, E and K) can have a toxic effect, and although extra water-soluble vitamin (B-complex and C) intake will mostly end up being excreted in urine, excessive intake of these vitamins can have toxic effects as well. Additional vitamin C and vitamin E intake, however, might be worth considering. Both of these vitamins have been shown to have beneficial antioxidant and other health-related properties. Moreover, there is evidence that athletes may need more vitamin C compared to those that do not exercise regularly and additional vitamin E intake may reduce exercise-related muscle tissue damage.

Minerals are necessary for growth, metabolism and a variety of other physiological processes. Like vitamins, a tennis player's mineral requirements generally can easily be met by a well-balanced diet; although, certain minerals may need special attention by some players. These typically include calcium and iron and sometimes zinc. In addition, excessive and repeated sweating may cause a progressive sodium deficit—this issue is comprehensively addressed in Chapter 6. Calcium and iron deficits can be encouraged by low caloric intake (which often includes low intake of protein and dairy products), other dietary influences, and excessive sweating. In women, iron status can be further challenged by menstrual bleeding. But, unless a player is restricting calories, mineral status is usually not a problem. As a guide, all players should regularly eat foods that are rich in calcium and iron (e.g. meat, chicken, fish, milk, yoghurt, dark, leafy green vegetables, wholegrain breads and fortified cereals, etc.); this will probably ensure adequate intake of these and most other minerals. Importantly, arbitrary excessive mineral supplementation can also have deleterious effects on health and can interfere with the absorption of other minerals.

For tennis players, like many athletes, it is sometimes a challenge to maintain a well-balanced diet, especially when travelling and playing a lot. So, to prevent a potential vitamin or mineral deficiency, it is safe and probably prudent to regularly take a one-a-day multivitamin/mineral supplement that provides *no more than* 100% of the recommended dietary allowance (RDA) (National Research Council

1989) for any one vitamin or mineral. Slightly higher amounts of vitamins C and E can be supplemented, although it is probably better to obtain these through careful food selection (e.g. fruits, vegetables, legumes).

Summary

Proper nutrition is important in any tennis player's quest to reach peak performance. When integrated with proper training and adequate rest, a well-balanced and varied diet, coupled with a dietary strategy that optimizes prematch and during-play hydration and carbohydrate availability and promotes timely and sufficient postmatch rehydration and restoration of carbohydrate stores and other nutrients, will greatly enhance a tennis player's opportunity to be a regular winner on the court.

Lastly, all players differ in what foods and which nutritional strategies they can tolerate and perform well with. New foods, drinks or other dietary protocols should be experimented with well prior to any important tournament or match.

Acknowledgement

A very sincere thank you goes to my good friend and colleague Stella L. Volpe, for her valuable thoughts and comments in reviewing this chapter.

References

Bergeron, M.F., Maresh, C.M., Kraemer, W.J. *et al.* (1991) Tennis: a physiological profile during match play. *International Journal of Sports Medicine* **12**, 474–479.

Brouns, F. (1993) *Nutritional Needs of Athletes.* John Wiley & Sons, Chichester.

Chen, J.D., Wang, J.F., Li, K.J. *et al.* (1989) Nutritional problems and measures in elite and amateur athletes. *American Journal of Clinical Nutrition* **49**, 1084–1089.

Evans, W.J. (1993) Exercise and protein metabolism. In: Simopoulos, A.P. & Pavlou, K.N., eds. *World Review of Nutrition and Dietetics, Nutrition and Fitness for Athletes,* Vol. 71, pp. 21–33. Karger, Basel.

Faber, M., Spinnler-Benade, S.-J. & Daubitzer, A. (1990) Dietary intake, anthropometric measurements and plasma lipid levels in throwing athletes. *International Journal of Sports Medicine* **10**, 140–145.

Ferrauti, A., Weber, K. & Strüder, H.K. (1997) Metabolic and ergogenic effects of carbohydrate and caffeine beverages in tennis. *Journal of Sports Medicine and Physical Fitness* **37**, 1–9.

Foster-Powell, K. & Brand Miller, J. (1995) International tables of glycemic index. *American Journal of Clinical Nutrition* **62**, 871S–893S.

Grandjean, A.C. (1989) Macronutrient intake of the US athletes compared with the general population and recommendations made for athletes. *American Journal of Clinical Nutrition* **49**, 1070–1076.

Hargreaves, M., Angus, D., Howlett, K., Marmy Conus, N. & Febbraio, M. (1996) Effect of heat stress on glucose kinetics during exercise in trained men. *Medicine and Science in Sports and Exercise* **28** (Suppl.), 58.

Heinemann, L. & Zerbes, H. (1989) Physical activity, fitness, and diet: behavior in the population compared with elite athletes in the GDR. *American Journal of Clinical Nutrition* **49**, 1007–1016.

Henriksson, J. (1991) Effect of exercise on amino acid concentrations in skeletal muscle and plasma. *Journal of Experimental Biology* **160**, 149–165.

Lemon, P.W.R. (1991) Effect of exercise on protein requirements. *Journal of Sports Sciences* **9**, 53–70.

National Research Council (1989) *Recommended Dietary Allowances,* 10th edn. National Academy Press, Washington, DC.

Sears, B. (1993) *Essential Fatty Acids, Eicosanoids, and Dietary Endocrinology.* Eicotec Foods, Marblehead, MA.

Strüder, H.K., Hollman, W., Duperly, J. & Weber, K. (1995) Amino acid metabolism in tennis and its possible influence on the neuroendocrine system. *British Journal of Sports Medicine* **29**, 28–30.

Vergauwen, L., Brouns, F. & Hespel, P. (1998) Carbohydrate supplementation improves stroke performance in tennis. *Medicine and Science in Sports and Exercise* **30**, 1289–1295.

Zawadzki, K.M., Yaspelkis, B.B. III & Ivy, J.L. (1992) Carbohydrate-protein complex increases the rate of muscle glycogen storage after exercise. *Journal of Applied Physiology* **72**, 1854–1859.

Chapter 6

Playing tennis in the heat: fluid and electrolyte balance

Introduction

The toughest opponent that tennis players often face cannot be seen across the net. Yet, its presence is constantly felt from anywhere on the court. A hot environment can be a dangerous and unrelenting enemy, especially to those who are unprepared. Even for players who are fit and take the necessary precautions, the heat can be oppressive, making it very difficult to perform at all, let alone win. At a recent Australian Open, many prominent professional players readily proclaimed their displeasure about the extreme climatic conditions with comments such as 'It's so hot, it's a joke', 'My feet were on fire', 'It was unbelievable', 'The conditions were inhumane', 'It was like an oven', and 'I had the feeling that my brain was cooking' (Finn 1997). Not all hot weather tournaments have the reputation that follows the Australian Open. Still, many tennis events can be as challenging or even worse for the players, especially when the combination of heat and humidity lingers throughout the week.

As with any vigorous physical activity, playing tennis, *in itself*, produces a considerable amount of heat, which will cause body temperature to rise. Fortunately, players normally have several means for dealing with this. For example, even a gentle breeze can prompt significant convective heat loss. Also, especially in a cool environment, there is a certain degree of dry heat exchange that occurs as heat is simply radiated from a player's body. However, sweating is typically the most effective and utilized on-court method for dissipating heat in hot weather. This poses a significant fluid balance challenge for many tennis players. Furthermore, if it is hot, sunny, still and *humid*, a player can be in real trouble. With these conditions, all ways for dissipating heat are

much less effective; plus it is even worse if adequate hydration is not maintained. If fluid balance and thermoregulation are not effectively managed on the court, and a tennis player becomes dehydrated and overheated, at the very least, the player will fatigue prematurely and possibly lose the match. More severely, heat exhaustion, heat cramps or, at worst, heat stroke may ultimately ensue.

This chapter will address several important aspects related to the fluid–electrolyte and thermoregulatory challenges that tennis players routinely encounter while competing in a hot environment (Bergeron *et al.* 1995a,b; Bergeron 1996). In addition, specific recommendations for prior, during and after play on how to maintain fluid–electrolyte balance, optimize performance and minimize heat-related problems will be presented.

Sweating rate

In warm to hot conditions, most adult tennis players will lose between 1 and 2.5 l of sweat during each hour of competitive singles play or on-court training. Even more impressive, sweat rates of up to 3.5 $l \cdot h^{-1}$ have been observed with some well-conditioned, high-level players who were competing in very hot and humid climates. Clearly, it would not be difficult for some tennis players to lose 10 or more litres of fluid in one long match.

The degree to which one sweats depends on a number of factors. As environmental heat stress (i.e. temperature, humidity and solar radiation) increases, the potential for a high sweating rate goes up as well. Likewise, as the intensity of play increases, sweating will correspondingly increase to offset the progressive rise in core body temperature as a result of a higher metabolic rate. Still, why doesn't every player sweat a lot when competing or training in warm to hot conditions? As with other physical characteristics, genetics has an important influence, and some players will always sweat more or less than others.

Acclimatization is another factor. Players who have been training and playing in a hot climate for several weeks or more (thus, are acclimatized to the heat) may sweat more compared to those who are not accustomed to such conditions. The same goes for cardiorespiratory fitness. Such training can improve sweat-gland function and increase plasma volume, which can help to maintain a higher sweating rate. One must keep in mind that a higher sweating rate is a good adaptation, because it gives a player a thermoregulatory advantage. Although, at the same time, more extensive sweating will be a greater challenge to offset with fluid intake, especially during play.

Senior tennis players typically experience a progressive decline in sweating rate, as they get older. In part, this is often due to a reduced intensity of play. However, there can also be age-related changes in the skin and sweat gland function. Boys and girls have lower sweating rates than men and women, due to a number of growth- and maturation-related factors; but these differences gradually decrease as adolescents reach their late teen years. Overall, women generally sweat less than men; however, this is not always the case.

Electrolyte losses

Sweat is mostly water, but it also contains a number of other elements found in the blood, including a variety of minerals in varying concentrations. The major mineral ions found in sweat are sodium (Na^+) and chloride (Cl^-), although the concentration varies with a number of factors. For example, well-conditioned tennis players, who are fully acclimatized to the heat, often have sweat sodium concentrations in the range of 5–30 mmol·l^{-1} (i.e. 115–690 mg of sodium per litre of sweat), whereas heat non-acclimatized players typically lose much more sodium through sweating (e.g. 40–100 mmol·l^{-1} or 920–2300 mg·l^{-1}). Nevertheless, some players can have a relatively high concentration of sodium in their sweat, no matter how fit or heat acclimatized they are, which again suggests a strong genetic influence. Sweat sodium and chloride concentrations also vary with sweating rate. As sweating rate goes up, the concentration of these minerals in sweat usually increases as well. Thus, men ordinarily lose much more sodium and chloride during exercise in the heat compared to women. Sweat sodium and chloride losses are characteristically low in boys and girls, but these electrolyte losses tend to increase progressively with age up until adulthood.

Even though the concentrations of sodium and chloride are much lower than their respective concentrations in blood (i.e. sweat is relatively hypotonic), extended tennis play in hot and humid weather can lead to sizeable sodium and chloride losses (Bergeron *et al.* 1995b; Bergeron 1996). Without adequate salt replacement, the cumulative effect of such electrolyte losses can bring about a progressive sweat-induced sodium deficit after several days of playing or training in the heat. This can readily lead to incomplete rehydration, poorer performance, heat-related muscle cramps (see below) (Bergeron 1996), and possibly put a player at a higher risk for developing heat exhaustion. In contrast, potassium (K^+) and magnesium (Mg^{2+}) sweat losses, for example, are typically much lower. In fact, players will generally lose 3–10 times as much sodium as potassium during play. With regard to calcium and trace minerals, such as iron and zinc, their concentrations in sweat are also very low; however, repeated extensive sweating can lead to a deficit of one or more of these elements (Tipton *et al.* 1993; Clarkson & Haymes 1995; Bergeron *et al.* 1998). Such deficits will not have a direct effect on fluid balance, *per se*, but a chronic dietary deficiency of any one of these nutrients (i.e. not enough consumed to offset sweat and other excretory losses) can clearly have a negative impact on overall health and performance.

Effects of hypohydration

While the majority of tennis players usually manage fluid and electrolyte losses well enough to avoid serious heat-related problems, such as cramps or heat exhaustion, most players probably compete regularly with some degree of a body water deficit. A number of these same players often begin matches somewhat dehydrated (Bergeron *et al.* 1995b; Bergeron 1996). This is not uncommon, especially in tournaments when players must compete in two or more matches on a single day. So, does a 2–3% body water deficit matter that much? Will it make a difference in a player's ability to compete or train? To date, very little research has specifically examined varying levels of a body water deficit (i.e. hypohydration) on tennis performance. However, the effects of hypohydration on physiologic function and exercise performance, using activities other than tennis, have been comprehensively investigated (Sawka 1992) and certain similarities should be assumed.

During exercise, blood flow from the heart (i.e. cardiac output) increases, so that the vital areas of the body (e.g. brain, heart, liver, etc.) and the active muscles receive an adequate and continuous supply of blood. Under most circumstances the body is very capable of meeting the additional cardiovascular demands of exercise, by primarily increasing heart rate. But, as a tennis player's body heats up, a larger portion of the central blood volume must go to the skin, in response to a greater need for thermoregulation via evaporative (sweating) and dry (radiation and convection) heat exchange. To compensate, heart rate goes up even more to maintain cardiac output. At first, play may just seem a little more difficult. However, as sweating continues and fluid is not fully replaced, the player readily becomes increasingly dehydrated. Eventually, with a reduced blood volume, the competition between central blood flow (i.e. to the muscles and organs, etc.) and circulation to the skin is too great. Consequently, both cardiac output and temperature regulation are adversely affected. Skin blood flow is reduced, despite an increase in core temperature. Core body temperature continues to go up and symptoms of fatigue rapidly become more apparent. Under these conditions a player is also at a much higher risk for developing heat illness. In addition, gastric (stomach region) emptying will decrease, which may eventually cause sensations of discomfort, nausea and bloating.

With respect to the other many physiological and psychological demands of tennis, it may only take a marginal (i.e. 1–2% of bodyweight) to moderate body water deficit to significantly reduce a player's strength, power, endurance, physical work capacity and even mental performance during play in the heat. Inadequate fluid intake during exercise can also affect muscle metabolism. As one's core and muscle temperature are consequently elevated, muscle glycogen will be used at a faster rate and muscle lactate production will increase (Hargreaves *et al.* 1996). Thus, fatigue occurs earlier. So, *any* degree of hypohydration will challenge a player's on-court cardiovascular, muscular, metabolic, thermoregulatory and psychological capacities and may readily lead to a decrease in performance. Unfortunately, it is also a challenge, and often impossible, to keep up with extensive sweating rates over the course of an entire match. Therefore, it is critical that players prepare and manage as best they can by following a predetermined and comprehensive hydration plan before, during and after play (see 'Recommendations', below).

Heat tolerance and age

For the most part, a tennis player's capacity to compete effectively and safely in the heat is largely based on that individual's heat tolerance, which is primarily determined by his or her ability to adequately regulate body temperature on the court. Thermoregulatory capacity, and thus core body temperature during play, is influenced by a variety of interrelated determinants, including cardiorespiratory fitness, electrolyte balance, sweating rate, blood volume, state of health, and even certain medications. Age is also a major factor.

Older people generally have a decreased sensitivity for thirst, along with a reduced ability to conserve water. Consequently, older people are generally at a higher risk for being chronically dehydrated to some degree. For this reason, it is important for many senior tennis players to particularly emphasize additional fluid intake prior to competing in the heat. Further, because of the lower capacity for sweating often associated with people over 60, there may be, for some senior tennis players, a lower tolerance of the heat, as well as a higher risk of overheating; although, importantly, overall thermoregulatory capacity and heat tolerance can be maintained or improved if senior players (or anyone else, for that matter) stay regularly active, fit, and well hydrated and give themselves an adequate opportunity to get acclimatized to the heat (see section 'Prior to play' under 'Recommendations', below). In other words, cardiorespiratory fitness and adequate hydration can offset these age-associated changes.

On the other hand, children will often experience a low level of tolerance for exercising in the heat, even if they are fit and well hydrated. With a much higher surface area to mass ratio and lower capacity for sweating, children depend more on dry heat exchange (i.e. convection and radiation) than evaporative cooling (i.e. sweating). Under some environmental circumstances, these methods work fine for children. But, if it is hot and sunny, a relatively larger exposed surface area can lead to a higher rate of heat absorption from solar energy. Plus, with a lower blood volume (relative to body size and surface area), children typically experience a higher degree of cardiovascular strain during exercise in the heat. Blood pressure, central circulation and thermoregulation can easily be compromised, as a limited blood supply must be additionally distributed to the skin and muscles. This situation is rapidly worsened, as a child becomes progressively dehydrated. Perception of effort increases and performance, of course, goes down. Add to all of this the fact that children generally produce relatively more heat as they exercise, due to a higher metabolic cost of locomotion (i.e. movement). Overall, in similar environmental conditions and with the same relative playing or training intensity, a child's core body temperature will probably be higher than an adult's. Thus, parents, coaches, tournament directors and medical support personnel should be particularly attentive to children playing tennis in the heat, because of their higher potential for incurring severe cardiovascular strain and developing heat-related illness.

These age-related characteristics of responses to thermal stress during rest and exercise are well outlined in two recent reviews (Pandolf 1997; Falk 1998).

Heat cramps

Tennis players who experience heat-related muscle cramps (usually males) know the following familiar scenario all too well. It is hot, humid, and the match has been going on for a while. Both players have been working hard for every point, and are feeling tired, but each feels that a win is within grasp. One of the players has been sweating a lot (and seemingly quite a bit more than his opponent), as he did during the previous match that day, but he has been very attentive to drinking water at every changeover. Then it happens. What began as only very subtle, hardly noticeable twitches in the legs several games ago, has now (usually 20–30 min later) evolved into completely debilitating, full-blown muscle cramps. The player can no longer continue the match, and now, once again, must default. What happened? Why do so many other players never have the same problem?

Heat-related muscle cramps (heat cramps) often occur during prolonged exercise when there have been previous *extensive* and *repeated* fluid and sodium losses. Such is often the case in a tennis tournament, especially by the time a player reaches a later round. Drinking plenty of water helps; but, to completely restore fluids, the salt lost through sweating must be replenished as well (Nose *et al.* 1988; Maughan *et al.* 1997). Otherwise, with a significant body water and sodium deficit, the fluid spaces around selected motor nerve terminals (where the nerves contact the muscles) could become contracted and the associated neuromuscular junctions might then become hyperexcitable and sensitive, resulting in seemingly spontaneous muscle contractions (i.e. cramps). Importantly, a sodium deficit is not often reflected in serum electrolyte measurements. Postplay serum sodium concentration might be slightly elevated, owing to hypotonic sweat secretion and renal sodium conservation. But otherwise, serum sodium should be normal after a match, once a player has a chance to rehydrate and replace electrolytes. This explains why players, who cramped on the court, often do not present with abnormal electrolytes in follow-up physician evaluations.

So why do all players not have cramp when they play several matches and sweat a lot? The key seems to be related to sodium balance differences. Those who are susceptible to (and are often afflicted by) heat cramps sweat considerably, lose an extensive amount of sodium and chloride through sweating, and typically have a relatively low (or at least inadequate) daily dietary salt intake. Other mineral deficiencies (e.g. calcium, magnesium and potassium) can also cause muscle cramps and various neuromotor problems, but they are not typically the culprits when a tennis player has cramps in the heat. Lack of conditioning and fatigue can cause a muscle cramp, but the cramp is usually localized and passive, stretching, massage or icing can often resolve it. Such is not the case with heat cramps. Fluid and salt intake (orally or intravenously) is necessary. So does this mean that all players should load up on salt? For some, extra salt intake *is* appropriate when playing or training in hot conditions or any time that sweating is expected to be extensive. Importantly, any plan for increasing dietary salt intake should include appropriate and adequate fluid intake. Also, such a dietary plan should be individually designed.

In other words, it is best to determine a player's specific sweating and electrolyte loss rates, so that a suitable and sufficient strategy can be implemented to ensure adequate rehydration and electrolyte balance; although, for most people with normal blood pressure, even excessive salt intake is not likely to pose a health threat (Taubes 1998). Thus, for the majority of healthy and active tennis players, adding a little more salt to foods and fluids, during periods of training or competition in the heat, will, at worst, be harmless and may indeed help.

For a more comprehensive description of a particular player's experience with heat cramps and how he was ultimately able to prevent further occurrences during training and competition by increasing his daily dietary intake of salt, see the case report by Bergeron (1996). The recommendations below also include some appropriate ways to increase fluid and salt intake prior to a match, during play and in recovery.

Recommendations

In order to manage all prematch, during-play and postmatch dietary aspects well, the information and suggestions described here should be integrated with the nutrition guidelines presented in Chapter 5. As with Chapter 5, the following match play recommendations are generally appropriate for on-court training and practice as well. However, these are only general guidelines. To obtain optimal effectiveness, all strategies for managing fluid and electrolyte losses should be based on player-specific requirements and considerations, and any new routine should be practised *prior to* an important match or tournament. In addition, the recommendations outlined here are specific to adults. While generally similar, the most appropriate and beneficial guidelines for children and adolescents may be different in some respects. It is also important to keep in mind that proper training (particularly regular endurance training), good health and adequate rest can greatly enhance *any* player's tolerance and performance in the heat.

Prior to play

When playing tennis in a hot environment, being acclimatized to the heat can be a tremendous

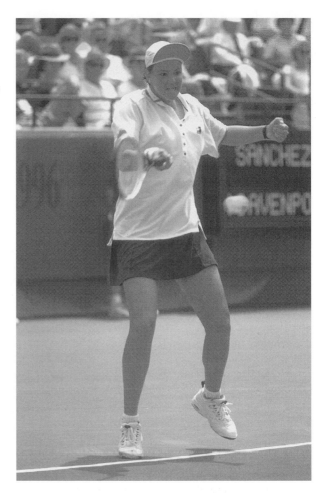

Fig. 6.1 Heat acclimatization is an important issue for tennis players competing in hot and/or humid environments. Photo © Allsport/G.M. Prior.

advantage (Fig. 6.1). For a non-acclimatized player, nearly full heat acclimatization can take 7–14 days, so long as the player trains or exercises daily for 1–2 h in the same heat. Importantly, the intensity and duration of training or exercise should be considerably reduced at first and then progressively increased throughout most of the acclimatization period. This assures gradual exposure to the heat and lessens the potential for excessive physiological heat strain and heat injury. Ideally, players should finish a heat-acclimatization period with several days of normal intensity and duration training/practice followed by a short taper period (see below). The resultant effects of the heat-acclimatization process include an earlier onset of sweating, a greater distribution of sweating over the body, an increased sweating rate and a decreased concentration of sodium and chloride in the sweat. These and other adaptations will improve a player's thermoregulatory capacity, cardiovascular stability during play, and tolerance of heat stress. Because an acclimatization process of 7–14 days (or more) is not always possible or practical, players with less acclimatization time should be especially attentive to fluid replacement and possibly increased salt intake, especially if they are prone to heat cramps. Moreover, cardiorespiratory (aerobic) fitness helps a tennis player achieve heat acclimatization more quickly and maintain heat acclimatization longer. Players who arrive at an event (that is in a hotter climate) with a high level of cardiorespiratory fitness and a less-than-optimal degree of heat acclimatization, may require much less time to adjust to the heat. This advantage might also be very helpful to a player who must leave a hot climate for a period of time between tournaments or when the weather is variable in a particular region during a series of events.

An obvious way to improve one's level of prematch hydration is, of course, to drink more fluid, beginning at least the night before. Players should make a special effort to do this, because it is easy to let oneself become unknowingly dehydrated, particularly in a new climate that is hotter than the one previously accustomed to. Generally speaking, if sufficient carbohydrates and electrolytes are provided by food intake, then water alone can serve as a primary or sole prematch beverage. However, other fluids, such as milk, juice and sport drinks can be used as well, and their consumption should be encouraged, as part of any well-balanced and varied dietary plan. Alcohol and excessive caffeine should be avoided, as they can accelerate fluid loss. As stated in Chapter 5, before a tennis match begins, a player's carbohydrate (i.e. glycogen) stores should be at or near capacity. Besides providing a readily available source of energy, muscle glycogen also has a fair amount of water stored with it. Thus, by replenishing carbohydrates (even partially), a tennis player can improve hydration status as well. Plus, concomitant food and fluid consumption has an effect on fluid retention, because of the inherent electrolytes and water in the food. Prematch

carbohydrate and hydration status can be further enhanced (at least for the first round of play) by a short taper period (e.g. 2–3 days). By progressively reducing training volume (and intensity somewhat) just prior to a tournament, a player has a better chance to restore carbohydrates, improve fluid and electrolyte balance, and adequately rest and recover prior to competition. (Note: A taper period might need to be longer (e.g. 7–10 days) to maximize performance, if a player has been training particularly hard.)

To achieve better restoration and retention of fluids, and to improve electrolyte balance (primarily sodium) prior to competition, tomato juice and/or a salted sport drink (e.g. up to 3 g of salt per litre), for example, can be consumed the night before and again on the morning of play. Importantly, this is in addition to one's regular intake of water and other appropriate drinks. Also, a variety of foods (e.g. cheese, tomato sauce, soup and certain prepared foods) contain moderate to high levels of sodium; these can be appropriate and nutritious choices in a dietary plan that emphasizes higher salt intake.

Approximately 1–1.5 h before the match begins, about 500 ml of a sport drink should be consumed, along with a small snack (see Chapter 5), in order to 'top off' carbohydrate stores and body water. Again, if extra salt is needed, a small amount (e.g. 1.5 g) can be mixed with the 500 ml of sport drink. Players can, of course, have more fluids (e.g. water, juice, sport drinks) right up to their match, but too much can prompt the need to urinate during the first set, although, just before play, one should be able to urinate, and the urine should be fairly clear or light coloured. This can be interpreted as a fairly good indication of adequate prematch hydration. However, frequent urine production, induced by diuretics or excessive consumption of beverages containing caffeine, does not imply that a player is well hydrated.

Many players are careful about consuming fluids during play, but they neglect to drink regularly during practices and their prematch warm-ups. Players and coaches should appreciate that the quality of practice or warm-up can be readily improved if hydration (and carbohydrate intake) is adequately maintained during these times. Moreover, for obvious reasons, the prematch warm-up is definitely not a time to let players get fatigued, dehydrated or carbohydrate depleted. Therefore, fluid and carbohydrate intake, during practice or while warming up for a match, should be similar to the rate of intake that is desirable and appropriate for play in the same conditions. Furthermore, it is often better to shorten and reduce the intensity of prematch practices and warm-ups when competing in a hot and stressful environment.

During play

Ideally, tennis players should ingest, during play, enough fluid, electrolytes and carbohydrate to fully support all circulatory, metabolic and thermoregulatory requirements, and to offset all fluid losses, so that 'normal' body water status (i.e. euhydration) is maintained. But, even with relatively short matches (e.g. less than 75 min), it is not unusual for some players to end up with a significant body water deficit (i.e. a loss greater than 2% of their prematch bodyweight). In fact, because many tennis players often *begin* matches dehydrated to some degree (Bergeron *et al.* 1995b; Bergeron 1996), a postplay body water deficit may be even worse than is indicated solely by one's pre- and postmatch bodyweight difference. Why do certain players not do a better job at maintaining hydration on the court? One reason is that thirst is not a rapidly responding indicator of body water loss; thus, thirst may not be a sufficient stimulus for maintaining good hydration during exercise (Greenleaf 1992). For some people there could be a fluid deficit of more than 1 litre before thirst is distinctly perceived. Plus, during play, it is a challenge to keep up with high sweating rates (e.g. greater than 1.5 l·h^{-1}). Consequently, it is not always feasible to avoid a body water deficit during play. For example, numerous tennis players often lose sweat at a rate faster than 2 l·h^{-1}. Yet, few of these players would feel comfortable consuming 2 or more litres per hour during a 2-h match. Even if someone did drink that much, it is likely that such a high rate of fluid intake would readily exceed maximal gastric emptying and intestinal absorption rates. Consequently, the player would probably inevitably feel somewhat bloated and uncomfortable. However, many players could do a much better job at keeping up with their on-court fluid losses, even with high sweating rates.

So exactly how much fluid should one consume during play? This primarily depends on the current rate of sweating. Generally, players should drink enough at each changeover to feel comfortably full. Up to 200 ml, or so, during each changeover is a typical upper limit for most adult players. For some, this might seem like too much, and it may very well be too much. On the other hand, players can become accustomed to higher rates of fluid intake. Besides, a larger volume of fluid in the stomach will assist gastric emptying and, thus, fluid delivery.

What should a player drink on the court? Water may be fine for short matches, but, as emphasized in Chapter 5, carbohydrate–electrolyte drinks (i.e. sport drinks) can have several distinct advantages over water alone. Besides providing energy and electrolytes, some carbohydrate–electrolyte drinks may be absorbed a little faster than water. They also tend to increase voluntary fluid intake (Boguslaw & Bar-Or 1996; Wemple *et al.* 1997b). All of these factors are especially important when playing in the heat. For someone who is prone to sweating considerably and getting heat cramps, a little bit of salt (e.g. up to 1.5 g·l^{-1}) can be added to most sport drinks. In addition, if a player drinks much more than 1 l·h^{-1}, a combination of a sport drink and water might be better tolerated and more appropriate than consuming that much sport drink alone. This scenario and rationale are detailed in Chapter 5 (see section on 'Nutrition during play').

Should tennis players continue to wear a wet shirt during play? Changing a sweat-soaked shirt not only feels better, it may help the body to better regulate temperature by reducing the effective vapour barrier against the skin. An insufficient vapour pressure gradient between the skin and air could inhibit evaporative cooling. In other words, leaving a wet shirt on might result in a higher body temperature and a greater fluid loss.

After play

After a match is completed, a tennis player's primary nutritional concern should be the restoration of fluid, electrolytes and carbohydrate. If the match was long and intense, and if there was a large sweat loss, a special emphasis must be made regarding each of these nutrients to ensure that recovery is complete. Particularly if another match must be played on the same day, rehydration and carbohydrate intake should be aggressive and begun immediately (appropriate carbohydrate restoration procedures are presented in Chapter 5). Also, it is very helpful to recover in a cool area (preferably indoors and air-conditioned). If this is not possible, most importantly, players should at least get out of the sun.

While most players probably appreciate the importance of rehydration, very few are likely to realize the actual extent of their own on-court fluid losses that must be replaced. So, how much does a player need to drink after a match? The answer, of course, depends on how much sweating occurred. It is often said that a player should put back exactly what was lost. For example, a 2-kg pre- to postmatch body-weight decrease would then suggest, in this case, that the player should drink two additional litres after play. Would that be enough? Research shows that fluid ingestion after prolonged exercise needs to be greater than the volume of fluid that was lost via sweating, because, during the rehydration process, there is still an obligatory production of urine—whether or not rehydration is complete (Maughan et al. 1997).

What should tennis players drink after a match? Again, generally speaking, if sufficient carbohydrates and electrolytes are provided by food intake, then water alone can serve as a primary or sole postmatch beverage, especially if the next match is not until the following day or later. However, unless adequate sodium and chloride are replaced, rehydration will remain incomplete (Nose et al. 1988; Maughan & Shirreffs 1997). Fortunately, after a long match and extensive sweating, players are typically very thirsty and often develop an enhanced salt appetite, in response to a fluid and sodium deficit. Consuming enough salt, fluids and certain foods, in combination with the body's normal physiological fluid and sodium conservation efforts, helps a player to readily restore and retain much of the lost water and electrolytes that will be required for the next match. Previously described dietary examples of several salt-loading options (e.g. salted sport drinks, tomato juice and other high-sodium foods) can be similarly useful during the postmatch recovery period. Moreover, Chapter 5 describes several aspects of postplay carbohydrate restoration that need to be considered as well when choosing a rehydration beverage. Plain water alone will rehydrate a player to a point, but it

also readily prompts increased urine production and premature elimination of the thirst drive (Nose et al. 1988). Notably, excessive water intake for several hours or more can even lead to severe problems (see section on 'Hyponatraemia', below). Players should also keep in mind that alcohol and caffeine can reduce the rate and amount of postplay plasma volume restoration and net fluid retention (Maughan et al. 1997; Wemple et al. 1997a).

Hyponatraemia

Given the strong emphasis in this chapter on fluid intake and the importance of adequate hydration, the concept of 'water intoxication' or 'overhydration' might seem somewhat inconceivable. Yet, ingesting more water than the body can excrete *is* possible. Following the advice of tournament medical personnel, in response to experiencing heat cramps, nausea and weakness, a 17-year-old, nationally ranked tennis player overzealously ingested water after playing a 4-h match in the heat (>38°C). In his hotel room, this player developed a seizure, slipped into a coma, and spent 2 days in the hospital before he recovered and his serum electrolytes were stabilized. An initial blood chemistry profile revealed a serum sodium level that was well below 120 mmol·l^{-1} (normal range at rest: 136–145 mmol·l^{-1}). He was classified as severely hyponatraemic. Although hyponatraemia *per se* implies only that there is a relative excess of water compared to sodium, this particular tennis player also probably had a sweat-induced sodium deficit from the previous match (M.F. Bergeron, unpublished observations). The precise mechanism underlying hyponatraemia is somewhat unclear, but it seems to be brought on by extensive sweating followed by ingesting low-sodium or sodium-free fluids (e.g. water) at a high rate for several hours or more. This scenario can readily occur in tennis.

So how does a tennis player avoid developing hyponatraemia? First, it is important to recognize several potential predisposing factors. Those with high sweating rates and extensive sweat sodium losses may be at greatest risk. Such players are those most likely to develop a sodium deficit that is fostered by these characteristics in combination with an inappropriately low salt intake. However, excessive drinking of water before, during and after play may be the most important determining factor. To prevent hyponatraemia, adequate salt intake before, during and after play is important (see the recommendations above for examples of appropriate food and sodium-containing fluid selections), particularly when playing multiple, long matches on successive days in the heat.

Compared to marathons, triathlons and other ultra-endurance events, the reported incidence of hyponatraemia in tennis is very low. However, a low reported incidence does not preclude its existence, and the case described above should not be considered unique. Furthermore, the degree of severity covers a wide spectrum. With some mild cases of hyponatraemia, a player might only experience fatigue, apathy, slight nausea and a headache. These symptoms are not uncommon during a hot-weather tournament. Hyponatraemia is a dangerous and potential threat to any tennis player—its seriousness and likelihood should not be underestimated.

Conclusions

Even if a tennis player is well hydrated, physiological function, thermoregulation and physical and mental performance will be challenged during play in the heat. However, many of the more serious performance- and health-related problems associated with playing tennis in the heat can be avoided by (besides not playing in such conditions) maintaining better water and electrolyte balance. The requirements to accomplish this are not difficult to incorporate into most match preparation and during-play routines. In addition, adequate heat acclimatization and cardiorespiratory fitness can further alleviate the thermal and cardiovascular strain imposed by high environmental temperatures. But once again, an improved heat tolerance and the thermoregulatory advantage provided by acclimatization and fitness can be readily offset by a water and sodium deficit. Therefore, it is critical that players, coaches, parents and trainers emphasize a commitment to the hydration recommendations outlined in this chapter and elsewhere (Bergeron *et al.* 1995a; American College of Sports Medicine 1996; Bergeron 1996; Maughan *et al.* 1997), as they do to overall practice and conditioning, so that playing tennis in the heat can be competitive, enjoyable and safe.

References

American College of Sports Medicine (1996) Position stand on exercise and fluid replacement. *Medicine and Science in Sports and Exercise* **28**, i–vii.

Bergeron, M.F. (1996) Heat cramps during tennis: a case report. *International Journal of Sport Nutrition* **6**, 62–68.

Bergeron, M.F., Armstrong, L.E. & Maresh, C.M. (1995a) Fluid and electrolyte losses during tennis in the heat. *Clinics in Sports Medicine* **14**, 23–32.

Bergeron, M.F., Maresh, C.M., Armstrong, L.E. *et al.* (1995b) Fluid–electrolyte balance associated with tennis match play in a hot environment. *International Journal of Sport Nutrition* **5**, 180–193.

Bergeron, M.F., Volpe, S.L. & Gelinas, Y. (1998) Cutaneous calcium losses during exercise in the heat: a regional sweat patch estimation technique. *Clinical Chemistry* **44** (Suppl.), A167.

Boguslaw, W. & Bar-Or, O. (1996) Effect of drink flavor and NaCl on voluntary drinking and hydration in boys exercising in the heat. *Journal of Applied Physiology* **80**, 1112–1117.

Clarkson, P.M. & Haymes, E.M. (1995) Exercise and mineral status of athletes: calcium, magnesium, phosphorus, and iron. *Medicine and Science in Sports and Exercise* **27**, 831–843.

Falk, B. (1998) Effects of thermal stress during rest and exercise in the paediatric population. *Sports Medicine* **25**, 221–240.

Finn, R. (1997) Sampras's 5-setter: 'It's so hot, it's a joke'. *The New York Times*, January 21, B11.

Greenleaf, J.E. (1992) Problem: thirst, drinking behavior, and involuntary dehydration. *Medicine and Science in Sports and Exercise* **24**, 645–656.

Hargreaves, M., Dillo, P., Angus, D. & Febbraio, M. (1996) Effect of fluid ingestion on muscle metabolism during prolonged exercise. *Journal of Applied Physiology* **80**, 363–368.

Maughan, R.J. & Shirreffs, S.M. (1997) Recovery from prolonged exercise: restoration of water and electrolyte balance. *Journal of Sports Sciences* **15**, 297–303.

Maughan, R.J., Leiper, J.B. & Shirreffs, S.M. (1997) Factors influencing the restoration of fluid and electrolyte balance after exercise in the heat. *British Journal of Sports Medicine* **31**, 175–182.

Nose, H., Mack, G.W., Shi, X. & Nadel, E.R. (1988) Role of osmolality and plasma volume during rehydration in humans. *Journal of Applied Physiology* **65**, 325–331.

Pandolf, K.B. (1997) Aging and human heat tolerance. *Experimental Aging Research* **23**, 69–105.

Sawka, M.N. (1992) Physiological consequences of hypohydration: exercise performance and thermoregulation. *Medicine and Science in Sports and Exercise* **24**, 657–670.

Taubes, G. (1998) The (political) science of salt. *Science* **281**, 898–907.

Tipton, K., Green, N.R., Haymes, E.M. & Waller, M. (1993) Zinc loss in sweat of athletes exercising in hot and neutral temperatures. *International Journal of Sport Nutrition* **3**, 261–271.

Wemple, R.D., Lamb, D.R. & McKeever, K.H. (1997a) Caffeine vs caffeine-free sports drinks: effects on urine production at rest and during prolonged exercise. *International Journal of Sports Medicine* **18**, 40–46.

Wemple, R.D., Morocco, T.S. & Mack, G.W. (1997b) Influence of sodium replacement on fluid ingestion following exercise-induced dehydration. *International Journal of Sport Nutrition* **7**, 104–116.

Chapter 7
Medical care of tennis players

Introduction

In this chapter, most common medical ailments will be discussed, including tennis-specific medical problems. There will be specific emphasis on the effects a particular disease may have on a tennis player. For each ailment the cause, incidence and symptoms are described. At the end of every section the preventative and treatment measures for the specific ailment are summarized. The following areas will be discussed:
- Brain and nervous system.
- The eye.
- Heart and blood vessels.
- Respiratory system.
- Digestive system.
- Endocrine system.
- Blood.
- Skin disorders.
- Infectious diseases.
- Overtraining and burnout.
- The female athlete's triad.
- Medical care during tournaments.

Brain and nervous system

Headaches

Headaches are very common in the general population; a headache is the seventh leading presenting complaint for ambulatory care encounters, even though most headache sufferers do not even seek medical care. Headaches can be classified into two main groups: headaches with an organic lesion (e.g. intracranial tumour, viral illness, heatstroke) and headaches with no organic lesion (migrainous and non-migrainous). Tennis players suffer from the same types of headache as the general population. In this

section we discuss the types of headache that are most relevant to tennis players: migraine, tension headache, headache related to neck problems, and benign exertional headache.

Migraine

Migraine is characterized by periodic headaches that are typically localized on one side of the head, often associated with visual disturbances (e.g. loss of vision, flashing lights) and vomiting. The pain is usually severe and throbbing, and may last from a few hours to several days. The attacks occur at intervals ranging from days to several months. The condition is believed to be caused by narrowing of the vessels of the brain, followed by widening of the vessels. It affects 3% of the male and 7% of the female population.

Treatment consists of rest and medication (sumatriptan is the drug of choice in 1998; propranolol, pizotifen and flunarazine may be used prophylactically). Precipitating factors that have been identified are stress, premenstrual changes, alcohol consumption, certain foods or hunger. Tennis players need to identify these triggers in order to gain more control over their migraine.

Tension headache

This is the most common type of headache, with a dull or pressure-like pain in the scalp, temples or back of the head. The pain is localized on both sides of the head and not accompanied by nausea or vomiting. It can be caused by stress, anxiety, poor posture, sudden strain or lack of sleep, possibly resulting in contraction of facial muscles.

Treatment: the pain generally responds well to massage, hot and cold showers, relaxation training and over-the-counter analgesic painkillers.

Neck-related headache

Cervicogenic or neck-related headache is a term used to describe a mechanically provoked headache. The anatomical substrate is formed by the upper three vertebrae of the cervical spine, which are innervated by the nervous roots of C2. Symptoms may be caused by inflammation, degeneration or functional blocking. The pain is usually localized in the back of the head, and may last hours or days, with varying intensity. The headache can be provoked or aggravated by rotation or flexion of the head, sneezing, coughing or straining, and by pressure on the nervous roots of C2. In tennis, the pain may be provoked while extending the neck during serving, worsening as a result of increased muscle tension.

Treatment can consist of massage, heat, analgesics or gentle mobilization techniques.

Benign exertional headache

This has been described as 'headache provoked by any type of exercise'. The headache is sudden in onset, with a rapid peak and decrescendo throbbing pain. This type of headache has been described in both tennis and squash players. The headache is thought to be caused by repeated traction of the brachial plexus, leading to a transitory leakage of cerebrospinal fluid and intracranial hypotension.

Treatment consists of rest.

Seizures

The prevalence of seizure disorders (formerly known as epilepsy) varies in different studies, but is estimated to be 0.5% in Western European countries. Up to 10% of the population suffers a single seizure episode. A seizure occurs when the electrical discharges by the brain cells become disorganized. Three main seizure types can be distinguished: the generalized seizure (grand mal), absence seizures (petit mal) and complex partial seizures (temporal lobe).

The generalized, or tonic–clonic seizure is characterized by a loss of consciousness and falling down, followed by a 15–20-s period of muscle rigidity (tonic phase) and then a 1–2-min period of violent, rhythmic convulsions (clonic phase). The seizure ends with a few minutes of deep, relaxed sleep before consciousness returns. A headache and drowsiness or confusion may be experienced afterwards, with no memory of the seizure. In the absence seizure, there is transient loss of contact with the environment, lasting only seconds, but it may occur as much as 100 times per day. The person does not move during the attack, apart from a fluttering of the eyelids or a twitching of the hand. Full recovery takes only seconds, with no memory of

the incident. Complex partial seizures are preceded by a characteristic sensation (aura) and are followed by physical movements and/or abnormal behaviour.

The incidence of seizures is generally reduced during exercise. However, in susceptible people, seizures may be provoked during tennis, due to fatigue, sleep deprivation (jet lag), hypoglycaemia, hyperthermia, hyperventilation, dehydration or stress. Prevention should be geared towards controlling these factors as much as possible.

Treatment of recurrent seizures consists of antiepileptic medication.

Tinnitus (ringing in the ear)

Phantom auditory perception—tinnitus or ringing in the ear—is a symptom of many pathologies. It is hypothesized that most tinnitus results from the perception of abnormal activity, defined as activity that cannot be induced by any combination of external sounds. It occurs in a surprisingly high proportion: 35% of the general population, and 85% of patients with ear problems.

Treatment: the prospects are rather pessimistic. A full oto-rhino-laryngologic (ear, nose and throat) examination with audiometry (hearing test) should be performed, and if possible, the underlying problem should be treated. For tennis players, it is important to know that high noise levels (air travel), salicylates (painkillers such as aspirin) and quinine (an antimalaria drug) have tinnitus-inducing properties.

The eye

Racket sports can lead to serious eye injury if the ball impacts with the eye. In tennis, the risk is increased by rushing to the net or when playing doubles. A prospective study conducted in Britain in 1989 demonstrated that even though sports accounted for only 2–3% of total eye injuries, they were responsible for 42% of all cases involving hospital admissions. All eye injuries, even those that appear to be minor, require thorough examination, and all serious eye injuries should be referred immediately to an ophthalmologist (eye doctor). The eye and its protective structures are shown in Fig. 7.1(a). The following problems may occur.

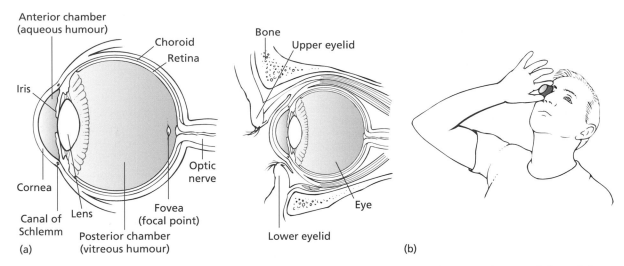

Fig. 7.1 (a) The delicate workings of the eye are protected by the bony structures of the orbit, the eyebrows and the eyelids. (b) To remove a small object from the eye, flush the eye with a small amount of clean water. (From Larson, D.E. (ed.) (1994) *Mayo Clinic Family Health Book*, 2nd edn, pp. 520 and 521. William Morrow and Company, New York.)

Lid lacerations

These can result from contact with the racket head or the tennis ball. Direct trauma to the eyelids can cause heavy bruising.

Treatment: cold compresses in the first 24–48 h. Lacerations of the eyelids require meticulous primary repair by an ophthalmic surgeon.

Corneal erosion

Corneal erosion can result from scratches caused by clay, twigs, the ball, the racket or other foreign bodies. The player complains of pain, sensitivity to light, a foreign body sensation, tearing, squeezing of the eye and blurred vision if the central cornea is involved. Inspection involves simple eversion of the lower lid and double eversion of the upper lid to find any foreign bodies. When a light is shone into the eye, the otherwise smooth corneal surface reveals a sharply circumscribed dull area, which stains green with 2% fluorescein.

Treatment: antibiotic eye drops and padding of the eye in order to prevent friction from movement of the lids.

Conjunctivitis

This can be caused by a foreign body, resulting in irritation of the eye, by a viral infection or by an allergic reaction. Symptoms may include pain, tearing, secretion and itching of the eye. The most common cause of conjunctivitis is a viral infection of the eye. This can result in severe symptoms and may take a long time to heal, but is usually harmless.

Treatment of irritation by a foreign body such as clay, a fly, sand, etc. involves removal of the foreign body by flushing the eye with a small amount of clean water, temporary removal of contact lenses, and treatment as described under corneal erosion if there is damage of the corneal surface (Fig. 7.1b). Allergies can be treated by removal of the allergen, decongestants, cromolyn and antihistamines.

Blood in the fluid of the eye (vitreous liquid)

Blood in the vitreous liquid, the fluid behind the lens, indicates damage to the retina, choroid or ciliary body. Ophthalmoscopic examination reveals a loss of the red reflex and a hazy appearance.

Treatment generally consists of bed rest, but more severe cases may require removal of the blood and vitreous fluids.

Commotio retinae

A commotio retinae can result from a direct blow to the eye by a tennis ball (Fig. 7.2). The contusion injury causes spastic contraction of retinal arteries, leading to poor circulation of a circumscribed retinal area. The player may remain asymptomatic if peripheral areas of the retina are affected, whereas involvement of the central retina will produce blurred vision. On ophthalmoscopic examination, the retina becomes opaque and develops a transient, white–grey colour.

Treatment consists of rest.

Retinal detachment

Retinal detachment may result from a blow or perforation of the globe; it may also result from indirect trauma, such as physical exertion or head and body trauma. Symptoms include flashes of light and visual field loss. Ophthalmoscopic examination may reveal elevation and folding of the detached retina, although the accompanying vitreous haemorrhage sometimes prevents a good view of the fundus.

Treatment: immediate referral is advisable, to determine whether laser therapy or bed rest is indicated.

Orbital injuries

Orbital injuries may result from direct trauma caused by a tennis ball, leading to orbital haemorrhage with bulging of the eye. A blow-out fracture may occur, because portions of the eye socket are paper thin (Fig. 7.2).

Treatment: bed rest and binocular patching. When a blow-out fracture has occurred, prophylactic antibiotics should be given to decrease the incidence of infection as a result of communication between the orbit and paranasal sinuses. Surgery is sometimes necessary to resolve double vision caused by extraocular muscle entrapment and to correct a sunken eye for cosmetic reasons.

Prevention of eye injuries

Experience offers no protection to eye trauma: most eye injuries occur at the highest level of play. Spectacles with hardened glasses do not offer any protection against ocular injuries, because they may shatter on impact. Contact lenses offer no protection either. Hard lenses should never be worn, because the lenses themselves may cause injury; soft lenses are reasonably safe. There are approved eye guards available, made of polycarbonate, which can be used by tennis players (Fig. 7.3). Players with the following eye problems are strongly recommended to wear protection: one functional eye only; severe myopia; Marfan's syndrome; and previous retinal detachment.

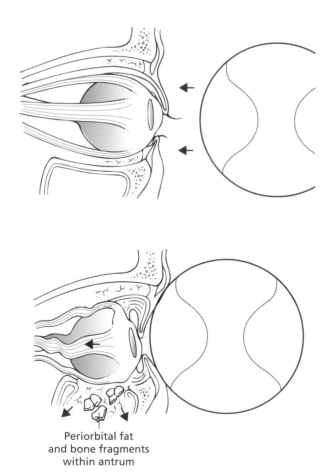

Periorbital fat and bone fragments within antrum

Fig. 7.2 Racket sports can lead to serious eye injury if the ball impacts with the eye. Soft tissues may be forced through the weak bony floor of the orbit into the maxillary sinus. (From Forrest, L.A., Schuller, D.E. & Strauss, R.H. (1989) Management of orbital blow-out fractures. *American Journal of Sports Medicine* **17**, 217–220.)

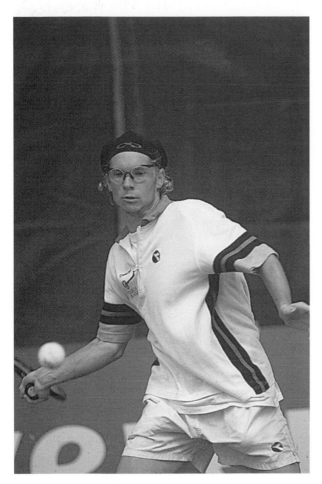

Fig. 7.3 Tennis player wearing safety goggles. The polycarbonate lenses are 2–3 mm thick and mounted in a sturdy frame. Photo © Henk Koster.

Heart and blood vessels

Cardiovascular risks

Tennis is a sport that can be played both as a recreational and as a competitive sport into old age. The International Tennis Federation organizes tournaments and championships for veterans, starting at the age of 35 and going up to 80 years and older (women up to 70 years and older). What are the risks of tennis for the elderly? The main concern with the elderly is the possibility that exercise may precipitate an acute episode of insufficient blood supply to the heart muscle, resulting in a heart attack or sudden cardiac

death. In the older age groups, there is an increased risk of underlying cardiovascular disease.

The prevalence of atherosclerotic heart disease in asymptomatic men in the 30–39 age group is 1.9% (women 0.3%), rising to 12.3% in those aged 60–69 (women 7.5%). Most epidemiological studies have shown that the risk of a heart attack or sudden cardiac death may indeed be increased during and immediately after exercise. However, regular exercise does decrease the risk of sudden cardiac death in the long term. Generally speaking, therefore, tennis players can be encouraged to continue playing into old age.

However, it would be preferable to be able to identify those with underlying cardiovascular diseases, so the necessary precautions can be taken. Exercise testing is often recommended for the over-35s who wish to play competitive tennis. Routine exercise testing in asymptomatic players is not warranted, however, due to the uncertainties associated with positive or negative multistage exercise testing (see 'Sudden cardiac death', below). A thorough clinical assessment, including exercise testing, is only recommended for players with multiple cardiovascular risk factors, premonitory symptoms and those with proven ischaemic heart disease.

Irregular heart beat

Most people experience an occasional skipped heart-beat or minor palpitation. Generally, such an event is not an indication of a problem. Extra heartbeats can be precipitated by triggering factors such as alcohol, chocolate, certain spices, tobacco or caffeine-containing foods and beverages. In those cases, the use of these substances should be avoided. Players may worry that palpitations or irregular heartbeats are caused by excessive stress on the cardiovascular system, caused by exercise. However, it has been shown that the prevalence of atrial and ventricular ectopia in athletes is no higher than in untrained normal individuals, which means that playing competitive tennis does not lead to excessive strain of the heart.

This does not mean that all rhythm disturbances in tennis players are innocent. Tennis players can suffer from the same diseases as the general population, and if the discomfort is severe or the problem recurs, a cardiologist should be consulted. The diagnosis is generally made using 24-h electrocardiographic (Holter) monitoring and/or stress testing. Echocardiography, angiography or electrophysiological testing may also be helpful.

Treatment consists of explanation of the benign nature and the avoidance of triggering factors.

Syncope (loss of consciousness)

Syncope is a sudden, transient loss of consciousness. Syncopal episodes are usually benign, but some causes can be life threatening. Seventy-five per cent of all syncopal episodes result from a vasovagal reaction, with venous dilatation, hypotension, and bradycardia. Such events typically occur in ballboys or girls, who have to stand still in the sun after sudden bursts of activity. It may follow a prodrome of light-headedness, dizziness, profuse sweating, and nausea. Vigorous tennis in hot, humid weather may lead to syncope due to fluid losses caused by excessive sweating. Players recovering from gastroenteritis with associated vomiting and diarrhoea are at increased risk.

Treatment of a vasovagal episode consists of rest, cooling and rehydration.

Syncope due to rhythm disturbances is much less common, and can be difficult to diagnose. Patients suffering from syncope who present without an obvious aetiology need an extensive examination with a complete history, physical examination and careful diagnostic tests to reveal potentially serious underlying heart disease.

High blood pressure

High blood pressure or hypertension is diagnosed when blood pressure is consistently 160/90 mmHg or higher. Specific diseases or health problems, such as the use of oral contraceptives, aortic coarctation, renal artery stenosis or adrenal gland problems (secondary hypertension), are identified in fewer than 5% of cases. If no specific cause can be identified, the high blood pressure is categorized as essential hypertension. High blood pressure is generally without symptoms, but may lead to long-term complications, as a result of accelerated athero-sclerosis, stroke, kidney failure, myocardial infarction and peripheral artery disease.

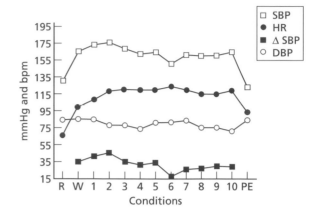

Fig. 7.4 Blood pressure and heart rate responses to tennis. (From Jetté, M., Landry, F., Tiemann, B. & Blumchen, G. (1991) Ambulatory blood pressure and Holter monitoring during tennis play. *Canadian Journal of Sport Sciences* **16**, 40–44.)

Generally, there is no objection against playing tennis with mild hypertension. A game of tennis leads to an increase in systolic blood pressure and a mild decrease in diastolic blood pressure. In a study of 21 middle-aged and older men (Jetté *et al.* 1991; see Fig. 7.4), an average increase of blood pressure was found from 130/90 mmHg at rest to 170/80 mmHg during singles play, with a heart rate ranging from 140 to 180 bpm (average 160 bpm). This is not considered to be in the danger zones. In addition, the game of tennis has been shown to have a mild lowering effect on blood pressure in the long run, comparable to aerobic exercise such as running or cycling. Therefore, tennis is generally considered beneficial to people with mild to moderate hypertension.

Treatment of hypertension includes medication (diuretics, β-adrenergic blockers, calcium-channel blockers and angiotensin-converting enzyme inhibitors), in addition to lifestyle changes such as weight loss, dietary changes and exercise.

Inflammation of the heart muscle (myocarditis)

Inflammation of the heart muscle usually occurs as a complication during or after various infectious diseases (rheumatic fever, coxsackie virus, influenza), exposure to certain chemicals or drugs. The diagnosis is made by electrocardiography, radiographic examination and heart muscle tissue examination (biopsy). In most cases, the inflammation clears and the patient is restored to good health.

Therapy consists of avoiding vigorous exercise until heart activity has returned to normal.

Heart attack

A heart attack occurs when a blood clot blocks the flow in one or more of the coronary arteries (Fig. 7.5). The result is that the heart muscle in the affected region dies. Patients who have recovered after a heart attack require careful screening in order to assess the risks and potential benefits of sport. Sport can be indicated in patients who have healed well and are rehabilitated from an acute episode, asymptomatic, in good muscular form and in stable condition. Tennis is contraindicated when symptoms or signs of clinical instability or abnormal results of laboratory investigations are found. Bulging of the heart chamber or diffuse alterations of the contraction pattern of the heart also contraindicate sport.

A stress test should be obtained, to determine the maximal heart rate that can be attained and to verify if there is no additional coronary insufficiency or electrical instability (ventricular tachycardia).

Treatment: as a general rule, maximal heart rate during play should not initially exceed 90% of the maximum heart rate attained during exercise ECG, or

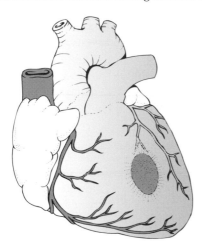

Fig. 7.5 A myocardial infarction or heart attack occurs when a blood clot blocks the flow in one or more coronary arteries, resulting in an area of damaged tissue. (From Netter, F.H. (1978) The heart. In: Yonkman, F.Y., ed. *The Ciba Collection of Medical Illustrations*, Vol. 5. CIBA, New York.)

80% of the maximum oxygen uptake. It is therefore preferable to start playing doubles rather than singles, because the average heart rate obtained during doubles play is lower than during singles play. There should be a gradual and progressive increase in the length and intensity of play. In most cases, unrestricted play is allowed after a couple of months if there are no complications.

Percutaneous coronary intervention (PCI)

Balloon dilatation of a coronary artery is indicated in cases of severe coronary stenosis (> 70% of the luminal diameter). If balloon dilatation is insufficient, additional stent implantation may be performed. After this procedure, which is performed through puncture of the great artery in the groin (usually the right), a 2-week period of rest is warranted to allow healing of the puncture site.

Treatment: after a successful PCI, tennis play is allowed without restrictions.

Coronary bypass surgery

Recommendations on tennis after coronary bypass surgery are similar to those for a heart attack. All non-invasive investigations like stress tests and echocardiography must be performed before sports activities begin. Healing of the sternum must be complete before resumption of play (6–12 weeks).

Treatment: there should be a gradual increase in intensity and length of play. Again, doubles play is initially preferred over singles play.

'Athlete's heart'

'Athlete's heart' is the term used to describe the adaptations of the heart associated with long-term physical training. It is a physiological (healthy) adaptation of the heart, characterized by a low resting heart rate, a soft systolic murmur, a variety of non-specific ECG abnormalities and an increased left ventricular mass. In contrast to the pathologically enlarged heart due to cardiac diseases such as diseases of the heart muscle (cardiomyopathy), valve disease or high blood pressure, an athlete's heart is not associated with an increased risk of cardiovascular morbidity or sudden cardiac death.

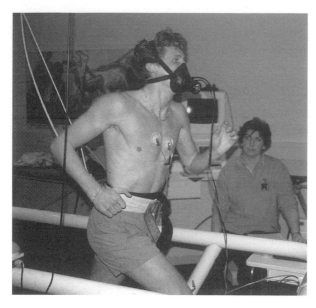

Fig. 7.6 Treadmill running is a reliable way to determine maximum oxygen consumption in tennis players.

In the past, tennis was generally considered a technical and tactical type of sport with relatively low cardiovascular demands. However, modern tennis has evolved into a sport with high physical demands, reflected by powerful strokes, fast rallies and long hours of play. It is therefore not surprising that most professional tennis players develop an athlete's heart. Other reflections of the increased physical demands of modern tennis are the increased maximum oxygen uptake found in top players: the average maximum oxygen uptake of the German Davis Cup Team increased from 54.6 ml·kg^{-1}·min^{-1} in 1982 to 63 ml·kg^{-1}·min^{-1} in 1991.

Sudden cardiac death

Sudden cardiac death in the young age group (under 35) is primarily due to structural cardiac disease that is congenital in nature. Examples are hypertrophic cardiomyopathy (thickened heart muscle due to disease), right ventricular dysplasia, long QT syndrome and Wolff–Parkinson–White syndrome. Therefore, the ATP Tour installed mandatory stress testing and echocardiographic screening as a preventive measure for sudden cardiac death for all ATP Tour players in 1996. No players were

excluded from competition as a result of screening (Fig. 7.6).

The most prevalent diagnosis in athletes over 35 who die suddenly is ischaemic heart disease. Identification of cardiac risk factors should be undertaken in all tennis players over age 35. These include personal and family history of coronary artery disease, smoking history, high cholesterol levels, inactivity, high blood pressure, and a history of diabetes and obesity. A thorough clinical assessment, including exercise testing, is recommended for players with multiple cardiovascular risk factors and/or premonitory symptoms.

Respiratory system

Nosebleeds

A nosebleed can be caused by a hard impact with the nose, such as a blow from a tennis racket or ball, but may also occur as a result of the common cold, sinus infection, allergy, dry air, hypertension or for no apparent reason. Most nosebleeds arise from the nasal septum, which contains many fragile blood vessels.

Treatment: nosebleeds can be stopped by first blowing the nose to remove all blood clots, and then pinching the nose with the index finger and thumb for 5–10 min with the player sitting upright. If necessary, a nasal tampon can be applied. Cold compression is not really helpful because the cold does not penetrate deep enough to reach the vessels on the septum. If bleeding continues, cotton wool soaked in adrenaline (epinephrine) 1 : 1000 should be applied to the nasal septum. If the bleeding still persists, chemical or electric cauterization may be applied to the bleeding site.

Rhinitis

Allergic rhinitis, either seasonal or perennial, can cause problems with nasal function depending upon the type and quantity of allergen exposure. Rhinitis may also be caused by other factors, such as infection, circulatory instability, nasal polyposis or medication.

Treatment: in allergic individuals, antihistamines may be appropriate. Topical spraying with nasal cromolyn may be useful to prevent reactions to inhalant allergens. In athletes with pollen, mould, dust and dander allergies, immunotherapy should be considered if the nasal symptoms are significant and cannot be controlled by environmental measures or acceptable drug therapy. Both topical and systemic decongestants are approved in the anti-doping regulations for tennis players (see also Chapter 21). Drugs that reduce congestion by vasoconstriction of the mucosa should not be used longer than 1 week, because long-term use causes development of rebound nasal congestion. Short-term use of nasal topical steroids may be helpful in athletes with vasomotor rhinitis and perennial rhinitis.

Sinusitis

Chronic sinusitis is one of the most prevalent chronic conditions in both athletes and non-athletes. Most commonly, the maxillary sinus is affected (Fig. 7.7). Infection, allergies and vasomotor rhinitis/sinusitis are the usual causes. Approximately 50% of infections are due to *Haemophilus influenzae* or *Streptococcus pneumoniae*. Specific factors that may predispose tennis players to this condition include traumatic injury of the eardrums and sinuses due to the sudden changes in air pressure when travelling by aeroplane. Clinical features of acute sinusitis include facial pain, headache, toothache, pain when tapping on the sinus, postnasal drip, cough, rhinorrhoea, nasal obstruction, a fever and nose bleeds. Chronic sinusitis may be more subtle in its presentation, with symptoms such as vague facial pain, postnasal drip, cough, nasal obstruction, dental pain, malaise and a mouth odour. The diagnosis is confirmed by the presence of a purulent nasal discharge for at least 3 weeks. Findings that may be seen on a plain radiograph include the presence of a fluid level and/or opacification of a sinus. Computed tomographic scanning may be helpful when radiological findings are unclear.

Treatment should start with nasal steam inhalation, followed by intranasal corticosteroids and/or brief courses of local decongestants. If this is not helpful, systemic therapy, including decongestants, anti-inflammatory agents, antibiotics and antihistamines (in case of nasal allergy) should be applied. As a last resort, the establishment of sinus drainage through the release of obstruction and the stimulation of mucus flow can be performed. The antibiotic of first choice is amoxycillin (amoxicillin), either alone or in combination with clavulanic acid. Penicillin-allergic patients should use cefaclor, cotrimoxazole or doxycycline.

Viral upper respiratory tract infection

In 1994/95, upper respiratory tract infections were responsible for 8% of the on-site withdrawals in the ATP Tour. Three or four colds per year per person is typical. Acute respiratory illnesses can be caused by more than 200 different viral strains, but most often the rhino-, corona- or enteroviruses are responsible. Most colds primarily affect the nose and throat, although the same viruses can cause bronchitis and laryngitis. More serious bacterial infections of the throat, ears and lungs can follow a viral cold.

Colds are spread by direct contact with infected secretions (shaking hands, kissing) or indirect inhalation of the virus in the air. Contrary to common belief, exposure to cold temperatures, damp environments or draughts does not seem to enhance vulnerability. Either a single bout of exhausting exercise or persistent over-training or stress can increase the susceptibility to and severity of upper respiratory and other viral infections, although resistance to bacterial infections is apparently unaltered. This is because strenuous exercise has a depressant effect on the immune system, which may persist for a week or more.

Symptoms of a viral upper respiratory tract infection can range from a runny nose, sneezing and congestion to sore throat, hoarseness and a non-productive cough. Patients often feel weak and occasionally have sore muscles, despite little or low-grade fever. Infections

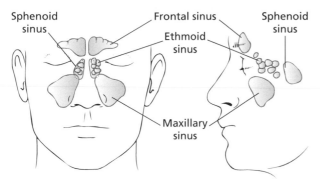

Fig. 7.7 The sinuses. (From Larson, D.E. (ed.) (1994) *Mayo Clinic Family Health Book*, 2nd edn, p. 591. William Morrow and Company, New York.)

may greatly affect performance. Exercise during the prodromal and early acute phase of some infections may worsen or prolong the illness. Therefore if signs and symptoms indicate that viral infection is impending, the player should greatly reduce volume and intensity of heavy training for 1–2 days.

Treatment: because a cold is caused by a virus, antibiotics are not helpful. A cold usually lasts 3–4 days but can persist up to 10–14 days. Non-prescription cold remedies, decongestants, cough syrups, cough drops and gargling with warm salty water may help to relieve some of the symptoms. Coxsackie virus infection can produce symptoms of the common cold but may also invade heart muscle and produce inflammation of the heart muscle. This is a potentially serious disease with an increased risk of acute arrhythmia's leading to sudden death during exercise.

It is therefore advisable to abstain from tennis with a temperature of over 38°C!

Exercise-induced asthma

Exercise-induced asthma is a particular manifestation of asthma characterized by a variable degree of bronchoconstriction minutes after strenuous exercise. It is the most common pulmonary syndrome seen in young athletes, with a 10–15% incidence in competitive athletes. In the 1984 Summer Olympic Games in Los Angeles, 67 of 597 (11.2%) participants were affected. Groups at high risk are those with asthma (70–80%) and allergic rhinitis (40%). Classic symptoms are wheezing, chest tightness and/or shortness of breath during exercise, with a cough in the post-exercise period. Maximal air flow obstruction typically occurs 5–15 min after cessation of exercise, with spontaneous remission within 20–60 min. There is usually a refractory period with symptom-free exercise 2–4 h after the episode of bronchospasm. Some athletes have a secondary delayed-phase obstructive period 4–10 h after initial bronchospasm, typically manifested as night-time coughing.

The strongest trigger for an attack is cold, dry air. The rapid breathing during exercise tends to cool and dry the bronchial tubes, resulting in hyperirritable bronchial systems. Exercise-induced bronchospasm can be diagnosed by demonstrating a decrease in pulmonary function (forced expiratory volume at 1 s or peak expiratory flow rate) after exercise. This can be done by using an exercise challenge test, consisting of 6–8 min of strenuous treadmill running and spirometric measurements at 3-min intervals for at least 15 min after exercise.

Treatment: certain measures may help to prevent or minimize exercise-induced bronchospasm, such as avoiding exercise in cold, dry environments or wearing a scarf or face mask when having to do so. Breathing through the nose also helps. A gradual, prolonged warm-up period before the event should be performed. Conditioning may reduce the severity of attacks, and interval training is a good way to build up stamina, as this type of training has been shown to provoke fewer attacks. Smog increases the risks of bronchospasms, and because smog is usually worse in the afternoon and early evening, players with a tendency to exercise-induced asthma may wish to avoid practising or competing at those times.

The majority of players can be successfully managed by using antiasthmatic drugs. Most clinicians would start with a selective β_2 agonist such as salbutamol or albuterol used 5–10 min pre-exercise. This usually provides effective prophylaxis against the development of exercise-induced bronchospasm (Fig. 7.8).

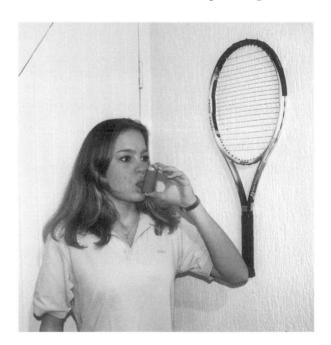

Fig. 7.8 The use of an inhaler 5–10 min before play usually provides effective prophylaxis against the development of exercise-induced bronchospasm.

If the patient becomes wheezy later in the exercise session, the dose can be repeated.

Alternatives to therapy include cromoglycate or inhaled steroids and/or theophylline. Regular medication helps diminish lung hyperactivity, reducing the risks of asthmatic attacks. The medications mentioned above are not prohibited by the anti-doping programme; β_2 agonists used in aerosol form are allowed, and inhaled or oral corticosteroids are allowed if prescribed by physician. For further details, see Chapter 21.

Digestive system

Viral gastroenteritis

Gastrointestinal problems were responsible for 13.5% of the on-site withdrawals in the ATP Tour in 1994/95. Viral gastroenteritis is commonly transmitted through the oral–faecal route, and possibly by respiratory transmission. Hand washing is a key to prevention. The symptoms consists of diarrhoea, nausea and vomiting, along with fever, abdominal cramps and muscle pains.

Treatment: although the course of gastroenteritis is normally self-limited, fluid replacement during the illness is essential. Clear fluids, especially those containing electrolytes (oral rehydration salts) are suggested, along with caffeine-free soft drinks, fruit juices, broths and bouillon. Antimotility drugs such as loperamide (Imodium) can be effective in reducing abdominal cramps and diarrhoea, but must be used with caution because they can prolong the gastrointestinal infection. The athlete may return to play as soon as the physical symptoms, such as diarrhoea, have resolved and he or she is well rehydrated.

Food poisoning

This is caused by the ingestion of contaminated food, most commonly the toxin of the *Staphylococcus* bacterium. Dairy products and meats are frequently contaminated, often through the hands of a food handler. Outbreaks may occur during warm weather, when the bacterium multiplies rapidly in foods outside the refrigerator. Symptoms are vomiting and diarrhoea 1 or 2 h after the food is ingested. Discomfort usually subsides after a few hours.

Treatment is not necessary except for rehydration of the player. Antimotility drugs are not recommended, because they may prolong or worsen the illness.

Traveller's diarrhoea

Athletes going to Latin America, Africa, the Middle East and Asia are at highest risk of traveller's diarrhoea. Symptoms usually begin during the first week of a stay and last 48–72 h, although peak physical performance may not be regained for a week or more. *Escherichia coli* accounts for approximately 50% of the cases, but *Salmonella*, *Shigella*, *Giardia lamblia* and rotavirus can also produce the illness, which is passed on through the oral–faecal route. Symptoms include diarrhoea, cramps, nausea and malaise.

Treatment: for preventive purposes, tap water and iced beverages should be avoided, as well as food from street vendors, fresh leafy greens and fruits that cannot be peeled before eating. The most important treatment once again is rehydration. In the absence of fever or bloody stools, loperamide can be used to help control the diarrhoea, in a dosage of 4 mg initially followed by 2 mg after each unformed stool. Patients with moderate to severe traveller's diarrhoea can be treated with a combination of 160 mg trimethoprim and 800 mg methoxazole twice a day for 3 days, with ciprofloxacine 500 mg twice a day for 3 days, or with doxycycline 100 mg twice a day for 3 days.

Heartburn

Heartburn is a deeply placed burning retrosternal pain caused by reflux oesophagitis. This is a common complaint among athletes. The increased incidence of upper gastrointestinal symptoms with exercise may be caused by the delay in emptying gastric contents from the stomach. Increased stomach content may increase the athlete's susceptibility to gastro-oesophageal reflux as well as the likelihood of nausea and vomiting.

Treatment: players suffering form heartburn should eat a small pre-exercise meal that is high in carbohydrate and low in fat, because fatty foods tend to delay gastric emptying and promote reflux. Most tennis players are able to eat solid foods, such as bananas, oranges or sandwiches during the course of a match. If this causes problems, however, sports drinks should be used instead. If additional measures are required, the use of antacids or H_2-receptor antagonists such as cimetidine may reduce the incidence of heartburn and upper abdominal pain associated with exercise.

Stitch in the side

Many athletes complain of a sharp, colicky pain in the left or the right upper quadrant of the abdomen during strenuous exercise. This is commonly referred to as a 'stitch'. The exact cause is unknown, but it may be due to muscle spasm of the diaphragm or trapping of gas in the hepatic or splenic flexure of the colon.

Treatment: avoidance of a solid meal prior to exercise, drinking small quantities of liquid, or reducing the intensity of training may be helpful.

Irritable bowel syndrome

The irritable bowel syndrome, also known as spastic colon or nervous diarrhoea, is one of the commonest gastrointestinal disorders, causing lower abdominal pain and constipation or diarrhoea. Other symptoms include abdominal distension and rumbling of the stomach. It is a dysfunction of the large intestine, for which no organic cause can be found. Attacks may be induced by anxiety or stress.

Treatment: the most important aspect involves explaining the physiological basis of the symptoms. The player should be encouraged to increase fibre levels in his or her diet. High-fibre foods include wholegrain products, fruits, vegetables and legumes. In addition, hydrophilic colloids (metamucil) may be prescribed. Pain and diarrhoea can be relieved by an anticholinergic drug such as mebeverine (duspatal).

Endocrine system

Diabetes mellitus

Diabetes mellitus is a clinical syndrome characterized by hyperglycaemia, due to deficiency or diminished effectiveness of insulin. The disease is chronic and affects the metabolism of carbohydrate, protein, fat, water and electrolytes. In insulin-dependent diabetes mellitus (IDDM), most common in those aged below 30, the body fails to produce the hormone insulin. In non-insulin-dependent diabetes mellitus (NIDDM), occurring mainly in the middle-aged and elderly, there is a depressed sensitivity to insulin at the cellular level. Patients with IDDM must receive exogenous insulin (Fig. 7.9). NIDDM (90% of diabetics) is usually managed by diet and/or tablets, but approximately 20% of individuals may require exogenous insulin.

Treatment: tennis players suffering from diabetes should be encouraged to monitor their blood glucose level before, during and after exercise to learn their own response pattern. Control of blood glucose can then be achieved by adjusting carbohydrate intake and insulin dosages. Athletes with IDDM need to be flexible and are recommended to use a short-acting insulin before every meal, supplemented with a long-acting insulin to cover the night-time period. The dose can be adjusted, depending on the length and intensity of exercise. Moderate exercise of less than 30 min (1 set of tennis) rarely requires any insulin adjustment, although a small snack just prior to exercise may be needed, especially if the blood glucose level is less than 5 mmol·l^{-1}. If short-acting insulin is used, the dose may need to be reduced if exercise lasts more than 45–60 min.

An approximately 20% reduction in the short-acting component is usually enough for a prolonged exercise session, although a decrease in total daily insulin dose may ultimately be required. The patient with IDDM is at greatest risk of developing dangerously low blood sugar levels 6–14 h after strenuous exercise (nocturnal hypoglycaemia); this can be avoided by adjusting insulin and caloric intake after strenuous exercise.

Athletes with NIDDM and diet therapy alone do not usually need to make any adjustments for exercise. However, they are also advised to carry some glucose with them.

• *Benefits of exercise*: exercise in NIDDM may constitute an important component of treatment because of the beneficial effects on increasing insulin sensitivity and the rare occurrences of hypoglycaemia. In IDDM, exercise does not improve glycaemic control. However, in both IDDM and NIDDM, exercise does lead to other long-term positive changes, such as a reduction in blood pressure, lowering of body fat, increased fitness level and an improved serum lipid profile.

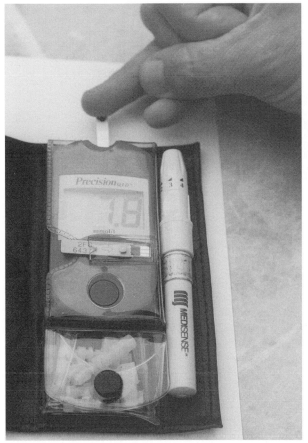

(a)

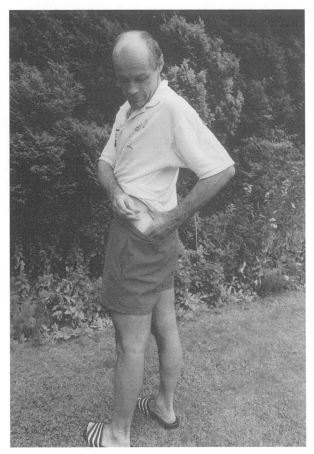

(b)

Fig. 7.9 Self-administration of insulin. (a) Apparatus; (b) technique.

• *Risks of exercise*: low blood sugar level is the major problem for athletes with IDDM. Symptoms include sweating, nervousness, tremor and hunger. If the low blood sugar level is not corrected, confusion, abnormal behaviour, loss of consciousness and convulsions may occur. At the first indication of a low blood sugar level, the athlete should ingest carbohydrate in solid or liquid form. A semiconscious or unconscious diabetic patient requires intravenous glucose administration. Athletes should be alerted to the possibility of delayed exercise-induced low blood sugar levels several hours after completion of exercise. Exercise may cause diabetic ketoacidosis when diabetes is poorly controlled, with insulin deficiency at the beginning of exercise.

Long-term complications of diabetes include ischaemic heart disease, damage to the retina, damage to the nerves, and peripheral vascular disease. A full examination is therefore advisable before starting any exercise programme or an increase in the intensity of exercise, paying particular attention to the cardio-vascular system, the feet and the eyes. For those over 35 years of age or those with 15 years of diabetes, an exercise ECG should be considered, as diabetics are vulnerable to 'silent ischaemia'.

Blood

Anaemia

Sports anaemia is the term used to describe both dilutional pseudo-anaemia and the true anaemia of athletes, in which haemoglobin is diminished. Dilutional pseudo-anaemia is a beneficial adaptation to endurance training, due to the expansion of the plasma volume. The haemoglobin and haematocrit levels seem to be decreased, but in reality there is an increase in the absolute amount of circulating haemoglobin. The most common cause of true anaemia is iron deficiency, because without enough iron the body cannot produce enough haemoglobin. There are several primary causes of the deficiency, including insufficient consumption of iron-containing foods, poor iron absorption in the intestines, loss of blood (menstruation) and excessive transpiration (iron bound to transferrin).

The symptoms of anaemia tend to appear so gradually that they often go unnoticed, but their severity increases as the condition progresses. The player may feel tired and less tolerant of exercise. The skin, gums, nail beds and eyelid linings may be pale. Eventually, anaemia may become so severe that the heartbeat seems more rapid and noticeable. Various blood tests can be used to diagnose iron-deficiency anaemia, including measurement of haemoglobin, haematocrit and serum ferritin values. Other types of anaemia, such as folate deficiency, B_{12} deficiency and anaemia secondary to chronic diseases, should be ruled out.

Treatment: an important measure to prevent iron-deficiency anaemia that is not due to disease is adequate nutrition. Foods rich in iron include meats (especially liver), fish, poultry, eggs, legumes (peas and beans), potatoes and rice. The iron in many vegetables is poorly absorbed. The body's absorption of iron can be enhanced by drinking citrus juice when taking a supplement or eating iron-rich food. Milk, tea and coffee decrease iron absorption. Players with low serum ferritin levels (<20 ng·ml^{-1}) may be treated with oral iron supplementation (ferrous sulphate or ferrous gluconate).

Skin disorders

Blisters

Blisters can develop at any site of prolonged friction, causing fluid to accumulate between the layers of the skin. Preventive measures are to wear clean, well-fitting socks and shoes. If a particular toe or foot area is prone to increased shoe contact, it should be covered with adhesive tape. This barrier between the skin and the irritant prevents friction and thus blistering. Blister formation is treated with a horseshoe-shaped felt or a skin-care pad (second skin).

Treatment: to avoid inflammation, blisters should not be punctured unless they are so painful that the player cannot run or hold a racket. After disinfecting the area, the blister should be punctured at several points along the base with a sterile needle, leaving the overlying skin intact. It can then be covered with a gauze pad or second skin.

Bunion

When hallux valgus is present (abducted hallux and adducted metatarsal), a bony protrusion—a bunion—may develop at the outside of the first metatarsophalangeal joint. The bunion is often subjected to constant rubbing, resulting in an overlying bursitis.

Treatment consists of padding, appropriate foot-wear both on and off the court (no narrow shoes with high heels!) and correction of excessive pronation with orthotics. Surgery is occasionally indicated.

Corns (clavi)

A corn is a circumscribed, conical hyperkeratotic thickening of the skin with the apex pointing inwards. Corns are smaller (3–10 mm) than calluses. These lesions often develop over the skin covering the distal head of the metatarsals.

Treatment: a corn can be treated with silver nitrate solution or a salicylic acid plaster. Soaking the area with warm water before rubbing helps to soften it. Improperly fitting shoes are a common cause.

Calluses

Callus is a diffuse thickening of the skin over bony protrusions, where there is increased pressure and repeated friction. It usually forms under the central part of the heel and under the second and third meta-tarsal heads. In athletes who continually press down along the medial aspect of the foot (pronated feet), callus will also occur beneath the first metatarsal head (Fig. 7.10). Callus is a protective response of the skin to increased pressure or irritation over a long period of time.

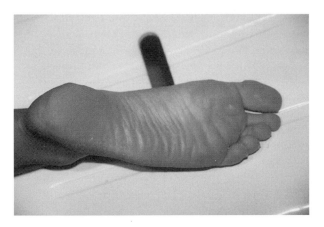

Fig. 7.10 Excessive callus formation under the forefoot.

Treatment: if calluses are painful, they should be reduced in size by rubbing with pumice stone, sandstone, a callus file or sandpaper, after soaking the thickened area in warm water. Cushioned pads are helpful to reduce pain and pressure.

Tennis toe

This can occur as a result of 'starting and stopping' in tennis, leading to repetitive trauma of the toe against the front side of the shoe and bleeding under the toenails. It usually affects the hallux or second toe, whichever is longer. Pain may be experienced due to the increased pressure under the toe, but is not always present. The nail may turn blue or, in cases of repetitive trauma, black.

Treatment: in cases of severe pain, drilling a hole in the nail with a heated needle or paper clip, enabling the blood to escape, can relieve pressure. Properly fitting shoes and socks, tight lacing and retying of shoes, as well as trimming the toe nails short, are all beneficial preventive measures.

Ingrown toenail

An ingrown toenail is usually the result of poor nail cutting (round instead of straight). Patients often present in acute pain with tenderness on gentle palpation.

Treatment: when no infection is found, a small piece of cotton can be placed under the edge of the nail to encourage it to grow past the skin. If the nail is infected, with redness and swelling of the perionychium, treatment with soaks and antibiotic therapy for 5–7 days is recommended. Resection of the outer aspect of the nail may be performed to prevent the nail border injuring the soft tissue. To prevent recurrence of the problem, shoes with tight toe boxes should be avoided and the nail should be cut straight across.

Excessive sweating

Excessive sweating in the palms of the hands can be a problem for tennis players, particularly on hot, humid days. The racket grip becomes slippery and the player starts to lose grip.

Treatment consists of topical application of aluminium chloride solution, or drying the hands with sawdust or magnesium oxide before serving.

Insect stings

Insect stings such as ant, bee and wasp stings are common, painful, but rarely deadly. Each year, 10% of the population are stung by bees and wasps.

Treatment: remnants of insect parts, such as the sting, should be removed as quickly as possible. The sting continues to inject venom, and the faster the removal, the lower the dose of venom received. Suction devices are available that are thought to keep envenomation to the minimum. Local reactions can be treated by cold compresses and analgesics. Oral antihistamines decrease the oedema and pruritus that may accompany stings.

Rarely, an anaphylactic reaction may occur, leading to major systemic reactions such as upper airway obstruction, severe bronchospasm, central cyanosis and a marked fall in blood pressure with syncope (anaphylactic shock).

Treatment: the immediate treatment goal is to maintain an adequate airway and support the blood pressure. Intramuscular adrenaline (epinephrine) should be given quickly. The standard dose is 0.03–0.05 ml·kg^{-1} of a 1 : 1000 solution (0.01–0.15 ml·kg^{-1} in children). This dose can be repeated at 5- to 10-min intervals according to the response. In addition, supplementary oxygen and intravenous fluids should be administered. Antihistamines and corticosteroids are useful as second-line therapy. Because stinging

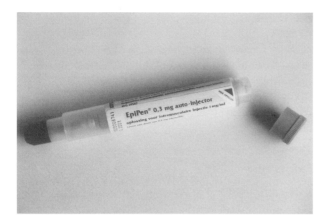

Fig. 7.11 The Epi-Pen auto-injector.

insects cannot be consistently avoided, venom im-munotherapy offers an effective means of preventing life-threatening reactions. All players at risk should be given a prescription for an emergency adrenaline (epinephrine) syringe (Fig. 7.11).

Sun-related disorders

During the outdoor season, tennis players are unable to avoid regular sun exposure. Prolonged exposure to sunlight can produce acute reactions in the epidermis (sunburn) and more serious long-term damage to the dermis.

Sunburn is induced mainly by ultraviolet B (UVB, 290–320 nm). Players most likely to develop sunburn are those with fair skin, who tan minimally. A tan has a protective effect against UVB exposure by acting as a neutral density filter, absorbing and scattering ultraviolet radiation and probably by trapping free radicals. The clinical manifestations of sunburn include erythema, heat, oedema and vesicle formation.

Treatment: cool compresses of tap water will help to relieve the pain and heat of sunburn.

Prevention: if prolonged exposure is anticipated, a sunscreen with a skin protection factor of 15 or more is recommended. This is particularly important during hours when the sun is strongest (2 h before or after noon), or in regions where the ozone layer is thin. Sunscreen products that do not have an oil or gel base will minimize any decrease in the evaporation

of sweat from the skin surface. Sun-blocking agents such as zinc oxide or titanium dioxide provide good protection for vulnerable areas such as the nose, lips or helix of the ear.

The potentially harmful long-term effects of sun exposure include premature ageing of the skin and skin cancer. UVA was once considered to be fairly innocuous because it causes 1000-fold less burning than UVB. However, UVA penetrates far more deeply. Sunlight contains 500–1000 times as much UVA as UVB, and UVA is thought to be largely responsible for the ageing effect of sunlight, leading to looseness, wrinkling, loss of elasticity and atrophy of the skin. In addition, growing clinical, experimental and epidemiological data link ultraviolet radiation to skin cancer, in particular basal cell carcinoma and squamous cell carcinoma. The evidence linking melanoma with sun exposure is not as strong. Sun-sensitive players should be aware of these risks and use sunscreens that are effective in both the UVB and the UVA range.

Infectious diseases

Infectious mononucleosis

Infectious mononucleosis (glandular fever) occurs as a result of infection with the Epstein–Barr virus. The incidence is highest in the 15–30 age group. It is believed to be spread by infectious saliva (which is why it is known as 'kissing disease'). The incubation period varies with age: from 7 to 14 days in children and adolescents to as long as 30–50 days in adults. Symptoms include fatigue, fever, sore throat, headache and nausea. Clinical examination may reveal a throat infection, swollen lymph nodes and enlargement of the spleen.

The illness lasts between 5 and 15 days, but it may take several months before the fatigue and weakness completely disappear.

Treatment: management of a player with infectious mononucleosis involves rest from sporting activity until all acute symptoms have disappeared. If the liver is involved (hepatitis), a low-fat diet should be prescribed. Training is allowed as soon as blood tests show improved liver function. Training should be resumed gradually, first increasing duration and then intensity, with adequate periods of rest.

Folliculitis

Folliculitis may occur after a vigorous massage as a result of a staphylococcal infection, especially when insufficient lubricants are used, or after leg shaving. Symptoms are a pustular rash, sometimes accompanied by a low-grade fever, generalized malaise and headache.

Treatment: the rash is usually self-limiting and disappears in 1 to 2 weeks. In serious cases antibiotics may be prescribed.

Athlete's foot

Fungal skin infections are very common among tennis players, because the fungi thrive in the warm, moist and dark conditions in tennis shoes. The symptoms of athlete's foot (tinea pedis) are irritation and itching between the toes, sometimes accompanied by cracking and peeling of the skin. The term onychomycosis is used when the fungus infection has spread to the nails (Fig. 7.12). These infections are mildly contagious and may spread to other areas (crotch, armpit). Common means of transmission include contact in public showers and swimming areas, shared towels or contaminated bath mats.

Preventive measures consist of keeping the feet dry, regular changes of socks, the use of foot powders and bringing two pairs of shoes to the court.

Treatment: the toes and feet should be dusted with antifungal drying powders two to three times a day. An antifungal cream can be applied in the morning

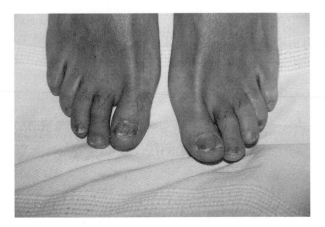

Fig. 7.12 Fungal infection of several toenails.

and evening. Every morning clean socks should be worn, and shoes should be changed every day, in order to let the other pair dry. If the nails are infected, correct diagnosis by fungus culture or potassium hydroxide preparation is extremely important before beginning prolonged therapy. Oral griseofulvin or trisporal will give the highest cure rate.

Pityriasis versicolor (yeast infection)

This infection is caused by a yeast, *Pityrisporon furfur*. It appears as salmon-pink, finely scaling maculae, that fail to tan with sun exposure.

Treatment consists of an overnight application of selenium sulphide (dandruff shampoo), and a reapplication a week later. Another method is daily 15-min applications of selenium sulphide, followed by a rinse for 7–14 days.

Cold sores

Cold sores, also known as fever blisters, are caused by the herpes simplex Type 1 virus. They usually appear on the gums and the outside of the mouth and lips, nose, cheeks or fingers. They are single or clustered, small, fluid-filled blisters on a raised, red, painful area of the skin. Symptoms usually last for 7–10 days. The blisters form, break and ooze; then a yellow crust forms and finally sloughs off to uncover pinkish, healing skin.

The infection is transmitted by contact with another person's active infection, by touching or kissing. Eating utensils, drinking bottles, towels and razors are other common sources. The virus reverts to a latent form within the nerve cells, but emerges again as an active infection on or near the original site. Preceding the attack, itching or heightened sensitivity may be felt at the site. Recurrences are generally milder than the initial infection and are triggered by menstruation, sun exposure, stress or any illness with fever.

Treatment consists of local application of aciclovir, an antiviral medication, five times a day. Early application of aciclovir may prevent a recurrence. Because recurrences can be triggered by sun exposure, a sunblock should be used during hot weather conditions. Needless to say, players should bring their own clean drinking can and towels to prevent an initial infection.

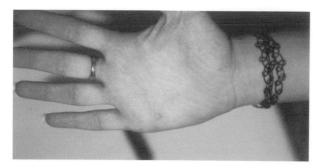

Fig. 7.13 Even a small wart on the hand may be very painful when gripping the racket.

Warts

Warts are benign viral epithelial tumours caused by the human papillomavirus. They range in size from 1 to 2 mm to large tumours. On the hands, they present as circumscribed, firm, cauliflower-shaped raised areas, which are irregular and rough (Fig. 7.13). Plantar warts tend to grow inward because of weight bearing; they can then become painful. They can be distinguished from calluses by gentle paring with a scalpel, which will reveal soft, granular, elongated mounds of dermis.

Both common and plantar warts may turn into more than a cosmetic problem for tennis players, if holding a racket or running becomes increasingly painful. Their course is self-limiting, but they can be very resistant to treatment.

Treatment consists of destructive techniques such as caustic acids, cryotherapy, liquid nitrogen and electrodesiccation. Occasionally, treatments such as daily applications of salicylic acid plasters or topical gels are successful. Excision and radiotherapy are not recommended. Aggressive therapy should be postponed when preparing for important tournaments, because it can seriously disable the player.

Overtraining and burnout

Overtraining is a state of prolonged fatigue and chronically depressed performance as a result of too much physical or mental stress. It occurs when the body's capacities to adapt are chronically exceeded. Other common symptoms are loss of motivation, a lack of desire to train or compete, weight loss, decreased appetite, sleep disturbances, emotional instability and depression. Physiological signs are an increased resting and exercise heart rate, with a slow recovery time. Blood tests may show a decreased plasma testosterone to cortisol ratio. An increased susceptibility to viral infections and increased injury rate may also raise suspicion that the athlete is overtrained. A few days of rest are not enough to make an overtrained athlete feel better: recovery from overtraining may take weeks or months.

Burnout is the term often used in conjunction with young tennis players who retire at an early age because of physical or mental complaints. Overtraining particularly affects tennis players who are highly motivated and/or who compete in too many matches and tournaments without adequate rest intervals, especially with the added stress of environmental changes such as excess heat or cold, altitude, crossing of time zones, strange environments and unfamiliar food. Viral illnesses may also add to the risk of overtraining. In order to prevent overtraining, it is important to vary the intensity and duration of the training load and to balance the intensity and volume of stress with the intensity and volume of recovery, with attention to non-tennis activities and competition-free periods (periodization).

Management consists of rest and stress reduction through a regeneration programme, which may involve relaxation therapy and counselling. Recovery takes several weeks to months. Because burnout seems to occur more often in younger players, the WTA has introduced the age eligibility rule for young female players. This rule prohibits female players from turning professional before the age of 14 and restricts the number of tournaments in which they may compete until they reach the age of 18. In addition, a player development programme has been introduced to minimize the physical, psychological and developmental risks of female athletes.

The programme consists of player–parent seminars offered on-site at tournaments, using retired players as mentors, annual physical examinations, extensive medical coverage at tournaments and career counselling.

The female athlete's triad

Eating disorders and menstrual dysfunction have been shown to occur at an increased rate in athletes. Along with osteoporosis, these have become known as 'the female athlete's triad' and are discussed below.

Eating disorders

Eating disorders affect between 1% and 10% of adolescent and college-age women, with a higher prevalence among female athletes. Women account for 90–95% of patients with eating disorders. Factors involved in the development of eating disorders in female tennis players are the importance attached to becoming lean, the belief that leanness improves performance (thinner is better), and the general sociocultural demand placed on all women to be thin.

Anorexia nervosa is diagnosed when there is severe weight loss (more than 15% below ideal bodyweight) by self-starvation, an intense fear of gaining weight, and primary or secondary amenorrhoea. Obsessive preoccupation with food, strict monitoring of food intake, a disturbed body image and excessive exercise are common symptoms.

Bulimia nervosa is diagnosed in patients with recurrent episodes of binge eating, with a minimum of two episodes per week for at least 3 months, a sense of lack of control over eating behaviour, over concern with body shape and weight and regular use of self-induced vomiting, laxatives, diuretics, strict dieting or exercise to prevent weight gain.

Menstrual dysfunction is common in players with bulimia nervosa, with fewer than 10% having normal menses. The risks associated with both types of eating disorder are nutritional deficiencies, decreased bone density, infertility, decreased immune function, electrolyte disturbances, low blood pressure, slow heart beat, gastrointestinal problems and psychiatric problems. Clinicians should suspect the presence of eating disorders in young players who appear excessively thin, who have a distorted body image (i.e. they are convinced they are too fat when in fact they are extremely thin) or who present with absence of menstruation.

Treatment may consist of individual, behavioural, group or family therapy with, possibly, psychopharmaceuticals.

Menstrual dysfunction

There is a higher incidence of delayed menarche in athletes than in non-athletes.

It has been suggested that each year of high-intensity participation in sport prior to menarche retards the onset of menstruation by 5 months. However, it is not clear to what extent exercise is responsible for the delay. The studies may be biased, because late menarche could also reflect delayed physical maturation in athletes, the late maturer having a more linear physique and motor skill characteristics suited to sporting success.

The prevalence of menstrual cycle alterations such as oligomenorrhoea or amenorrhoea is considerably higher in athletes (12–66%, depending on the study) than in sedentary controls (2–5%). The normal menstrual cycle is 23–35 days, with 10–13 cycles per year; this is called eumenorrhoeic. Oligomenorrhoea is defined as three to six cycles per year at intervals greater than 36 days. Primary amenorrhoea is the absence of menstrual periods by age 16. Secondary amenorrhoea is the absence of three to 12 consecutive menstrual periods, after normal menarche has occurred.

Factors that seem to play a role are intensive training, nutrition (low-calorie diets, low fat and protein content), body composition changes (weight loss, low percentage of body fat), hormonal changes with exercise (altered secretion of the luteinizing hormone), changes in the 24-h rhythm due to intercontinental flights, psychological stress and reproductive immaturity (nulliparity, delayed menarche, oligomenorrhoea). Menstrual dysfunction, especially amenorrhoea, is associated with low oestrogen levels and low bone mineral density.

Treatment of amenorrhoea in the athlete requires thorough evaluation, firstly in order to rule out serious pathological conditions. If the diagnosis is athletic or hypo-oestrogenic amenorrhoea (amenorrhoea due to low oestrogen levels), the athlete needs education about the aetiology. The main objective of treatment in hypo-oestrogenic amenorrhoea is to ensure adequate oestrogen levels. This may be achieved by the athlete by reducing the level of exercise or increasing the percentage of body fat. If the athlete is unwilling to reduce the level of exercise, oestrogen replacement should be commenced. This can be given in the form of the oral contraceptive pill or as combined oestrogen/progesterone therapy. If the first presentation of the amenorrhoeic athlete is with a stress fracture, bone density examination should be considered.

Osteoporosis

Osteoporosis is defined as a decrease in bone mass and strength that leads to an increase in fractures, particularly the vertebral bodies, proximal femur and distal radius. A series of vertebral compression fractures over time can produce a stooped posture, commonly called dowager's hump. Most studies have found lower bone mass among women with exercise-induced oligomenorrhoea and amenorrhoea compared with eumenorrhoeic control women. This may seem strange, because exercise is known to increase bone density as a result of the increased cortical stress on the bone, which enhances remodelling. Excessive exercise, however, may result in an hypo-oestrogenic state with an opposite, negative effect on bone mass, increasing the risk of osteoporosis.

Primary prevention of osteoporosis relies on obtaining a maximal bone density by adequate calcium intake (1200–1500 mg·day^{-1}) and an adequate, but not excessive, amount of exercise. Athletes with osteopenia and amenorrhoea may be advised to decrease training intensity and volume, and drink three glasses of skimmed milk per day. Oestrogen replacement therapy may be indicated for those athletes who are not willing to make changes in their exercise or dietary patterns or who suffer recurrent stress fractures.

Medical care during tournaments

Tennis has evolved into a truly global sport, with more than 80 ATP and nearly 60 WTA tournaments organized each year. In addition, there are the Olympics, the Davis Cup and Federation Cup ties, junior events and a huge number of smaller professional events. This places heavy demands on the sport's medical care provided during these professional tournaments. The ITF, representing all national tennis federations, the WTA Tour and the ATP, representing the professional players, have all recognized the need to protect and promote the health and well-being of their players. The ITF Medical Committee meets on a regular basis.

The ATP's Medical Services Committee consists of two medical directors (orthopaedic/sports medicine doctors), five full-time sports medicine trainers (physical therapists/sports trainers), and an ATP staff liaison. The Committee is responsible for maintaining the standards of on-site medical facilities at ATP events and ensuring that ATP players receive consistent high quality care all year round. The Committee has established a network of ATP tournament physicians who communicate with the ATP's sports medicine trainers and one another. Members of the network attend a ATP sponsored Sports Medicine Conference every 2 years to discuss player care issues and hear presentations from experts in the field.

The WTA Tour has a Sport Sciences and Medicine department that aims to provide optimal health care to all players on the women's professional tennis circuit. The staff consist of a director, a chief medical advisor (sportsmedicine doctor), primary health care providers (physical therapists/certified sports trainers), and licensed massage therapists. The Sport Sciences and Medicine staff are directly involved with the professional women tennis players and attend each tournament on the WTA Tour, supported by local physicians.

The physiotherapists are the first point of contact for the player. This has the advantage of providing continuous care for the player, because they travel with the players to the same events. The physiotherapists manage the daily medical needs of the players. They have extensive background training in physical therapy and physical training. Their functions are both on-court and off-court, both of which are vitally important to the health of the athlete. On-court functions focus on immediate, emergency-type treatment. Off-court care focuses on the prevention of injuries and incorporates a variety of preparational, evaluational and rehabilitative skills and methods. They work in close relation with the tournament physicians and all staff on-site.

For every event a local physician, preferably a specialist in sports medicine or orthopaedic surgery, is hired as tournament physician. The standards and duties of the tournament physician are patient confidentiality, familiarity with tennis-specific injuries, establishment of communication with the staff, treatment of musculoskeletal injuries and minor medical illnesses on-site, access to medical specialists as needed, and up-to-date certification in basic life support.

The ITF is responsible for the medical care of the players at the Olympic games, the Davis Cup and the Federation Cup ties. The ITF sends physiotherapists to smaller tournaments, like the qualifying of the Federation Cup and the ITF Women's circuit ($50 000 and $75 000 prize money). The ITF Medical Committee meets on a regular basis and advises the national federations.

At the Grand Slams both the ATP and WTA Tour medical staff is present, complemented by physiotherapists, massage therapists and local physicians, generally including specialists from several fields.

Preferred working conditions

The preferred working conditions are to have separate rooms for the physician, ATP sports medicine trainer or WTA Tour primary health care provider, and the massage therapist. These rooms should be close to the locker rooms and to the courts. The rooms should contain massage tables, preferably with adjustable head ends or hydraulic tables, 10 m^2 working space per table, one knee roll per table, one work table (drug table), one medicine chest (lockable), hot and cold water, sufficient light, electric connections, waste bins, sheets for the tables, towels and one to two chairs. A refrigerator for ice and medication should be nearby. Basic hygienic standards, daily cleaning and daily replacement of used linen are required for all medical working places.

Recommended reading

Balaban, E.P. (1992) Sports anaemia. *Clinics in Sports Medicine* **11**, 313–325.

Chester, A.C. (1996) Chronic sinusitis. *American Family Physician* **53**, 877–887.

Consensus Conference (1985) Travellers' diarrhoea. *Journal of the American Medical Association* **253**, 2700–2704.

Fahey, P.J., Stallkamp, E.T. & Kwatra, S. (1996) The athlete with Type I diabetes: managing insulin, diet and exercise. *American Family Physician* **53**, 1611–1617.

Garcia-Albea, E., Cabrera, F., Tejeiro, J., Jimenez-Jimenez, F.J. & Vaquero, A. (1992) Delayed postexertional headache, intracranial hypotension and racket sports (letter). *Journal of Neurology, Neurosurgery and Psychiatry* **55**, 975.

Hannon, D.W. & Knilans, T.K. (1993) Syncope in children and adolescents. *Current Problems in Pediatrics* **23**, 358–384.

Hooper, S.L. & Mackinnon, L.T. (1995) Monitoring overtraining in athletes. *Sports Medicine* **20**, 321–327.

Hough, D.O. & Dec, K.L. (1994) Exercise-induced asthma and anaphylaxis. *Sports Medicine* **18**, 162–172.

Jetté, M., Landry, F., Tiemann, B. & Blühmchen, G. (1991) Ambulatory blood pressure and holter monitoring during tennis play. *Canadian Journal of Sport Sciences* **16**, 40–44.

Keul, J., Stockhausen, W., Pokan, R., Huonker, M. & Berg, A. (1991) Metabolische und kardiozirkulatorische Adaptation sowie Leistungsverhalten professioneller Tennisspieler. *Deutsche Medizinische Wochenschrift* **116**, 761–767.

Kontulainen, S., Kannus, P., Haapasalo, H. *et al.* (2001) Good maintenance of exercise-induced bone gain with decreased training of female tennis and squash players: a prospective 5-year follow-up study of young and old starters and controls. *Journal of Bone Mineral Research* **16**, 195–201.

McMahon, M. & Palmer, R.M. (1985) Exercise and Hypertension. *Medical Clinics of North America* **69**, 57–70.

Pardhan, S., Shacklock, P. & Weatherill, J. (1995) Sport-related eye trauma: a survey of the presentation of eye injuries to a casualty clinic and the use of protective eye-wear. *Eye* **9** (Suppl.), 50–53.

Shephard, R.J. & Shek, P.N. (1994) Infectious diseases in athletes: new interest for an old problem. *Journal of Sports Medicine and Physical Fitness* **34**, 11–22.

Skolnick, A.A. (1993) 'Female athlete triad' risk for women. *Journal of the American Medical Association* **270**, 921–923.

Van Linschoten, R., Backx, F.J.G., Mulder, O.G.M. & Meinardi, H. (1990) Epilepsy and Sports. *Sports Medicine* **10**, 9–19.

Weber, K., Ferrauti, A. & Strüder, H.K. (1995) Hämodynamische und metabolische Beanspruchung bei Senioren tennisspielern (-innen): Nutzen oder Risiko? *Deutsche Zeitschrift für Sportmedizin* **46**, 521–529.

Williams, S.J. & Nukada, H. (1994) Sport and exercise headache: Part 2. Diagnosis and classification. *British Journal of Sports Medicine* **28**, 96–100.

Zerbe, K.J. (1996) Anorexia nervosa and bulimia nervosa. *Postgraduate Medicine* **99**, 161–168.

Chapter 8
Travel and jet lag

Introduction

Tennis is the widest played of all racket sports. Several million play on a regular basis. The Grand Slam tournaments are played in America, Australia, England and France. There are other major tournaments played in the Middle East. This involves crossing many time zones, which will affect the circadian (cycles recurring repetitively every 24 h) or endogenous daily rhythms resulting in jet lag, which is a desynchronization or disruption of the normal circadian rhythms. This may play a major role in a player's performance. The length of flight is not critical but it is the number of time zones crossed. They may also have to acclimatize to heat, humidity, cold or altitude.

Factors affecting jet lag

Personality types

Extroverts tend to have fewer problems with jet lag than introverts. People who are anxious suffer more from jet lag than those who are relaxed. Older people are often more affected. Fit people are less likely to feel the effects. People with a rigid routine or morning types have the most problems (Hill *et al.* 1993). Athletes who do not like travelling or who are apprehensive about flying tend to have difficulty sleeping both before and during the flight and are more likely to have problems with jet lag.

Circadian rhythms

These are endogenous daily rhythms controlled by environmental cues or *Zeitgebers*, e.g. light and dark, time and temperature. The important *Zeitgebers* in humans appear to be a mixture of bright light and social factors. Over 300 physiological and psychological rhythms have been identified and normally they work in harmony. These rhythms attain a maximum and minimum, occurring at a specific time of day, e.g. body temperature, cortisol production and the sleep–wake cycle. Morning types have their highest body temperature about 1 a.m. and the lowest at 2 p.m., while evening types have their highest temperature about 4 p.m. and their lowest at 4 a.m. Extroverts tend to have their peaks later in the day and adapt better to a delay, i.e. going west, than to an advance in time phase. Diurnal temperature variation is between 36° and 38°.

Temperature

Physical and mental performance appears to be optimal around the period of the highest temperature. Factors involved in performance such as nerve conduction velocity, metabolic enzyme reaction rates and psychomotor performance are all affected by body temperature rhythms (Fort *et al.* 1971).

The majority of the components of sports performance, e.g. flexibility, muscle strength and short-term high-power output vary with time of day in a sinusoidal manner. In evening types they peak in the early evening close to the maximum body temperature (Atkinson 1996). Swimmers had better times in the evening (Rodahl *et al.* 1976).

Plasma cortisol and adrenocorticotrophic hormone (ACTH) levels reach their maximum at or shortly before the subject's normal time of waking in the morning. Cortisol rhythm may be related to arousal and wakefulness and variations in steroid level to mood (Conroy & O'Brien 1973). It is of great concern to athletes that performance is temperature dependent, particularly if they have to compete before synchronizing to the new local time (Fort *et al.* 1971).

Both the absorption and action of some drugs and their breakdown products can vary dramatically according to the time of day. Reaction time, perception, mood, anxiety, motivation and well-being are all influenced by time of day (Wright *et al.* 1983). Disruption of mood states and reduction in dynamic strength, anaerobic power and capacity and dynamic strength are affected. The effects of travel do not usually last after 3–4 days but there are marked variations in the rate of adaptation of the body's own rhythms after time-zone transition to a new environment (Reilly *et al.* 1997). The body temperature rhythms adjust before corticosteroids, which take much longer.

The biological clock

There are thought to be two biological clocks near the hypothalamus (a part of the brain): one portion controls the sleep–wake cycle, the other, which consists of receptors for body temperature and the pineal gland (which is in the brain), may also play a role (Arendt & Marks 1982). Recent evidence favours that a part of the brain consisting of the hypothalamic suprachiasmatic nuclei is the site of the biological clock in humans, which is influenced by light and dark cycles (Joseph & Knigge 1978).

The pineal gland is the fulcrum of a complex neuroendocrine system which makes an interaction between light and the human body possible by means of the production of a number of biochemical substances of which melatonin is one (Kral 1995). Melatonin is secreted at a circadian rhythm characterized by high nocturnal serum levels and low diurnal levels (Brown 1994). The pineal transforms tryptophan through serotonin to the final end product of indolamine melatonin; this latter substance carries phase of day information to all peripheral tissues (Kral 1995).

Light

A pathway from the eye to the brain mediates the effects of light. The retinohypothalamic pathway and excitatory amino acids (substances released at the nerve endings) play a key role in the transportation of light information to the interpretative centre in the nucleus (Dijk *et al.* 1995), the site of the biological clock. The secretion appears to be correlated not only with the intensity of light but also with its spectrum and time exposure. Melatonin seems to be involved in stress-associated mechanisms and may be able to reduce the symptoms of jet lag.

Phase delays (changes in the timing of the body's rhythms) can be induced by light exposure before the minimum of the endogenous core body temperature, which is approximately 1–2 h before the habitual time of waking, while phase advances are induced when light exposure is scheduled after the minimum of the endogenous core body temperature (Lewy *et al.* 1995)—the alteration of the amount of dark and light. It is important to use eyeshades after you have taken melatonin to encourage sleep. In healthy young people light exposure schedules that do not curtail sleep but induce moderate shifts of the endogenous circadian phase have been shown to influence the timing of sleep and wakefulness without markedly affecting sleep structure (Dijk *et al.* 1995).

Environmental factors

Environmental factors facilitate the phasing of circadian rhythms. Travelling across time zones outstrips the ability of the synchronizers, and desynchronization then occurs which results in jet lag, as it produces an abrupt displacement of environmental time cues, and endogenous circadian timing resynthesizes slowly. In 1884 the globe was divided into 24 one-hour zones with the prime meridian at Greenwich. The time zones are wider at the equator, 1000 miles (1600 km), and only 180 miles (288 km) at the poles.

Jet lag

Jet lag occurs when there is desynchronization of circadian rhythms and refers to the mental and physical effects of travelling rapidly across several time zones. It is associated with fatigue, lack of motivation, insomnia, gastrointestinal disturbance and depression. It varies with each individual: 25–30% have no or very few difficulties, 25% do not adjust.

Most rhythms tend to be longer than 24 h and adapt more easily to the longer day of a westbound flight and thus recovery from a westbound flight is usually easier than from an eastbound trip where the time zones are earlier and the day is shortened. It is easier to adapt to three rather than to five time-zone changes. Athletes should plan so that they have time to acclimatize. They need at least 1 day for each time zone crossed, more if there will be major differences in climate or altitude. Some people think that a daytime flight causes less jet lag particularly if they arrive at their destination in the evening but others experience less jet lag after an evening flight if they can sleep on the plane.

Adjustment is less rapid after an advanced phase shift of an eastbound flight, compared to a phase delay of a westbound flight. Resynchronization speed is fastest during the first 3–4 days after a time zone trip. Complete adjustment after six time-zone changes is usually 13 days for an eastbound and 10 for a west. Eastbound flights (Dement *et al.* 1986) decrease the total sleep time and sleep efficiency. There is an increase in slow-wave sleep but a decrease in rapid eye movement (REM) sleep (Suvanto *et al.* 1990).

Westbound, there is a shorter sleep time and a decrease in sleep efficiency but it does not affect REM sleep. The amount of sleep decreases with age; the duration of time in bed and total sleep time and sleep latency increase and there is early wakening as well as waking after sleep onset; this is why there is a longer recovery time in the older person (Suvanto *et al.* 1990).

Factors affecting athletes

Athletes can lose their competitive edge by crossing a few time zones. Some athletes travel half way around the world to compete in an event lasting two or three days. They should be in the best possible physical and mental performance on arrival. Fatigue may be due to hypoxia, dehydration or lack of sleep. Any members of the travelling party on medication, e.g. asthmatics or diabetics, should always bring an adequate supply of medication for the period of their stay, just in case the particular brands they are accustomed to use are not available in the country they are visiting. They should be carried as part of their hand luggage not in a suitcase in case it is lost. They should also carry their running shoes and orthotics or bring a spare pair of orthotics in case their luggage is lost.

Preflight recommendations

Book a non-smoking airplane if possible. Before travelling there is a lot of essential information that is required in order to plan a successful trip. You must find out as much as possible about the destination and if possible visit it at the same time, a year before the major competition. It is essential to find out about medical facilities available at the local hospital and at the competition site and medical insurance. Voltage for physiotherapy and entertain-ment equipment may be different and you may have to hire local equipment, e.g. interferential equipment, videos, etc. Advise on the essential and routinely re-commended vaccines and their limitations. Tetanus, polio, hepatitis B and A should be up to date for most countries.

Infections

Malaria

Malaria prophylaxis may be required in some coun-tries. Advise about the possible risk from insect bites particularly in countries where malaria is endemic. In some countries if the temperature is very hot there may be a risk of amoebic infection in small private swimming pools.

Diarrhoea

Athletes and officials should be warned not to eat strange food or to eat food bought from street food stalls and to drink bottled water as they may get diarrhoea, which is a common problem. They should bring their own food and drink if they have special requirements.

Diarrhoea is a common complication of travel. There may be a variety of causes, which include: bacterial infections (*Escherichia coli*, *Salmonella*, *Shigella*, *Campylobacter*), which are confirmed by culture of the stool; viral infections, e.g. rotavirus; and protozoan infection such as *Giardia lamblia*. The symptoms of infectious gastroenteritis include nausea, vomiting, diarrhoea and there may be systemic symptoms of fever, malaise, weakness and anorexia. Viral gastroenteritis usually has an acute onset and is usually self-limiting. It is essential to ensure the patient is well hydrated. *Giardia lamblia* is an organism (protozoan) that may cause intestinal symptoms in those exposed to infected water. Treat-ment is with tindazole or metronidazole. Athletes may also develop gastritis by eating very spicy foods, particularly if they are not used to them.

Fungal infections

Athletes may develop fungal infections. Particular attention should be paid to hygiene. They should wear cotton socks that should be changed frequently. Feet should be dried thoroughly especially between the toes.

Sun exposure

Protection against excessive exposure to the sun is important particularly for people with fair skin. It is equally important to realize that sun block may prevent the evaporation of sweat and so increase core body temperature. Exposure to high temperatures may reactivate herpes virus so it is important to use a block on lips.

Effects of flying

Book a morning flight so that you arrive at your destination in the evening. Plan travel arrangements carefully. Fly westwards if possible. Make sure you are not sick with excitement or worry and not tired or hung over. Exercise in the days prior to departure and try to avoid illness. If you have a cold, flying will make it worse, so, ideally, delay the trip. Try and have a good night's sleep before flying. Do not have a going-away party.

If several time zones will be crossed, then prior to departure, if possible, adjustments should be made by going to bed either a few hours before or after the normal time, e.g. if three times zones are being crossed on an eastbound flight, then go to bed and get up 3 h earlier, but preadjustment of the sleep–wake cycle is largely ineffective due to other factors that are difficult to overcome (Reilly *et al.* 1997). Partial adjustment is accompanied by a drop in the mean value of the performance curve.

Diet

Consideration of diet may help in alleviating jet lag. Before travel, adapt diet. The correct timing of food is important. A high-protein meal (meat, fish, eggs, dairy products) stimulates the adrenaline (epinephrine) pathway and increases arousal (Hastie 1990). A high-carbohydrate meal (pasta, salad, fruit, dessert) increases insulin secretion and facilitates uptake of tryptophan resulting in drowsiness (Fort *et al.* 1971; Ehret *et al.* 1980). Alternating light and heavy meals before a flight continually empties the body's supply of glycogen and then replenishes it, allowing a person's circadian rhythms to quickly shift to the new time zone.

Preadjust the body clock to the new time zone and gradually adapt to arrival time and practice and training if practical. Arrive well in advance of the event, 1 day for every hour, longer if you have to adjust to temperature changes as well. Know as much as possible about the destination before you fly.

All athletes should have their teeth checked before flying, as a defective filling or an apical abscess may result in severe pain in the tooth due to exposure of trapped gases during the flight.

Menstrual problems

Crossing several time zones will affect the menstrual cycle and in some cases this will have a profound effect on the performance of female athletes.

Other considerations

Women on the pill risk thrombosis from prolonged immobilization during a long flight. Swollen feet are a common problem on long flights. It is important to prevent this condition by walking around the plane and at stopovers. Elevate legs when possible. People with varicose veins should wear support hose. People with sinusitis or colds may develop severe headache or earache. They should use decongestives before take off.

A plaster cast on a limb may result in severe compression and a case of gangrene has been reported. Avoid air travel for 40 h after the application of a cast or use a split cast. Patients should not fly until at least 10 days after surgery, as fresh bleeding may result.

Allow 12 h between the last scuba dive and flying, and if the dive has been deeper than 30 ft (9.1 m) allow 24 h before flying to avoid the risk of decompression.

Abnormal circadian rhythms associated with depressive and affective illness may be aggravated by time-zone changes. One hundred and eighty patients were admitted to a psychiatric hospital from Heathrow airport after long flights in a 2-year period (Harding & Mills 1983).

Recommendations during flight

At the beginning of the flight set your watch to the arrival time zone. Exercise by walking around the plane, avoid the smoking area, try to sleep as much as possible, use eyeshades. Wear a collar so that you do not wake up with a crick in your neck.

Dehydration

The relatively low moisture content in aircraft on long journeys causes dehydration and dryness of the eyes, throat and skin. Contact lenses tend to dry out. It is essential to drink plenty of fluids, water, mineral water and limited fruit juices. Excessive fruit juice may cause diarrhoea. Avoid alcohol, tea, coffee and drinks containing caffeine. Increase intake of high-fibre food to avoid constipation. Children are more susceptible to dehydration and pressure changes. They should be given small amounts of water frequently. Older children should also be given boiled sweets.

Use a moisturizer on the skin and apply contact lens solution to keep eyes moist. Dehydration can reduce muscular endurance as a result of the flight. Four to six per cent water loss results in a 3% reduction in muscle strength.

To promote sleep, use blindfolds, earplugs and wear a collar as a neck rest—this will help you to sleep better, and prevent you sleeping in an awkward position, which may result in neck pain and problems competing. Wear comfortable, loose-fitting clothes. Take off your shoes, recline the seat, make sure that you are comfortable and warm enough.

Some travellers use melatonin. Some people may require medication to help them sleep. Medication that decreases sleep latency and increases sleep duration and maintenance with no significant effect the next day should be taken. You should always try medication that you are going to use during the flight for the first time some weeks beforehand to make sure you have no side-effects.

Exercise as much a possible in the plane, get off the plane and walk around during the stopovers. If there is a long delay between flights, take a shower or swim.

Hypoxia or lack of oxygen

The reduction of oxygen pressure during a long flight results in more fatigue. This will affect performance and may also have adverse effects on people with chronic cardiovascular and pulmonary conditions.

Smoking will aggravate the hypoxia so passengers with potential problems and athletes who are going to compete should sit as far as possible from the smoking area.

Passengers who are afraid of flying may hyperventilate which causes lowering of the carbon dioxide in the blood, particularly if the cabin is hot and stuffy. This may result in muscle spasm, numbness and loss of consciousness. Treatment is to counsel before flying and if they hyperventilate, to breathe into a paper bag.

Sleep

Sleep disturbance is a major factor during flight. Lack of sleep will aggravate fatigue. Therefore, during the flight the passenger should try to sleep or at least doze as much as possible. On arrival adjust to the sleep pattern of the new country as soon as possible. Some people may need the help of short-acting sleeping tablets for the first few nights after arrival.

Medication

The effects of drugs may be increased when the patient is exposed to hypoxia in a pressurized cabin and the biological rhythms are desynchronized as a result of jet lag.

Hypoxia during flight results in more fatigue, and epileptics may need to increase their medication, as hypoxia and over-fatigue may precipitate an attack. Antihistamines should be avoided or a lower dosage used because of the side-effects, e.g. fatigue. Hypoxia and alcohol potentiate the effects of sleeping tablets.

Diabetes

Travel across time zones alters the normal time of meals, and diabetics may not have the opportunity to exercise which results in a physiological rise in glucose levels. Diabetics must adjust their insulin requirements to the meal times on the airplane and also on arrival. Increase insulin when flying west as the day will be longer but reduce it when flying east. Westbound travellers should continue taking normal insulin regime until departure. During long flights, administer one or two extra injections of short-acting insulin with each meal. On arrival continue insulin according to the local time. Travelling eastwards there should be a slight reduction in dose of insulin. A late evening meal on board the airplane should be covered with an extra dose of short-acting insulin 2–3 units. An extra breakfast dose of intermediate insulin should be reduced by 20–40%; late timing of breakfast means patients can skip lunchtime injection. Careful monitoring of glucose in the urine is required to protect against a sudden increase in blood glucose (Yudkin *et al.* 1990).

The rate of adjustment depends on many factors, which include the rhythms being measured, the number of time zones crossed, the flight direction, whether eastwards or westwards, and the strength of the *Zeitgebers* or time cues in the new time zones; some adapt quicker.

On arrival

Adapt to the local time of eating, training and sleeping. Spend as much time out doors in the daylight (Shiota *et al.* 1996). Do not take naps or stay in the bedroom. It is better to stay up until the local time to go to sleep. Have a high-carbohydrate diet the evening of the flight to induce sleep (increased secretion of serotonin makes people drowsy) and this also replaces glycogen. Eat a high-protein breakfast on arrival (increased tyrosine levels and the levels of catecholamines may increase arousal) (Hastie 1990). Socialize and do light training, not heavy training. If possible compete in the morning after a westbound flight and in the evening after an eastbound flight as this will harmonize more easily with the normal circadian rhythms. When allocating rooms on tour take into account which players require more sleep or which are light sleepers particularly if they have to share a room with someone who sleepwalks, snores or talks in their sleep. Insufficient sleep will affect performance. If they are sleep deprived they have a lower oral temperature and their time to exhaustion is decreased.

Short-acting sleeping tablets taken on the first few nights may help athletes who have difficulty with sleep.

Prevention of jet lag

- Time your travel. Allow at least 1 day per time zone to be crossed and longer if having to acclimatize to heat or cold.

- Fly west rather than east, as recovery time is shorter.
- Avoid late nights before travel. If feasible start to adjust to new time zone before flying.
- Pay attention to diet. Eat lightly before flying and avoid fatty foods on the plane.
- Eat little and drink a lot of water. Avoid alcohol for at least 6–8 h before the end of a long flight.
- If firm precautions are not taken to deal with the deleterious effects of jet lag, then all the hard training will be lost. Athletes who participate in international competition should definitely consider manipulating their precompetition schedules to offset circadian dysrhythm resulting from their long flight. Lack of sleep is a very important factor.

References

Arendt, J. & Marks, B. (1982) Physiological changes underlying jet lag. *British Medical Journal* **284**, 144–146.

Atkinson, G.T. (1996) Circadian variation in sports performance. *Sports Medicine* **21** (4), 292–312.

Brown, G.M. (1994) Light melatonin and the sleep wake cycle. *Journal of Psychiatric Neuroscience* **5**, 345–353.

Conroy, R.T.W.L. & O'Brien, M. (1973) Diurnal variation in athletic performance. In: *Proceedings of the Physiological Society*.

Dement, W.C., Seidel, W.F., Cohen, S.A., Bliwise, N.G. & Carskadon, M.A. (1986) Sleep and wakefulness in aircrew before and after transoceanic flights. *Aviation Space and Environmental Medicine* **57** (Suppl.), B14–B28.

Dijk, D.J., Boules, Z., Eastman, C. *et al.* (1995) Light treatment for sleep disorders. Consensus Report II, Basic properties of circadian physiology and sleep regulation. *Journal of Biological Rhythms* **10** (2), 113–125.

Ehret, C.F., Groh, K.R. & Meinert, J.C. (1980) Consideration of diet in alleviating jet lag. In: Scheving & Halberg, eds. *Principles and Application to Shifts in Schedule*, pp. 393–402. Sijithoff and Noordhoff, Rockville, MD.

Fort, A., Gobbay, J.A., Jackett, R., Jones, M.C. & Jones, S.M. (1971) The relationship between deep body temperature and performance on psychomotor tests. *Journal of Psychology* **219**, 12–18.

Harding, R.M. & Mills, R.F.J. (1983) *Aviation Medicine*. BMA, London.

Hastie, P. (1990) Dietary strategies for reducing travel fatigue. *Sports Coach*, Jul–Sept, 26–28.

Hill, D.W., Hill, C.M., Fields, K.L. & Smith, J.C. (1993) Effects of jet lag on factors related to sport performance. *Canadian Journal of Applied Physiology* **1**, 91–103.

Joseph, S.A. & Knigge, K.M. (1978) The endocrine hypothalamus: recent anatomical studies. In: Reichlin, S.,

Baldessarini, R.J. & Martin, J.B., eds. *The Hypothalamus*, pp. 15–47. Raven Press, New York.

Kral, A. (1995) The role of the pineal gland in circadian rhythm regulation. *Bratislavskae Lekarske Listy* **7**, 295–303.

Lewy, A.J., Sack, R.L., Blood, M.L. *et al.* (1995) Physical and mental performance: optimal period of highest temperature. In: *Ciba Foundation Symposium*, Vol. 183, pp. 303–317.

Reilly, T., Atkinson, G. & Waterhouse, J. (1997) Travel fatigue and jet lag. *Journal of Sports Sciences* **15**, 365–369.

Rodahl, A., O'Brien, M. & Firth, R.G.R. (1976) Diurnal variation in performance of competitive swimmers. *Journal of Sports Medicine* **16**, 72–76.

Shiota, M., Sudou, M. & Ohshima, M. (1996) Using outdoor exercise to decrease jet lag in airline crew members.

Aviation Space and Environmental Medicine **67** (12), 1155–1160.

Suvanto, S., Partinen, M., Harma, M. & Ilmairien, J. (1990) Flight attendants' desynchronosis after rapid time zone changes. *Aviation Space and Environmental Medicine* **61**, 543–547.

Wright, J.E., Vogel, J.A., Sampson, J.B., Knapik, J.J. & Patton, J.F. (1983) Effects of travel across time zones (jet lag) on exercise capacity and performance. *Aviation Space and Environmental Medicine* **54** (2), 132–137.

Yudkin, J.S.M., George, K., Alberti, M., Clarty, D.G. & Swai, B.M. (1990) Impaired glucose tolerance, is it a risk factor for diabetes or a diagnostic rat-bag? *British Medical Journal* **301**, 397–402.

Chapter 9

Strength training, flexibility training and physical conditioning

Introduction

No matter what your ability, you cannot play your best tennis if you are not physically fit. Being physically fit means that your heart, blood vessels, lungs and muscles can function at maximum efficiency. The physical demands of playing tennis stress all areas of the body. Proper conditioning can assist in the prevention of injury, as well as improvement of actual tennis performance. The ultimate goal will be to play tennis for as many years as possible without sustaining any injuries. Tennis is truly the sport for a lifetime, where players can train, compete and play tournaments year-round. Current research indicates that players achieve the best results when training methods replicate the actual demands of the sport. Therefore, in tennis, practice sessions should challenge the same energy systems, muscle groups and movement patterns stressed in competitive play. Aerobic and anaerobic capacity, muscular strength and endurance, power, response time, speed and agility, dynamic balance, coordination and flexibility, along with the development of gross and fine motor skills, are all important components in the development of a successful tennis game (Groppel & Roetert 1992). By identifying the performance characteristics advantageous to successful performance in tennis, you can design a training programme to optimize improvements in the desired trait. Moreover, special programmes can be developed to improve any deficient qualities (Roetert et al. 1995).

Lower body

Flexibility

Few people are as flexible around all of their joints as they need to be. Therefore, especially when playing tennis, which places tremendous demands on different body parts in their extremes of motion, a proper flexibility programme is vital. Throughout a match, the player is called on to generate force from a variety of body positions: changing direction, reaching for a shot, stopping quickly, and serving are just a few examples. Increasing flexibility through a stretching programme can help you enjoy injury-free tennis and improve your range of motion to enable you to play at your best. Flexibility is the degree to which the soft-tissue structures surrounding a joint—muscles, tendons and connective tissues—stretch (Sobel et al. 1995). Sobel et al. recommend the following procedures and safety precautions when improving flexibility for tennis:

1 A medical doctor should be consulted before beginning any flexibility/conditioning programme.
2 Before stretching, warm up 3–5 min or until you break into a light sweat to increase body temperature.
3 Emphasize slow, smooth movements and coordinate deep breathing while you stretch. Inhale deeply; then exhale as you stretch to the point just short of pain; then ease back slightly. Hold for 10 s as you breath normally; then exhale as you slowly stretch farther, again just short of pain. Hold again for 10–20 s. Repeat three times.
4 If a stretch hurts or if you feel a burning sensation, you are stretching too far.
5 Stretch to your own limits.
6 Stretch your tight side first.
7 Do not lock your joints.
8 Do not bounce.
9 Stretch large muscle groups first (e.g. your thigh, hamstring or calf muscles) and repeat in the same order every day.
10 Stretch the most inflexible areas of your body. Conversely, do not stretch only the most flexible areas, because you may decrease joint stability and exacerbate muscle imbalances.
11 Stretch daily and be consistent with the time of day you stretch. Avoid stretching in the morning, because that is when you are least flexible. An ideal time to stretch is after aerobic activity.

Most lower leg injuries in tennis competition are chronic in nature and occur from repetitive stress of the many quick starts, stops and changes of direction. Stretching the muscles of the lower extremities is critical in the prevention of both acute and chronic injuries

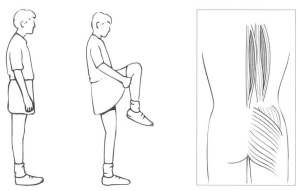

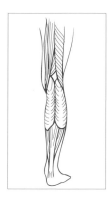

Bend one leg and grasp the back of the thigh just above the knee. Slowly pull the knee to your chest. Hold position.

Fig. 9.1 Flexibility exercise—knee–chest flex.

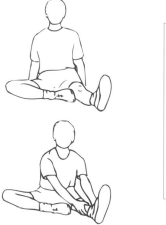

Try to bring the chest to the thigh by bending forward from the hips. Keep the back straight. Pull your toes back to point towards your face.

Fig. 9.3 Flexibility exercise—hamstring stretch.

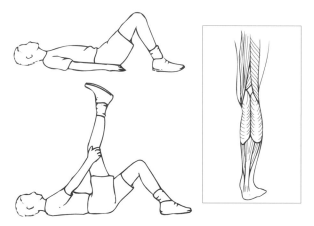

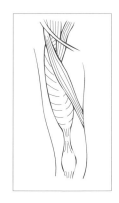

Straighten one leg and raise it towards the trunk. Use your hands to gently increase the stretch. Point your toes towards the face to stretch the calf.

Fig. 9.2 Flexibility exercise—hamstring stretch.

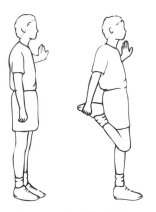

Stand on one leg. Bend the opposite knee while grasping the ankle. Keeping the back flat and the buttocks tucked under, bring your knee down as far as you can, trying to point it straight down to the floor. Do *not* point the knee out or twist it!

Fig. 9.4 Flexibility exercise—quadriceps stork stretch.

and aids in protecting the joints when placed in extreme positions. The important muscle groups affecting the knee joint include the hamstrings, gastrocnemius and quadriceps. Tightness of the quadriceps and hamstring muscles may result in an overload of forces at the level of the knee. Repeated stretching will reduce the load on the muscle tendon unit at a given strength. Figures 9.1–9.7 show some of the recommended flexibility exercises to help reduce the risk of injury to the lower extremity (they recreate exercises 1, 2, 3, 5, 6, 7 and 9 from the USTA 'Basic 10 Flexibility Exercises' card).

Strength (see pp. 121–123)

Strength is the amount of weight you can lift or handle at any one time. Muscular endurance is the number of times your muscles can lift a weight or how long your muscles can hold an amount of weight. Although maximal strength does decrease steadily with age,

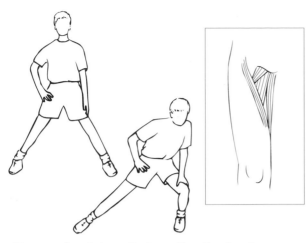

Place one hand above the knee, the other hand on the opposite hip. With toes pointing forward, slowly bend the knee your hand is on until you feel a stretch in the groin area. Roll your weight onto the inside of your foot.

Fig. 9.5 Flexibility exercise—groin stretch.

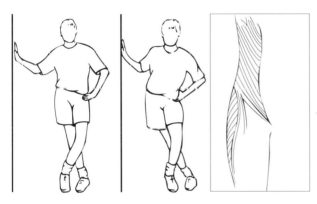

Stand with your right hand on the wall, your weight on your right leg, and your left leg crossed in front of it. Gently push the right hip towards the wall. Increase the stretch by standing farther from the wall.

Fig. 9.6 Flexibility exercise—hip stretch.

strength training can lessen the impact of ageing on performance. Performing strength-training exercises increases bone density, improves overall muscle strength and can be especially important in correcting muscle imbalances, due to the one-sidedness of tennis. Recent studies indicate that people, regardless of their age, gender or initial level of fitness, have

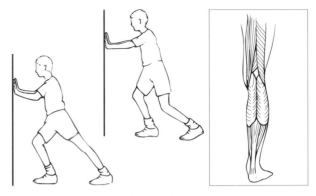

Keep the back knee straight, the heel on the floor, and the foot pointing forward. Bend the forward knee and lean your trunk forward. Do not arch the lower back. Then slightly bend the back leg, raise the heel 2 inches off the floor, and lean into the wall. This time, feel the stretch near the heel.

Fig. 9.7 Flexibility exercise—calf stretch.

considerable ability to increase strength with training. Even though in tennis, upper body strength deserves attention for achieving optimum stroke potential and injury prevention, coaches should include a proportionately significant amount of lower body strength and endurance conditioning in their tennis training design. By increasing muscular strength and endurance, a player will be able to move around the court as well at the end of a match as he or she did at the beginning. In addition, tennis requires that a player move with explosive movements. Greater power allows the player to respond quicker and produce forceful movements with less effort. Players with explosive first steps get into position quickly, set up well and hit effective shots. Moreover, an explosive first step will give the player the speed necessary to get to balls hit farther away.

Not only will a proper strength base allow a player to cover the court and reach many shots, a strength-training programme that minimizes structural and functional asymmetry may also allow the player to play injury free. Ellenbecker and Roetert (1995) found that, in contrast to the upper body, it appears that symmetrical lower extremity strength can be expected in the quadriceps and hamstring musculature of elite junior tennis players. The following exercises are recommended to strengthen the lower body.

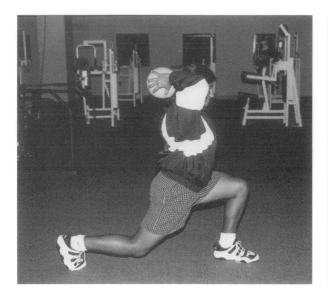

Fig. 9.8 Lunge exercise.

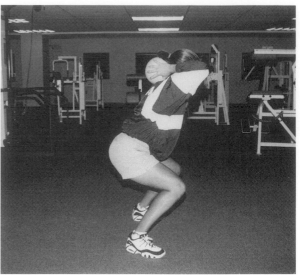

Fig. 9.9 Squat exercise.

Lunge (Fig. 9.8)

The lunge is a very tennis-specific movement pattern and can be performed as a 'straight-ahead' movement as pictured, or in a 45° diagonal (left and right) to increase application for tennis. The player begins standing with the feet shoulder width apart and can increase the resistance with this exercise by placing a medicine ball behind the neck, and securely holding the ball with both hands. While keeping the trunk erect, the player takes a step forward (as pictured), slowly lowering and absorbing the bodyweight. The front knee should be bending, reaching at most a 90° angle. For players with a history of knee problems, the front knee should not bend more than 45–60°. From the player's perspective, the knee should not protrude beyond the front toe at any time. From the lowered position, the player presses him- or herself back to the starting position.

Squat (Fig. 9.9)

Using the medicine ball again behind the head for resistance, or dumb-bells at the player's sides, the player descends in a controlled manner keeping the trunk erect. The knees should bend just short of 90°, with the tips of the knees being in line with the front of the toes as pictured.

Other recommended exercises

Other recommended exercises include:

- leg press;
- calf raises;
- step-ups;
- hip abduction/adduction;
- hamstring curls;
- knee extensions.

Aerobic and anaerobic endurance

Get fit to play tennis, do not play tennis to get fit. Even though this may be excellent advice for avoiding injury on the court, playing tennis does give fitness benefits. Physiological research shows that the aerobic capacity of relatively sedentary people decreases by about 10% per decade (Roetert 1996). However, if you play tennis, you can have significantly less of a decrease in aerobic capacity as you age. With training, our aerobic capacity only decreases 5% every two decades. Although singles may give you more of an aerobic benefit, playing doubles certainly qualifies under the American Surgeon General's recommendation of 30 min of moderate physical activity most days of the week. People who start playing at a young age and continue throughout their lifetime retain the highest level of fitness.

However, if someone has not played in a long time, he or she can still obtain significant benefits even if the sport is taken up again later in life.

Thus, even though the sport of tennis provides us with numerous fitness benefits, it is best to prepare properly before stepping onto the court.

What is the best way to train for the sport of tennis? To answer that question, we will take a look at the energy demands of the sport. The energy used to run in a long-distance race comes from the aerobic (with oxygen) system, while the energy utilized in short bursts of activity, such as an 18-m dash is called anaerobic (without oxygen). Although it is difficult to quantify the energy demands of tennis, we know that tennis is a sport that relies on both a strong aerobic as well as anaerobic system (Groppel & Roetert 1992).

Most points in tennis, even on a clay court, last less than 10 s, while the average point on a hard court between two equally matched players typically lasts less than 5 s. Within that time period, you may see up to four direction changes. Each of these short bursts of effort is an anaerobic activity. Obviously anaerobic training is very important.

This does *not* mean you can ignore aerobic training. In a tennis match you have 25 s rest between points and 90 s between games. If a player's aerobic fitness is low, it is difficult to recover between points and games and the player is more likely to tire at the end of a match. Another advantage of a strong aerobic base is that it provides a player with the endurance to have quality workouts. Therefore, because matches can last a long time, and to help players recover quickly between points, aerobic fitness is important as well.

One form of training that may help you achieve both aerobic and anaerobic benefits is interval training. Interval training involves periods of exercise interspersed with periods of rest. Emphasis can be placed on either aerobic or anaerobic fitness by manipulating training distance, training intervals, recovery intervals between exercise, and repetitions of the exercise. Tennis players should train intensely for 5–10-s bursts of activity, followed by 25–30-s rest periods. This closely mimics the demands of the sport. Keep in mind that training intensities may need to be modified several times, as there are many individual differences in players. Try

incorporating the following interval training programme into workouts:

Interval training programme for tennis

Components:
- A hitting partner or coach to feed balls. One coach can conduct this training sequence for a maximum of two players at once.
- One hour of work-out time. Each person will be drilled for 1 h. If you have a hitting partner, alternate every 30 min—you will need a 2-h time block.
- A minimum of 80 balls; 160 if a coach is working with two players.
- A stop watch.
- Realistic feeding. Remember the average distance covered per point is only 60 ft (18 m), therefore feeding continuously from corner to corner is unrealistic. Feeding rate should be approximately 1.3 s per feed. At that rate, feeding 15 balls should take around 20 s. The feeder can vary the placement of the balls based on the needs of the player. A waist-high ball basket will assist the coach with feeding. The player should not know how many balls will be fed during each point, thus simulating match situations.
- Targets. These designate hitting areas—cones, ball cans, boxes.
- The player is to hit balls at designated target areas.
- Except for warm-up, the player is to complete the entire series at maximum intensity.
- The feeder should follow a predetermined schedule of exercise/rest intervals spaced every 10–15 min, with 90-s breaks for the player to sit down, drink and towel off. The player must sit down.
- Heart rate monitor (optional). Heart rates should be taken before and after 90-s breaks to gauge work loads, intensity levels and recovery rates.

For a specific example of a work/rest interval schedule, see Table 9.1.

Speed and agility

Tennis is often described as a game of emergencies, because with every shot the opponent hits, a ball could have a different velocity, a different type and/or amount of spin, and it can be placed in many different parts of the court (Groppel & Roetert 1992). Tennis places acute demands on the ability of the player to move quickly

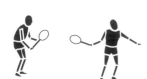

	Series 1 W/R*	Series 2 W/R	Series 3 W/R	Series 4 W/R	Series 5 W/R
1	2/15	7/20	8/20	3/25	7/20
2	6/15	2/20	8/20	3/25	5/20
3	3/15	2/20	8/20	3/25	1/20
4	10/15	16/20	8/20	3/25	10/20
5	8/15	4/20	8/20	3/25	6/20
6†	2/15	6/20	8/20	3/25	3/20
7	7/15	1/20	8/20	3/25	2/20
8	15/15	12/20	8/20	3/25	7/20
9	4/15	9/20	8/20	3/25	16/20
10	3/15	3/20	8/20	3/25	4/20

Table 9.1 Work (*W*)/rest (*R*) interval schedule. (From Loehr 1991.)

90-s sit-down break between each series. During the 90-s break, the feeder must pick up the balls and prepare for the next series. The feeder must also record heart rates before and after the break.
Note: Whenever possible, record the number of balls hit outside the designated target areas. The goal is to keep errors to a minimum during all sequences.
* '*W*' is the number of balls to feed (work) and '*R*' is the number of seconds of recovery (rest).
† Feeds 6 to 10 should occur in each series only after the player has served the ball.

in all directions, changing directions often, stopping and starting, while maintaining balance and control to hit the ball effectively. Therefore, speed and agility are important physical abilities in the sport of tennis. Good agility and speed allow the player to move around the court quickly and smoothly to position for a shot. In fact, Roetert *et al.* (1992) found that agility may be the most important physical ability (besides actual stroke technique) to influence the competitive level of young tennis players. Although some players are born with natural speed, all athletes can achieve good results by training their muscles and nervous systems. Training techniques should mimic the demands of the sport. Match analyses indicate that tennis requires approximately 300–500 bursts of energy over the course of a match (Deutsch *et al.* 1988). Therefore, quickness and agility drills should simulate the same movement patterns with many short sprints and direction changes (Fig. 9.10).

The mid-section

Introduction

We all know that it is important to have strong legs to help you get around the court as fast as possible, and that a strong arm is needed to provide a forceful swing. Equally important may be the muscles of the trunk. These muscles serve as an important link between the lower and upper body, as force is being transferred from the ground all the way up to the racket. Studies have shown that these muscles contract at a very high intensity while executing most tennis strokes. In addition, studies show that low back pain is fairly common in tennis players. Although in some players low back pain may be due to hereditary factors or disc degeneration, in most cases it can be avoided by performing appropriate strength and flexibility exercises.

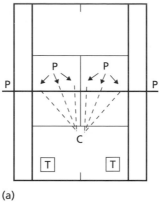

Purpose of the drill: Improves movement skills around the net.
Set-up: Player stands in the centre of one of the service boxes. Coach stands with basket of balls on the opposite side of the centre service line.
Action: Coach feeds balls rapidly from the opposite side service line, moving the player back and forth and side to side within the service box. If there is more than one player, the second player quickly jumps in when the first player misses.
Coaching tip: Split step to change direction quickly.

(a)

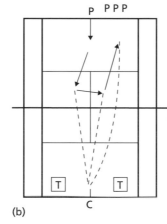

Purpose of the drill: Works on hitting a variety of shots as the player advances to the net to close out the point.
Set-up: Coach feeds balls rapidly from the opposite side baseline.
Action: Player shuffles along the baseline, then sprints forward to the centre service line, split steps and hits a forehand volley immediately followed by a backhand volley while closing in to the net. The final shot in the sequence is an overhead while backing up.
Coaching tip: Replicates common patterns of play.

Fig. 9.10 Tennis-specific drills to improve quickness on court. (a) Protect your turf. (b) Transition drill. P, Player; C, coach; T, target; →, path of player; ----, ball feed from coach.

(b)

Kinetic link

An important aspect of the sport of tennis is the ability to exert muscular force at a high speed. The components of muscular strength and power allow a player to run on the court and also to hit the ball with maximum impact. Hitting with power means that the player must optimize the action between the larger body parts to hit with high velocity and still allow the upper limb to maintain good control over the racket. A successive summation of forces is integral to successful performance of the tennis strokes. Transferring a ground reaction force up through the legs, hips, trunk and arm is critical in virtually all strokes. The timing of the transfer of these forces is crucial. When this movement is inefficient, it may not only cause an error, but also create the potential for injury. The muscles of the trunk are a vital link in the body's kinetic chain. Because the body is interconnected from top to bottom through the muscular system, the trunk muscles are as important as the arms and legs in the consideration of physical training.

Flexion and extension

Because a player must use abdominal muscles to some extent in all tennis strokes, it is important to strengthen these muscles to enhance performance and prevent injury. However, you should bring the low back strength up to a similar level to avoid an imbalance that could result in injury. Abdominal and low back strength should be relatively equal. A study of elite level junior tennis players compared abdominal strength to low back strength with a Cybex 6000 isokinetic dynamometer. Strength ratios revealed that these top-ranked players had significantly more strength in the abdominal musculature than in the low back muscles (Roetert *et al.* 1996). This is in contrast to the average population whose low back strength was found to be greater than the abdominal strength. By catching these weaknesses and imbalances early, exercise programmes can be designed to help reduce back injuries and pain.

Rotation

The ability to develop power in tennis is often a function of how well the upper and lower body are connected (Roetert *et al.* 1997). Rotation of the trunk is crucial to developing power in tennis players' groundstrokes, as well as serves. Strokes become more effective as the body is turned faster and with more control. Strengthening the muscles that rotate the trunk and increasing their range of motion assist in producing effective and efficient strokes. More range of motion means developing force over a longer period of time. This helps to develop greater impact forces against the ball.

Players appear to be hitting more often with an open stance and generating more forces as they turn. The rotational forces and involvement of the trunk in the open-stance forehand are greater than in the classic forehand of 30 years ago. Particularly, players step around the backhand to hit the 'inside-out' forehand more often. The idea of hitting the forehand with a large amount of upper body torque is to develop greater angular momentum, the result of which is a harder-hit ball.

The key muscles responsible for rapid trunk rotation are the internal and external obliques. They act as trunk rotators and help the rectus abdominus with trunk flexion.

Injury prevention

Preventing injuries to the lower back and trunk generally involves both flexibility and strengthening exercise. As mentioned previously, tennis players tend to have stronger abdominal musculature as

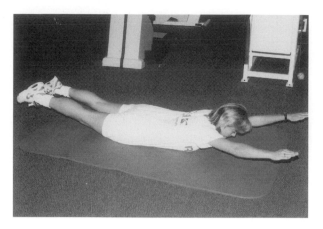

Fig. 9.11 Superman exercise.

compared to the strength of the muscles in the lower back. Because of this, it is important that exercises be performed to balance this relationship between the abdominals and low back musculature. Emphasizing exercises that will increase strength in the low back musculature, as well as the muscles that rotate and stabilize the spine are currently recommended. A low resistance (typically bodyweight or use of a 2–3-kg medicine ball) and high repetition format is recommended with these exercises as well. Due to the trunk muscles' integral role in all tennis specific movement patterns, failure to promote endurance through a repetitive programme of exercise could result in injury or suboptimal performance. Examples of exercises that would serve to promote balance and improve performance for the tennis player are listed below.

Superman exercise (Fig. 9.11)

The player lies on his or her stomach with arms and legs extended. Both arms and legs are simultaneously lifted or extended, holding for a count of 1–5 s. A variation of this exercise includes raising the left arm and right leg together, then switching to the right arm and left leg. By alternating the arm/leg combination that is raised, the muscles of the trunk are forced to stabilize the spine. This exercise primarily works the erector spinae muscles, and the gluteals.

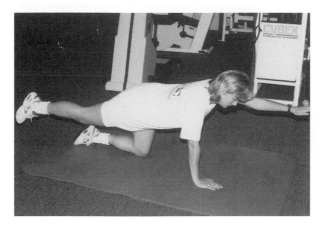

Fig. 9.12 Cat exercise.

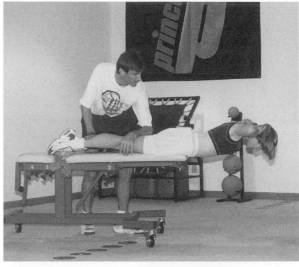

(a)

Cat exercise (Fig. 9.12)

The player begins this exercise in a quadruped position (on hands and knees). Keeping the back as firm as possible, by tightening the abdominals and squeezing the buttocks, raise the left arm and right leg in an alternating fashion. Slowly return the arm/leg pair to the starting position, then switch to raise the right arm and left leg. Small weights can be placed in the hands and around the ankles to increase the intensity of this exercise.

Back extensions (Fig. 9.13)

With a partner, the player lies on his or her stomach with the edge of a supportive surface at approximately waist level. The player begins bent at a 30–60° angle at the waist (the head would be pointing toward the ground). With the partner supporting the player's legs, the player extends the back to the neutral position (Fig. 9.13a), then slowly returns to the starting position. The arms can be raised and hands intertwined behind the head to add resistance. A 2–3-kg medicine ball can also be held by the player to add resistance. Another variation of this back extension exercise can be performed without the assistance of a partner (Fig. 9.13b). The legs are straightened together while the upper body supports the player's bodyweight. The legs are then slowly lowered to the starting position and the exercise is repeated.

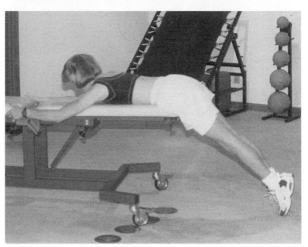

(b)

Fig. 9.13 Back extensions: (a) with partner; (b) without partner.

Machine exercises for the trunk

Both the back extension and rotary torso machine can be used by tennis players to promote lower back strength, and to work the oblique musculature, respectively. These machines are pictured in Figs 9.14 and 9.15.

Even though many tennis players have an imbalance in their trunk musculature, abdominal exercises are recommended as a complement to the other exercises applied to support the spine.

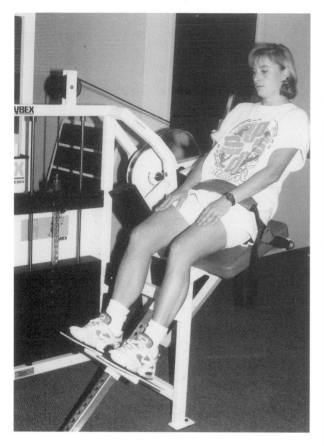

Fig. 9.14 Back extension machine exercise for the trunk.

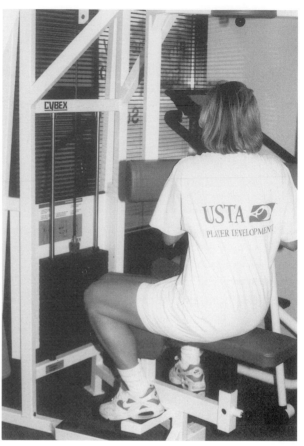

Fig. 9.15 Rotary torso machine exercise for the trunk.

Abdominal crunch exercise (Fig. 9.16)

The player lies on his or her back with feet raised and placed on a bench or box. The hands are placed behind the head or crossed over the chest. The hands should not pull the head forward but merely support the head and neck. The player curls up until the shoulder blades are no longer touching the ground. It is not necessary to curl up all the way until the chest touches the thighs, because the abdominals are most active early in the exercise.

Oblique exercise

Because tennis involves an excessive amount of repetitive rotation, it is important to train the oblique abdominal muscles. Figure 9.17 shows a crossover crunch, where the player lies on his or her back with

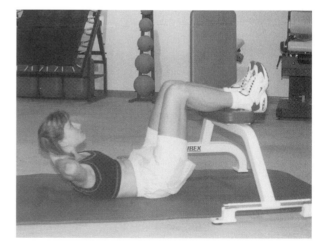

Fig. 9.16 Abdominal crunch exercise.

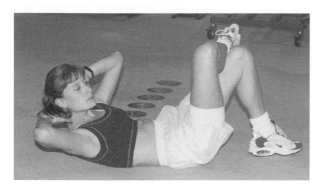

Fig. 9.17 Oblique exercise—crossover crunch.

one knee bent and foot flat on the floor. The opposite knee is bent so the heel rests on the other knee. The hands are held behind the head, but the hands are not used to pull the head forward. The upper body is then curled so the elbow on the opposite side of the elevated knee moves toward the knee in a diagonal

direction. This movement is repeated to the opposite direction as well. A variation of this diagonal sit-up can be performed using a 2–3-kg medicine ball (Fig. 9.18). The arms and trunk are brought up in a diagonal direction as pictured. These exercises stress the rotational component inherent in all tennis strokes.

Medicine ball exercises

Several additional medicine ball exercises can be used to strengthen the oblique musculature for tennis players. These exercises not only strengthen the required muscles, but also encourage trunk rotation. Figure 9.19 shows the partner backhand medicine ball toss. Standing approximately 15 ft (4.5 m) apart and using a 3–4-kg medicine ball, each player executes a simulated forehand or backhand stroke throwing the ball on a diagonal (like a cross-court tennis stroke) to a partner. The lower extremities and trunk produce identical movements simulating the rotation and footwork patterns of a tennis stroke. Again, sets of 30–50 repetitions are used to promote endurance of these muscles.

In addition to strengthening, proper flexibility is of the utmost importance in preventing back injuries in tennis players. Players with tight hamstrings place greater stress on the spine because the tight hamstrings limit rotation of the pelvis and force the spine to incur greater arcs of movement during aggressive sport-specific movements. Therefore, increasing hamstring flexibility will allow a more normal relationship of pelvis and spinal movement. Particular

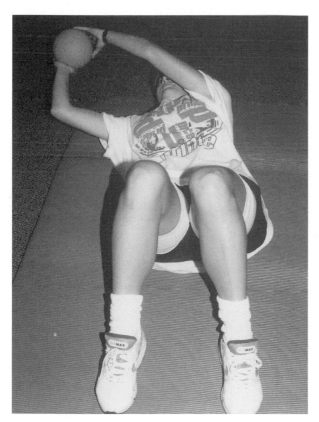

Fig. 9.18 Oblique exercise with medicine ball.

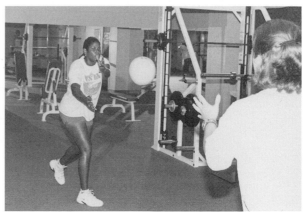

Fig. 9.19 Partner backhand medicine ball exercise.

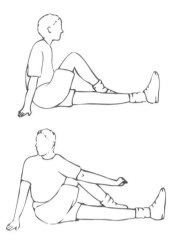
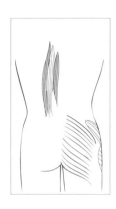

Place the right foot on the outside of the left knee.
Bring the left arm around the right knee, resting the
elbow above the outside of the right knee. Slowly turn
the head and upper body to the right. You'll end up
looking over your right shoulder.

Fig. 9.20 Flexibility exercise—spinal twist stretch.

stretches to emphasize for the tennis player to prevent
back injuries are:
• knee to chest stretch—see section on lower body,
above (Fig. 9.1);
• hamstring stretches—see section on lower body,
above (Figs 9.2 and 9.3);
• spinal twist stretch (Fig. 9.20).

Upper body

Introduction

The upper extremity in tennis has traditionally
been the most common site of overuse injuries. The
repetitive nature of the tennis-specific movement
patterns, as well as the explosive speed at which
they are carried out, require precise acceleration of
the arm to produce power and timely deceleration
of the arm to prevent injury. Additionally, research on
the upper extremity of tennis players clearly shows
muscular (Ellenbecker 1992) and skeletal (Priest &
Nagel 1976) adaptations or changes from the repeated
stresses playing tennis imparts to the human body.
A training programme that emphasizes proper
flexibility and muscular balance, as well as strength
and endurance, is required to prevent injury and
optimize performance.

Flexibility

Flexibility patterns of the upper extremity in highly
skilled tennis players have been extensively studied
(Ellenbecker *et al.* 1996). This research consistently
shows that shoulder internal rotation (Fig. 9.21)
on the dominant racket-playing arm is tighter than
the corresponding non-dominant side. Not only is
shoulder internal rotation limited on the dominant
side in elite-level tennis players, but this limitation
begins in players as young as 11–12 years of age,
and becomes progressively more limited (tighter) as
players age and continue to play competitive tennis
(Kibler *et al.* 1996).

Due to the findings of a consistent pattern of
limited shoulder internal rotation, current strategies
in rehabilitation and preventative conditioning utilize
stretches for the muscles and shoulder joint capsule
(posterior) that are responsible for limiting this important motion. Figure 9.22 shows the recommended
stretches for the shoulder in the tennis player that
address the tight areas and movement patterns. These
stretches should be performed consistent with the
general flexibility recommendations outlined in the
section on lower body.

One stretch that is not recommended is the anterior
(front) shoulder stretch. This stretch involves grasping
the fence or object behind the body and rotating
the body forward while keeping the hand and
arm fixed behind you. This stretch was previously
recommended to prevent tightness in the front of the

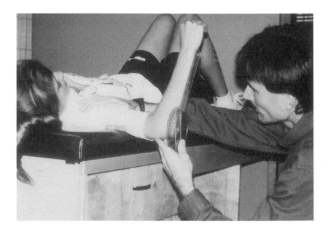

Fig. 9.21 Player having internal rotation measured with a
goniometer with scapular stabilization.

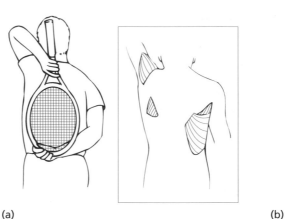

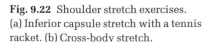

Fig. 9.22 Shoulder stretch exercises.
(a) Inferior capsule stretch with a tennis
racket. (b) Cross-body stretch.　　(a)

(b)

shoulder and increase shoulder external rotation.
Advances in research and a better understanding
of how the shoulder functions in overhead athletes
has identified that many of these overhead athletes
have too much flexibility (looseness) in the front of
the shoulder, which can lead to instability of the
shoulder and potentially injury. Therefore, this type
of stretching, with the arms behind the body as
mentioned above, or with a partner, is no longer
recommended for most tennis players.

In addition to stretches for the shoulder, current
preventative conditioning programmes also recommend stretches for the elbow, forearm and wrist.
Research on elite level tennis players has shown
that the dominant (racket-side) elbow does not fully
straighten. The muscles on the undersurface of the
forearm (flexors and pronators) are responsible for
stabilizing the elbow and are very active during
tennis strokes, and become tight with repetitive
tennis play. Tightness in these muscles limits motion
at the elbow and wrist and can place the player at
risk for development of elbow and wrist injury. The
stretches shown in Fig. 9.23 are used to address
the muscles in the elbow, forearm, wrist and hand.
These stretches should be performed with the elbow
as straight as possible to increase the effectiveness of
the stretch.

Muscular balance

One of the most important aspects in both rehabilitation and preventative conditioning programmes for
any athlete is muscular balance. Muscular imbalances

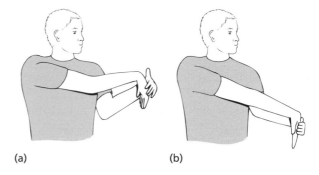

(a)　　　　　　　　　(b)

Fig. 9.23 Elbow, forearm and wrist stretches.

occur in the upper extremity of the tennis player
from selective activation of certain groups of muscles
required to generate power for serving and other
tennis-specific movement patterns. One of the
primary muscular imbalances found in the tennis
player is in the shoulder. Extensive research using
isokinetic machinery to measure strength in elite
tennis players has identified muscular imbalances
between the shoulder internal and external rotators on
the dominant, tennis-playing extremity (Ellenbecker
1992, 1995). The muscles that internally rotate the
shoulder (pectoralis major, lattisimus dorsi and
subscapularis) become significantly stronger on
the dominant arm from serving, hitting forehands,
and other tennis movements. These large, powerful
internal rotator muscles become so strong and
dominant that an imbalance occurs between these
muscles and their matching counterparts, the
external rotators.

The external rotators (infraspinatus and teres minor) primarily function to stabilize the humeral head (ball) in the glenoid (socket) and to decelerate the shoulder during the follow-through phase of the tennis serve following ball contact. In contrast to the very large internal rotator muscles, the external rotator muscles that perform these vital stabilizing functions are very small, and are located in the back of the shoulder. Therefore, a muscular imbalance occurs between the muscles in the front of the shoulder (internal rotators), and the muscles in the back of the shoulder (external rotators). The use of isokinetic machines in research has shown that the normal strength relationship between these important muscle groups is 3 : 2 with the internal rotators being the '3' and the external rotators being the '2'. However, in elite level tennis players, this relationship becomes more of a 2 : 1 relationship where the internal rotators become twice as strong as the external rotators. This type of muscular imbalance can lead to injury, and suboptimal performance.

Due to the presence of muscular imbalances in the tennis player, current strategies for performance enhancement and injury prevention/rehabilitation focus on balancing these muscular imbalances. In the next section on muscular strengthening, much emphasis is placed on the external rotators and muscles of the upper back which are, in most cases, underdeveloped in the tennis player, and do not appear to be strengthened simply from repetitive tennis play. The use of a supplemental set of exercises for the upper back and shoulder region is imperative to promote muscular balance and prevent injury.

Muscular strength and endurance

Several important concepts must be considered when implementing a programme to enhance strength and endurance in the upper extremity of tennis players. These concepts are specificity, muscular balance, and the kinetic link or kinetic chain. The specificity principle implies that conditioning and rehabilitation programming should specifically match the inherent demands of the sport in which the athlete is involved. As stated earlier in this chapter, tennis demands anaerobic bursts of energy and maximal level performances that must be repeatedly executed in an endurance or aerobic type of framework over the course of a tennis match or practice session that often lasts several hours. Therefore, strengthening exercises for tennis players must include a balance between muscular strength and endurance. Currently, most sport scientists and medical professionals recommend a lower resistance level and higher repetition format. Resistance training with up to three sets of 12–15 repetitions are commonly applied to foster local muscular endurance.

With specific reference to the upper extremity, muscular endurance is of paramount importance. Previous research conducted by these authors showed that the shoulder external rotators fatigued faster than the internal rotators in elite junior tennis players using a high-speed fatigue protocol on an isokinetic machine. This further exemplifies the importance of supplemental strength programming for the external rotators, since they are weaker and fatigue faster than the internal rotators of the shoulder.

The kinetic link principle, as described earlier in this chapter, is an important concept to apply, when dealing with conditioning of the upper extremity in tennis players. Inclusion of the upper back and scapular (shoulder blade) musculature in the training programmes of tennis players is required, due to the function of the shoulder as an important connection between the power generation from the lower body and trunk into the upper arm and, ultimately, the racket. Failure to include the upper back and scapular musculature in training programmes for the shoulder and elbow would prevent optimal transfer and application of the kinetic link system.

Evaluation of the upper back and shoulder region of elite tennis players reveals several important findings; the first is that the shoulder of the dominant racket arm is often lower than the non-dominant side. Additionally, the shoulder blade is often protracted or further away from the spine on the racket side. Kibler (1991) has devised a test called the lateral scapular slide test, to measure the position of the scapula. Kibler has determined that on healthy uninjured persons, less than a 1-cm difference should exist between sides. In tennis players, due to the repetitive stresses and eccentric loads placed on the muscles and structures in the back of the shoulder and scapular region, scapular position often approaches or mimics the scapular position seen in persons with shoulder dysfunction. The consistent finding of postural adaptations in tennis players has led to the develop-ment of the term 'tennis shoulder' (Priest & Nagel

1976). While this response is, in many cases, thought to be merely a response to the eccentric stresses and loads applied to the arm, exercises to enhance the muscular stabilization of this area are an important part of a comprehensive programme for tennis players and provides an example of how knowledge of the kinetic link system can be applied in conditioning programmes.

In addition to the development of strength and endurance in the shoulder and upper back, it is necessary that the tennis player have enhanced strength and endurance of the musculature that crosses the elbow, forearm and wrist. Research using electromyography (EMG) demonstrates the consistently high activation levels in the wrist extensor muscles during nearly all phases of tennis strokes. Research has also shown that lesser skilled players and players with tennis elbow have higher activation levels in the forearm and wrist musculature and for longer durations than more accomplished, healthy tennis players. Isokinetic testing of the wrist flexors and extensors and forearm pronators and supinators has shown 20–30% greater strength on the dominant arm for the pronators, flexors and extensors (Ellenbecker 1995). Inclusion of wrist and forearm strengthening and endurance exercise is an important part of a tennis player's programme, due to the repeated reliance and activation of these important muscles with tennis play.

Summarizing the principles of specificity, muscular balance and the kinetic link has led to the development of a recommended set of exercises for the upper extremity of the tennis player. For the purpose of this chapter, the exercises will be broken down into several groups. In general, these exercises can be initiated using a resistance level that allows the player to perform 12–15 repetitions per set without pain or muscular substitution (breaking form). Begin, in most cases, with two sets of each exercise, progressing to three to four sets, depending on player fitness level and the amount of time/emphasis placed upon strengthening, if the player is following a periodized training programme.

Recommended exercises

Rotator cuff exercises (Fig. 9.24)

Specific instructions: these exercises work the rotator cuff, which is a group of four muscles (supraspinatus,

infraspinatus, teres minor and subscapularis) that stabilize the shoulder joint. Consistent with the kinetic link principle, these exercises also work the muscles that stabilize the scapula (rhomboids, trapezius and serratus anterior). Very small weights are used with these exercises, because even the strongest athletes have very small and weak rotator cuff musculature. In most cases, a 0.5–1.5-kg weight is plenty of resistance for proper execution of these exercises.

Elastic tubing shoulder exercises (Fig. 9.25)

Specific instructions: elastic tubing serves as an excellent form of resistance for the tennis player and can easily be incorporated while travelling or training at multiple sites. For most players, medium resistance (blue—Theraband) is recommended.

• For exercising the external rotators in the neutral (arm at side) position (Fig. 9.25a), a towel is placed under the armpit to slightly bring the arm away from the side and ensure that the arm remains in that position during the exercise. The shoulder is then externally rotated away from the stomach until it is pointing directly in front of the player. The arm is then slowly brought back to the starting position, fighting the resistance of the tubing. The opposite hand is placed under the exercising arm's elbow, to ensure that the shoulder only rotates and does not substitute the movement pattern.

• To exercise in the 90° abducted position (Fig. 9.25b), the opposite arm is used to support the shoulder in the scapular plane (position just in front of the body on a 30° diagonal). The player is instructed to bring the back of the hand backward, externally rotating the shoulder until the arm is vertical and then, in a controlled manner, return the arm to the starting position that is pictured. Training the shoulder external rotators in this position more closely simulates the position the muscles work during the serving motion.

Scapula/upper back exercises

Seated row. This exercise can be performed using a variable resistance machine (Fig. 9.26) or using rubber tubing while sitting on the floor with the knees slightly bent. The primary benefit is to strengthen the muscles that stabilize the shoulder blade (scapula). While the arms are brought back as pictured, the player

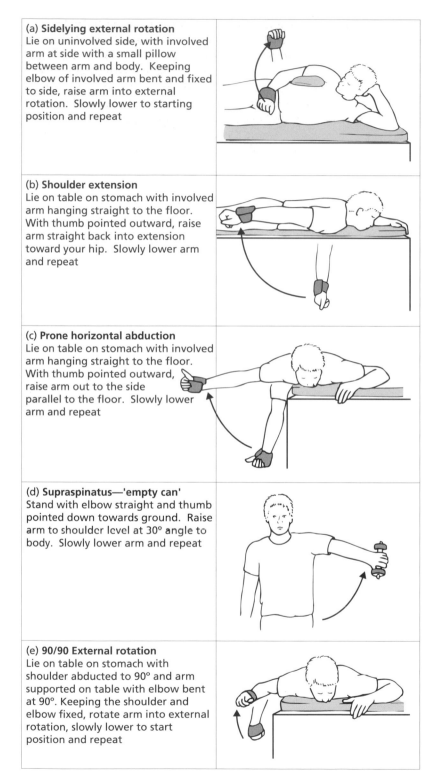

(a) **Sidelying external rotation**
Lie on uninvolved side, with involved arm at side with a small pillow between arm and body. Keeping elbow of involved arm bent and fixed to side, raise arm into external rotation. Slowly lower to starting position and repeat

(b) **Shoulder extension**
Lie on table on stomach with involved arm hanging straight to the floor. With thumb pointed outward, raise arm straight back into extension toward your hip. Slowly lower arm and repeat

(c) **Prone horizontal abduction**
Lie on table on stomach with involved arm hanging straight to the floor. With thumb pointed outward, raise arm out to the side parallel to the floor. Slowly lower arm and repeat

(d) **Supraspinatus—'empty can'**
Stand with elbow straight and thumb pointed down towards ground. Raise arm to shoulder level at 30° angle to body. Slowly lower arm and repeat

(e) **90/90 External rotation**
Lie on table on stomach with shoulder abducted to 90° and arm supported on table with elbow bent at 90°. Keeping the shoulder and elbow fixed, rotate arm into external rotation, slowly lower to start position and repeat

Fig. 9.24 Rotator cuff exercises.

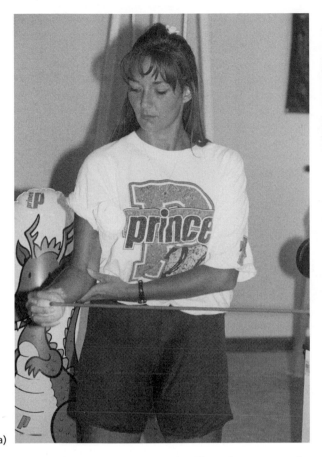 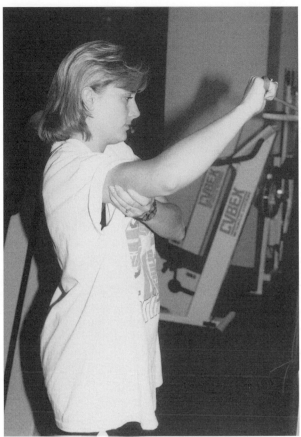

(a) (b)

Fig. 9.25 (a) External rotation with rubber tubing in neutral position. (b) External rotation with rubber tubing in 90° abducted position.

is instructed to squeeze the shoulder blades together. A slow return to the starting position is emphasized, due to these muscles' important eccentric action during tennis play.

Upright row. Using a dumb-bell and supportive surface, this one-sided or unilateral rowing exercise works similar muscles used in the above exercise, but at a different length and movement pattern. Care must be taken to only bring the elbow back even with the body as shown in Fig. 9.27, as further backward movement may stress the front of the shoulder. For side-to-side balance purposes, these exercises should be performed by both the racket and non-racket sides.

Lat. pull-down. The lattisimus dorsi is a very large muscle that spans the lower and mid-back. It provides

stability for the trunk, and also is an internal rotator of the shoulder. Most players know how to execute a Lat. pull-down exercise, but often pull the bar back behind the neck. For tennis players and overhead athletes in general, we recommend pulling the bar to the front of the chest near the sternum. This places less stress on the front of the shoulder.

Shoulder shrug. In a standing position, this exercise is performed with the player shrugging the shoulders up towards the ears with dumb-bells or rubber tubing in the hands. In addition to shrugging the shoulders upward, it is recommended that the shoulders then be moved backward, squeezing the shoulder blades together. Then the shoulders are relaxed back to the resting position. A forward roll of the shoulders is not generally recommended because that would

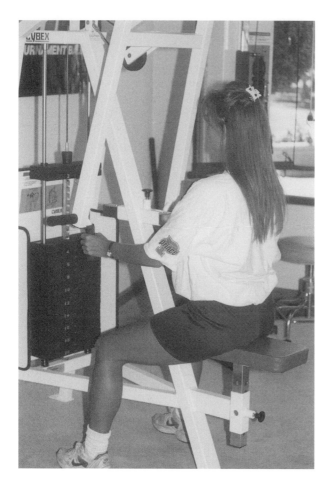

Fig. 9.26 Seated row exercise.

recruit muscles that are already overdeveloped in most tennis players.

Shoulder press. The shoulder press exercise (Fig. 9.28) can be performed using dumb-bells as pictured, a barbell, medicine ball, or using a chest press machine. The key movement to emphasize in the tennis player is the pressing out away from the body to as far as the hands can reach. This movement actually 'rounds' the shoulder blades and strengthens a very important muscle (serratus anterior). In most players, we recommend that the arms be brought down only half way to the chest (so the elbows stay in front of the body). This reduces strain on the front of the shoulder and prevents injury or aggravation. This exercise also works the triceps, and pectoral muscles as well.

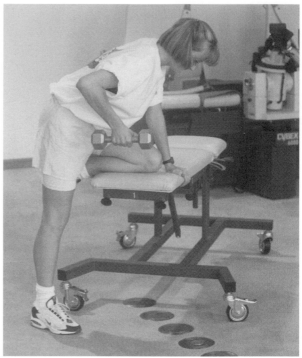

Fig. 9.27 Upright row exercise.

Medicine ball exercises. The use of a 2–3-kg medicine ball can be a beneficial addition to a tennis player's upper extremity strengthening programme. Typical patterns with the medicine ball are a chest pass, similar to the one used in basketball, as well as an overhead 'soccer throw in' type pass.

Additional exercises. Bicep and tricep curls are also recommended to stabilize the shoulder and elbow.

Wrist and forearm exercises. See Fig. 9.29.

Fig. 9.29 (*opposite*) Forearm and wrist strengthening exercises. (a) Wrist curl extension. Sit in a chair with the elbow flexed and forearm resting on a table or over the knee with the wrist and hand hanging over the edge. The hand is turned so the palm is down. Stabilize the forearm with the opposite hand and slowly curl the wrist and hand upward. Be sure to move only at the wrist, not at the elbow. Raise hand slowly, hold for a count and slowly lower weight. Repeat. (b) Wrist curl flexion. As in (a) but with the hand turned so the palm is up. (*continued p. 122*)

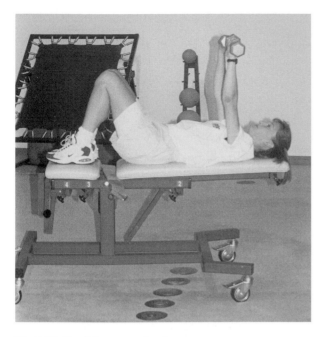

Fig. 9.28 Shoulder press exercise.

Addendum: Exercise intensity, exercise prescription and the RM system

Increases in strength and maximal power of the muscles are brought about through exercise programmes involving very high opposing force (also termed 'resistance') by means of free weights, exercise machines or gravity acting on the body. Such high opposing force would limit the number of repetitions that can be performed to exhaustion in an exercise 'set' to 20 or fewer and, therefore, a 'set' duration of less than 30 s. Exercise programmes based on higher repetitions per set (e.g. 30–50 repetitions before exhaustion) develop local anaerobic endurance but are not conducive to strength and maximal power development.

Strength training programmes around the world are routinely based on a system of exercise to a 'Repetition Maximum' (RM) as presented over 50 years ago by Thomas L. De Lorme (De Lorme 1945).

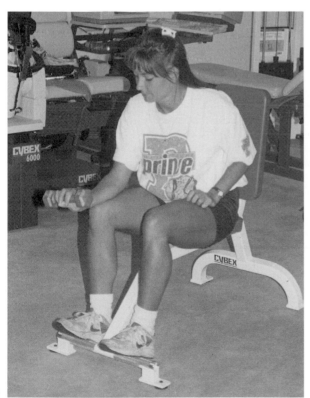

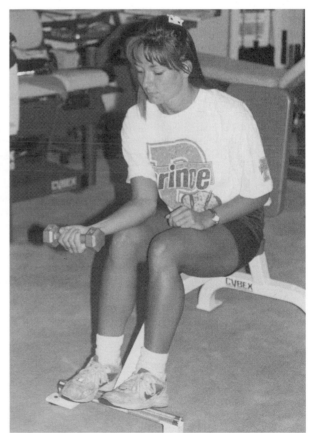

(a)

(b)

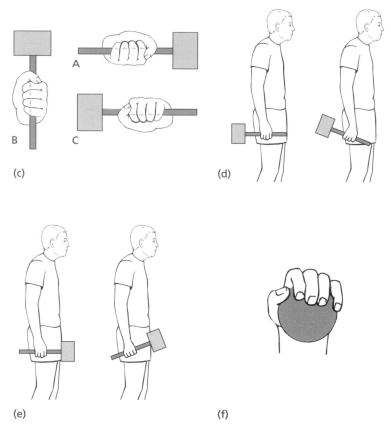

(c)

(d)

(e)

(f)

Fig. 9.29 (*cont'd*) (c) Forearm rotation (pronation/supination). Sit in a chair with elbow flexed and forearm resting on a table or your knee with the wrist and hand hanging over the edge. Using a dumb-bell with weight at only one end (i.e.) a hammer, begin the exercise with the palm-up position (A). Slowly raise the weight by rotating your forearm and wrist to the upright position (B). Hold for a count and slowly return to the starting position (A). When finished with the recommended number of repetitions of this exercise, begin with the exercises again in the palm-down position (C). Slowly raise the weight by rotating your forearm and wrist to the upright position (B). (d) Ulnar deviation. In a standing position with your arm at your side, grasp a dumb-bell with weight on only one end. The weighted end should be behind your exercising hand. With your forearm in the neutral position (thumb pointing straight ahead of you), slowly raise and lower the weight through a comfortable range of motion. All the movement should occur at your wrist with *no* elbow or shoulder joint movement. You will not be able to exercise through a very large arc of movement. *Repeat.* (e) Radial deviation. In the standing position with your arm at your side, grasp a dumb-bell with weight on only one end. The weighted end should be in front in the neutral position (thumb pointing straight ahead of you), slowly raise and lower the weight through a comfortable range of motion. All the movement should occur at your wrist with *no* elbow or shoulder joint movement. You will not be able to exercise through a very large arc of movement. *Repeat.* (f) Grip strengthening. Begin with elbow bent at 90° at your side. Place a tennis ball or putty in the palm of your hand. Squeeze firmly, hold for 3–5 s. Release pressure. Repeat until fatigue occurs. As pain allows, progress to performing this exercise with the elbow straight.

Every time the athlete performs a particular exercise, the bout (or 'set') is performed for the maximum number of repetitions possible (Repetition Maximum or RM) and this number is recorded along with the mass lifted or the opposing force recorded on an exercise machine. Repeated testing at increasingly higher opposing force will eventually lead to the determination of a '1 RM', a set in which the athlete can perform the movement only one time. In the RM system, the mass lifted or the opposing force recorded as the 1 RM is accepted as the athlete's 'strength' for the particular movement at the particular point in time in the training programme.

The weekly and daily programmes and the predicted RM for each set are then based on the curvilinear relationship between the mass lifted (or resistance provided) and the number of repetitions before exhaustion. This is determined for each muscle group and each individual exercise. The exercise sets can be identified as light, medium and heavy as follows:

Light: 12–15 RM
Medium: 7–10 RM
Heavy: 3–5 RM

The terms light, medium and heavy are relative terms for the exercise intensity in that the exercise performed in each of the three categories is both highly intense and stressful. The number of sets for a particular exercise and the intensity of each set as determined by the predicted RM for light, medium and heavy are then prescribed for each muscle group as based on the point in time in the competitive season, the physical condition of the player, and consideration of both physiological and psychological considerations (Kraemer & Häkkinen 2002). Varying the intensity among light, medium and heavy ('variation') is employed as much for diversion and psychological reasons as for the desired physiological adaptations of the musculature. Typically, the tennis player beginning a strength training programme performs one set of each exercise in a particular exercise session and, after a few weeks, advances to two sets and, eventually, three sets. Strength training should take place at least three times a week but the number of sessions and the time involved will vary according to the player's yearly competitive schedule.

The principal adaptation to strength exercise by the tennis player's musculature is an increase in size (hypertrophy) of the type II (fast-twitch) muscle cells. The total increase in size of the muscle then presents the possibility for the expression of greater force and power when making contact with the ball. As the player's strength for a particular movement increases, the number of repetitions before exhaustion (RM) increases and the exercise prescription is altered so as to present a higher resistance designed to result in the desired RM within the light, medium and heavy ranges.

References

De Lorme, T.L. (1945) Restoration of muscle power by heavy resistance exercises. *Journal of Bone and Joint Surgery* **27**, 645–667.

Deutsch, E., Deutsch, S.L. & Douglas, P.S. (1988) Exercise training for competitive tennis. *Clinics in Sports Medicine* **7**, 417–427.

Ellenbecker, T.S. (1992) Shoulder internal and external rotation strength and range of motion of highly skilled junior tennis players. *Isokinetics and Exercise Science* **2**, 1–8.

Ellenbecker, T.S. (1995) Rehabilitation of shoulder and elbow injuries in tennis players. *Clinics in Sports Medicine* **14** (1), 87–109.

Ellenbecker, T.S. & Roetert, E.P. (1995) Concentric isokinetic quadricep and hamstring strength in elite junior tennis players. *Isokinetics and Exercise Science* **5**, 3–6.

Ellenbecker, T.S., Roetert, E.P., Piorkowski, P.A. & Schulz, D.A. (1996) Glenohumeral joint internal and external rotation range of motion in elite junior tennis players. *Journal of Orthopaedic and Sports Physical Therapy* **24** (6), 336–341.

Groppel, J.L. & Roetert. E.P. (1992) Applied physiology of tennis. *Sports Medicine* **14** (4), 260–268.

Kibler, W.B. (1991) Role of the scapula in the overhead throwing motion. *Contemporary Orthopaedics* **22**, 525–532.

Kibler, W.B., Chandler, T.J., Livingston, B.P. & Roetert, E.P. (1996) Shoulder range of motion in elite tennis players. *American Journal of Sports Medicine* **24** (3), 279–285.

Kraemer, W.J. & Häkkinen, K. (eds) (2002) *Strength Training for Sport*. Blackwell Science Ltd, Oxford.

Loehr, J. (1991) Practice with playing intensity for peak performance. In: Roetert, P., ed. *USTA Sport Science for Tennis Newsletter*, Spring.

Priest, J.D. & Nagel, D.A. (1976) Tennis shoulder. *American Journal of Sports Medicine* **4**, 28–42.

Roetert, E.P. (1996) Why tennis is the sport for all ages. *Tennis*, August, 60–61.

Roetert, E.P., Garrett, G.E., Brown, S.W. & Camaione, D.N. (1992) Performance profiles of nationally ranked junior tennis players. *Journal of Applied Sport Science Research* **6** (4), 225–231.

Roetert, E.P., Piorkowski, P.A., Woods, R.W. & Brown, S.W. (1995) Establishing percentiles for junior tennis players based on physical fitness testing results. *Clinics in Sports Medicine* **14** (1), 1–21.

Roetert, E.P., McCormick, T.J., Brown, S.W. & Ellenbecker, T.S. (1996) Relationship between isokinetic and functional trunk strength in elite junior tennis players. *Isokinetics and Exercise Science* **6**, 15–20.

Roetert, E.P., Ellenbecker, T.S., Chu, D.A. & Bugg, B.S. (1997) Tennis-specific shoulder and trunk strengthening. *Strength and Conditioning* **19** (3), 31–39.

Sobel, J., Ellenbecker, T.S. & Roetert, E.P. (1995) Flexibility training for tennis. *Strength and Conditioning*, December, 43–50.

Chapter 10

Pre-participation profiling for tennis

Introduction

Traditionally, the goals of a sports participation fitness programme have been to prepare the athlete for safe participation in sports, to uncover any life-threatening conditions the athlete may have and to satisfy legal requirements set forth by various governing bodies (Kibler 1990). This chapter on pre-participation profiling for tennis players will specifically focus on the physiological aspects of assessment for the purpose of developing baseline information to help strengthen weaknesses and lessen the risk of injury. The main purposes, as outlined by Groppel and Roetert (1992), are to assess fitness levels, develop normative data and establish the basis for longitudinal tracking. In this case, the normative data will provide a base for tennis-specific conditioning. From the test results, players and coaches can determine which fitness areas need to be improved for players on an individual basis. Specific training programmes can then be designed based on the player's fitness testing results. Practically, the goals are to enhance a player's performance, reduce the risk of injury and design an appropriate training programme so that the athlete's playing career can be as long as possible.

Goals of testing

Performance enhancement

Because tennis has become a sport with year-round involvement, superior fitness and preparation is required. Every player wants to have that extra step of footspeed, hit more powerful shots with less effort, increase the speed of his or her serve and handle the power of a stronger opponent. In addition, it is great to last through a long match and still come back fresh the next day. Research indicates that players achieve the best results when their training activities replicate the actual demands of the sport (Groppel & Roetert 1992). Practice sessions should challenge the same energy systems, muscle groups and movement patterns stressed in competitive play. Testing the physiological variables of flexibility, strength, power, aerobic endurance and speed and agility will provide a baseline for designing appropriate training programmes. Proper flexibility will assist in reaching those wide shots, making quick direction changes and bending for low volleys. Another important aspect of the sport of tennis is the ability to exert muscular force at a high speed. Muscular strength and power allow you to run around the court, as well as to swing your racket forcefully. To be able to last those long matches, you want to make sure you have good aerobic endurance. However, throughout a match, you will also be asked to sprint around the court in every conceivable direction. Therefore, having excellent speed and agility is critical.

Injury prevention

Another important reason to utilize fitness testing with tennis players is to prevent injuries. Research using elite tennis players has consistently identified musculoskeletal adaptations from repetitive tennis play. An example of these adaptations include muscular imbalances in the shoulder and trunk (Ellenbecker 1991, 1992, 1995; Chandler et al. 1992; Roetert et al. 1996; Ellenbecker & Roetert 1999), as well as postural changes such as depression of the dominant shoulder (Priest & Nagel 1976). One of the most effective ways of monitoring the progression of these and other musculoskeletal adaptations is with the use of the testing protocol developed by the United States Tennis Association (USTA) Sport Science Committee outlined in this chapter.

In addition to the musculoskeletal tests described that clearly aim to prevent injury, the fitness tests and general physiological testing includes injury prevention aspects as well as the obvious performance enhancement benefits. Measuring a player's aerobic capacity may initially seem like a test geared only towards performance enhancement, but in the big picture has injury prevention goals as well. For example, if a player has a poor aerobic capacity, he or she will recover slower between points and have a greater potential to fatigue, thus, footwork and optimal biomechanics may be jeopardized and ultimately lead to a shoulder or elbow injury, due to improper positioning, kinetic link energy transfer, and early fatigue.

The use of a comprehensively developed testing programme with specific tests for tennis players will allow sports scientists and coaches to track and monitor all aspects of musculoskeletal and physiological function, and facilitate the design of programmes for both preventative conditioning and performance enhancement.

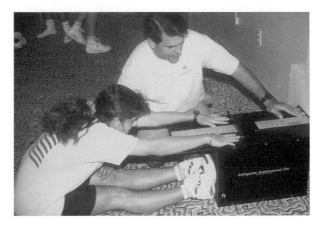

Fig. 10.1 Sit and reach exercise.

Fitness-testing protocol

What follows is a fitness testing protocol designed specifically for top-level junior tennis players by the USTA Sport Science Committee (Roetert *et al.* 1995). These tests emphasize critical elements necessary for optimal performance and the prevention of common tennis injuries. The starting positions and performance parameters required for performing these tests are outlined followed by a fitness data chart based on research collected over the past 10 years. These data are included to allow interpretation of the test results specific to each player being tested. The ranges provided in the charts are based on fitness testing information gathered at 120 USTA area training centres. Each training centre attracts the top 20 ranked junior tennis players in a specific geographical region of the USA.

Flexibility

Flexibility is the range of motion available at a joint. Because in tennis you may have to generate force from a variety of positions, it is critical to be as flexible as possible.

Sit and reach

Measure the flexibility of the hamstrings and lower back (Fig. 10.1).

Equipment	Sit and reach box, measuring stick or tape measure	
Start position	Athlete	Sit on the floor with legs extended out in front
	Examiner	Hold the knees down to the floor
Performance	Athlete	Place your hands next to one another with the index fingers touching, then lean forward with arms extended as far as possible out over the toes
	Examiner	Make sure the athlete holds the stretch without bouncing
Measurement	Examiner	Measure the distance from the toes to the fingertips • If the hands reach past the toes, the figure is expressed positively in cm • If the hands do not reach the toes, the figure is expressed negatively in cm **Record the best of 3 trials**

Sit and reach (cm):

	Excellent	Good	Average	Needs improvement
Girls				
14 and under	> 15	10–15	5–10	< 5
18 and under	> 20	17–20	12–17	< 12
Boys				
14 and under	> 7	2–7	0–2	< 0
18 and under	> 24	5–24	2–5	< 2

Hamstrings

Measure the flexibility of the hamstrings one leg at a
time using a goniometer.

Equipment	Training table, goniometer, two test examiners	
Start position	Athlete	Lie in supine position on training table
	Examiner 1	Stand next to the hip opposite of the side being tested
	Examiner 2	Kneel down facing the hip of the side being tested
Performance	Examiner 1	Hold the pelvis down at the hip with one hand, reach across the body and raise the leg with the other hand (keeping the knee straight) until tightness is felt in the hamstring
Measurement	Examiner 2	Use the lateral aspect of the leg and lateral border of the trunk as landmarks to align the arms of the goniometer. Measure the angle at the hip with a goniometer
		Record 1 trial

Shoulder rotation

Measure the internal and external range of motion
in the shoulders with a goniometer.

Equipment	Training table, goniometer, two test examiners	
Start position	Athlete	Lie in supine position on training table, with shoulder abducted at 90°, and the elbow bent at a 90° angle
	Examiner 1	Stand next to the hip of the side being tested. With the hands, hold down the front of the shoulder, not allowing it to roll forward during rotation. No scapular motion during this measure is allowed (Ellenbecker *et al.* 1996)
	Examiner 2	Kneel down facing the shoulder of the side being tested
Performance	Athlete	Shoulder is internally and externally rotated from a neutral position
Measurement	Examiner 2	Angle of rotation of the arm is measured by a goniometer
		Record 1 trial each for dominant and non-dominant arm

Normal patterns (ranges) of motion (°) for shoulder int/ext rotation with 90° abduction:

	Girls (ages 11–18)		Boys (ages 11–18)	
	Dominant	Non-dominant	Dominant	Non-dominant
External	95–105	95–105	95–105	90–100
Internal	45–55	55–65	40–50	50–60

Aerobic endurance

Aerobic endurance is the ability to take in, transport and use oxygen. Aerobic energy is used during prolonged, steady-paced activities mainly using the large muscle groups. A strong aerobic base will allow the tennis player to recover more quickly between points, and perform longer before getting tired.

1.5-mile (2.4-km) run

Measure aerobic endurance by recording the time to complete the run. (This test should be performed on a different day from all other tests. A practice run, on a different day, is recommended if time permits.)

Equipment	400-m (440-yard) track (Cinder or Tartan tracks recommended), stopwatch, 1 test examiner	
Start position	Athlete	Stand with toes behind starting line
	Examiner	Stand off the track, near the starting line. Use the command 'Ready—Go' to start the run
Performance	Athlete	Run 6 laps around the track as fast as possible
Measurement	Examiner	Record the time elapsed as the athlete crosses the finish line
	Record 1 trial	

1.5-mile (2.4-km) run (min : s):

	Excellent	Good	Average	Needs improvement
Girls				
14 and under	< 11 : 00	11 : 00–12 : 00	12 : 00–13 : 00	> 13 : 00
18 and under	< 10 : 30	10 : 30–11 : 00	11 : 00–11 : 30	> 11 : 30
Boys				
14 and under	< 10 : 00	10 : 00–11 : 30	11 : 00–11 : 30	> 11 : 30
18 and under	< 9 : 45	9 : 45–10 : 15	10 : 15–11 : 00	> 11 : 00

Agility and speed

Agility and speed are your ability to move around the court quickly and smoothly to position yourself for a shot. Agility is crucial to good court movement. It allows you to be in the correct position and provides a solid platform from which to hit the ball. Speed is important to get to the ball. The faster you can get to a ball, the more time you have to prepare for your shot.

18-m (20-yard) dash

Equipment		Stopwatch, masking tape, test examiner (*measuring stick optional)
Set-up		Using masking tape, mark off a start and finish line 20 yards apart. (The distance from one baseline to the opposite service line is 18 m (20 yards))
Start position	Athlete	Stand with toes behind starting line
	Examiner	Stand next to the finish line. Raise the arm with the stopwatch up in the air to give the runner a visual clue. Use the command 'Ready—Go', and on 'Go' drop the arm and start the stopwatch
Performance	Athlete	Sprint to the finish line as fast as possible
Measurement	Examiner	Record the time elapsed as the athlete crosses the finish line
		Record the best of 3 trials

18-m (20-yard) dash (seconds):

	Excellent	Good	Average	Needs improvement
Girls				
14 and under	< 3.30	3.33–3.40	3.40–3.60	> 3.80
18 and under	< 3.20	3.20–3.36	3.20–3.54	> 3.62
Boys				
14 and under	< 3.20	3.20–3.30	3.30–3.50	> 3.50
18 and under	< 2.90	2.90–3.00	3.00–3.30	> 3.30

Hexagon test (Fig. 10.2)

Equipment		Stopwatch, masking tape, goniometer or protractor, test examiner
Set-up		Using masking tape, create a hexagon (six sides) on the ground, with side 60 cm long, and an angle of 120° between each side. Designate one side to be the 'starting line'
Start position	Athlete	Stand inside the hexagon facing the starting line
	Examiner	Stand outside the hexagon facing the athlete. Use the command 'Ready—Go' and start the stopwatch
Performance	Athlete	1. Jump with both feet over the starting line to the outside of the hexagon 2. Immediately jump back inside the hexagon, then jump to the outside of the next adjacent side (remain facing forward) 3. Continue jumping in and out as you go around the hexagon 4. As quickly as possible, make three revolutions around the hexagon without touching any of the sides with your feet
Measurement	Examiner	Record the time elapsed as the athlete jumps back into the hexagon after three revolutions
		*Time penalties: 0.5 s for each line touch 1.0 s for jumping a side out of sequence
		Record the best of 2 trials

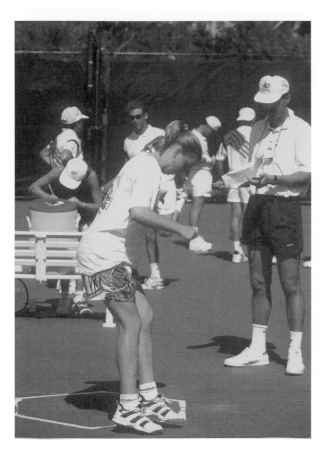

Fig. 10.2 Hexagon test.

Hexagon (seconds):

	Excellent	Good	Average	Needs improvement
Girls				
14 and under	< 10.90	10.90–12.00	12.00–12.90	> 12.90
18 and under	< 12.00	12.00–12.10	12.10–12.40	> 13.40
Boys				
14 and under	< 11.10	11.10–12.00	12.00–12.80	> 12.80
18 and under	< 11.80	11.80–13.50	13.00–13.50	> 13.50

Sideways shuffle

Equipment	Stopwatch, masking tape, tennis court, test examiner	
Start position	Athlete	Stand at the 'T' facing the net, with one foot on either side of the line
	Examiner	Stand a few feet in front of the athlete, with back to the net. Use the command 'Ready—Go' to start the test
Performance	Athlete	1. While facing the net, shuffle along the service line and touch the doubles sideline with one foot
		2. Immediately shuffle back across the service line and touch the opposite doubles sideline
		3. Shuffle back to the centre 'T' to finish
		4. No crossover steps are allowed
Measurement	Examiner	Record the time elapsed as the athlete crosses the centre 'T', after touching both doubles sidelines
		Record the best of 2 trials

Side shuffle (seconds):

	Excellent	Good	Average	Needs improvement
Girls				
14 and under	< 6.0	6.0–7.0	7.0–7.30	> 7.30
18 and under	< 7.0	7.0–7.10	7.10–7.40	> 7.40
Boys				
14 and under	< 6.40	6.40–6.70	6.70–7.00	> 7.00
18 and under	< 5.50	5.50–5.60	5.60–5.70	> 5.70

Spider test

Equipment	5 tennis balls, masking tape, stopwatch, tennis court	
Set-up	Use masking tape to mark off a 30 cm by 44 cm rectangle behind the middle of the baseline, using the baseline as one of the 44-cm sides	
	Position five balls as follows: Ball 1: baseline/sideline intersection, ad court Ball 2: sideline/service line intersection, ad court Ball 3: centre 'T' Ball 4: sideline/service line intersection, deuce court Ball 5: baseline/sideline intersection, deuce court	
Start position	Athlete	Stand facing the ball 1, with one foot touching the taped rectangle
	Examiner	Stand behind the taped rectangle, out of the court. Use the command 'Ready—Go' and start the stopwatch
Performance	Athlete	Sprint to ball 1, retrieve it and place (do not throw) it inside the taped rectangle. Continue to retrieve each ball, one at a time in sequence, and place them in the taped rectangle (anticlockwise pattern)
	Examiner	Remove each ball after it is placed in the rectangle to prevent the athlete from stepping on it
Measurement	Examiner	Observe the time elapsed after the last ball has been placed inside the rectangle
		Record the best of 2 trials

Spider test (seconds):

	Excellent	Good	Average	Needs improvement
Girls				
14 and under	< 17.52	17.52–18.14	18.14–18.60	> 18.60
18 and under	< 17.10	17.10–17.16	17.16–17.34	> 17.34
Boys				
14 and under	< 16.80	16.80–17.42	17.42–18.00	> 18.00
18 and under	< 14.60	14.60–15.00	15.00–15.40	> 15.40

Power

Power is the amount of work you can perform in a given time period. Power is required during activities requiring both strength (force) and speed. Tennis requires you to move with explosive movements. Greater power allows you to respond quicker and produce forceful movements with less effort.

Overhead medicine ball toss

Equipment		6-pound (2.7 kg) medicine ball, tape measure, masking tape
Set-up		Extend a tape measure in a straight line about 15 m. Secure each end of the tape measure to the court with tape. For a starting line, place a 60-cm piece of tape on the court perpendicular to the beginning of the tape measure
Start position	Athlete	Stand behind the starting line facing forward and, with both hands, hold the medicine ball behind your head
	Examiner	Stand a few feet to the side of the tape measure, near the centre
Performance	Athlete	With both hands, toss the ball over your head as far as possible down the tape measure. One step forward may be taken without crossing the starting line
Measurement	Examiner	Observe the point on the tape measure where the ball lands
		Record the best of 2 trials

Overhead medicine ball toss (metres):

	Excellent	Good	Average	Needs improvement
Girls				
14 and under	> 6.8	5.5–6.8	4.3–5.5	< 4.3
18 and under	> 7.1	5.8–7.1	4.6–5.8	< 4.6
Boys				
14 and under	> 8.3	6.8–8.3	5.2–6.8	< 5.2
18 and under	> 10.5	8.9–10.5	7.1–8.9	< 7.1

Reverse medicine ball toss

Equipment		6-pound (2.7-kg) medicine ball, tape measure, masking tape
Set-up		Extend a tape measure in a straight line about 15 m. Secure each end of the tape measure to the court with tape. For a starting line, place a 60-cm piece of tape on the court perpendicular to the beginning of the tape measure
Start position	Athlete	Stand behind the starting line, facing backward. Hold the ball in front of you with both hands at waist level
	Examiner	Stand a few feet to the side of the tape measure, near the centre
Performance	Athlete	Bend your knees keeping your back straight and thrust upward with the legs. Toss the ball using both hands backward over your head. No steps are allowed
Measurement	Examiner	Observe the point on the tape measure where the ball lands
		Record the best of 2 trials

Reverse medicine ball toss (metres):

	Excellent	Good	Average	Needs improvement
Girls				
14 and under	> 9.5	8.0–9.5	6.5–8.0	< 6.5
18 and under	> 10.5	8.3–10.5	6.1–8.3	< 6.1
Boys				
14 and under	> 12.6	9.8–12.6	7.1–9.8	< 7.1
18 and under	> 14.1	11.7–14.1	9.5–11.7	< 9.5

Forehand medicine ball toss (Fig. 10.3)

Equipment		6-pound (2.7-kg) medicine ball, tape measure, masking tape
Set-up		Extend a tape measure in a straight line about 15 m. Secure each end of the tape measure to the court with tape. For a starting line, place a 60-cm piece of tape on the court perpendicular to the beginning of the tape measure
Start position	Athlete	Stand behind the starting line, facing forward. Hold the ball with both hands in front of you, arms extended
	Examiner	Stand a few feet to the side of the tape measure, near the centre
Performance	Athlete	Using a forehand stroke motion, toss the ball as far as you can down the tape measure. One step is allowed. Concentrate on releasing the ball out in front of you
Measurement	Examiner	Observe the point on the tape measure where the ball lands
		Record the best of 2 trials

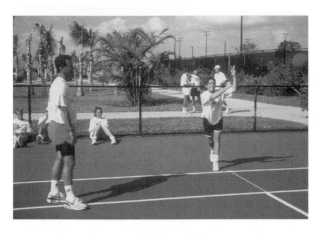

Fig. 10.3 Forehand medicine ball toss.

Forehand medicine ball toss (metres):

	Excellent	Good	Average	Needs improvement
Girls				
14 and under	> 8.9	7.4–8.9	5.8–7.4	< 5.8
18 and under	> 9.8	8.0–9.8	6.1–8.0	< 6.1
Boys				
14 and under	> 11.1	8.9–11.1	5.8–8.9	< 5.8
10 and under	> 12.9	10.8–12.9	8.6–10.8	< 8.6

Backhand medicine ball toss

Equipment		6-pound (2.7-kg) medicine ball, tape measure, masking tape
Set-up		Extend a tape measure in a straight line about 15 m. Secure each end of the tape measure to the court with tape. For a starting line, place a 60-cm piece of tape on the court perpendicular to the beginning of the tape measure
Start position	Athlete	Stand behind the starting line, facing forward. Hold the ball with both hands in front of you, arms extended
	Examiner	Stand a few feet to the side of the tape measure, near the centre
Performance	Athlete	Using a two-handed backhand stroke motion, toss the ball as far as you can down the tape measure. One step is allowed. Concentrate on releasing the ball out in front of you
Measurement	Examiner	Observe the point on the tape measure where the ball lands
		Record the best of 2 trials

Backhand medicine ball toss (metres):

	Excellent	Good	Average	Needs improvement
Girls				
14 and under	> 8.9	7.1–8.9	5.2–7.1	< 5.2
18 and under	> 9.5	7.7–9.5	5.5–7.7	< 5.5
Boys				
14 and under	> 10.1	8.3–10.1	6.5–8.3	< 6.5
18 and under	> 12.9	10.5–12.9	8.0–10.5	< 8.0

Vertical jump (Fig. 10.4)

Equipment		Measuring stick, tape
Set-up		1. Secure a measuring stick vertically to a gymnasium wall or the outside of a building. The athlete should be able to reach the **bottom** of the stick when reaching up over their head, with heels flat 2. Standing sideways to the wall, have the athlete raise the arm above the head, fingers extended, and touch the measuring stick as high as possible, with heels flat. Record this number as the 'standing reach'
Start position	Athlete	Stand sideways to the wall underneath the measuring stick
	Examiner	Stand on a ladder or chair next to the measuring stick to have a clear view of the point the athlete touches
Performance	Athlete	Bend the knees and jump upward with legs together, reaching with one hand as high as possible on the measuring stick
Measurement	Examiner	The difference between the standing reach and the highest point of the jump is the athlete's score
		Record the best of 2 trials

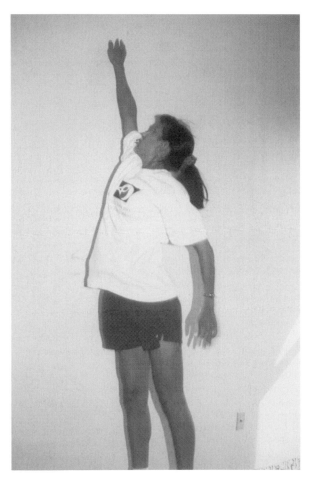

Vertical jump (cm):

	Excellent	Good	Average	Needs improvement
Girls				
14 and under	> 53	41–53	30–41	< 30
18 and under	> 56	43–56	33–43	< 33
Boys				
14 and under	> 69	56–69	43–56	< 43
18 and under	> 71	66–71	53–66	< 53

Muscular strength and endurance

Strength is the amount of weight you can lift or handle at any one time. Muscular endurance is the number of times your muscles can lift a weight or how long your muscles can hold an amount of weight. By increasing your strength you can increase the amount of force with which you hit the tennis ball. By increasing endurance, you will be able to perform movements as well at the end of the match as you did at the beginning.

Fig. 10.4 (*left*) Vertical jump test.

Sit-ups

The muscular strength and endurance of the abdominal muscles is measured. (Athletes with history of low back pain or injuries should not perform this test.)

Equipment	Stopwatch or clock	
Start position	Athlete	Lie in a supine position with hips flexed to 45° and knees flexed to 90°. Place hands on opposite shoulders, against the body
	Examiner	Place one knee between the feet of the athlete, and hold the feet stationary
Performance	Athlete	Elbows must touch the thighs on the ascent, shoulder blades must touch the mat on the descent, and hips cannot leave the mat
Measurement	Examiner	Record the number of sit-ups performed in 60 s or until exhaustion
		Record 1 trial

Sit-ups (number completed):

	Excellent	Good	Average	Needs improvement
Girls				
14 and under	> 53	46–53	42–46	< 42
18 and under	> 54	46–54	35–46	< 35
Boys				
14 and under	> 58	51–58	47–51	< 47
18 and under	> 63	56–63	50–56	< 50

Push-ups

Muscular strength and endurance of the upper body is measured.

Equipment	Stopwatch or clock	
Start position	Athlete	Start in the prone position with hands shoulder width apart and the weight of your lower body on your toes. Keep arms extended and the head, shoulders, back, hip, knees and feet in a straight line
Performance	Athlete	Bring your arms down so that they are parallel with the ground or below (form a 90° angle). Arms must be fully extended and body alignment straight on the way up to count as a full push-up
Measurement	Examiner	Record the number of complete push-ups in 60 s or to exhaustion
		Record 1 trial

Push-ups (number completed):

	Excellent	Good	Average	Needs improvement
Girls				
14 and under	> 44	36–44	27–36	< 27
18 and under	> 42	34–42	20–34	< 20
Boys				
14 and under	> 49	40–49	33–40	< 33
18 and under	> 52	49–52	35–49	< 35

Grip strength

The grip strength of the dominant and non-dominant hand is measured using a grip strength dynamometer.

Equipment	Lafayette grip strength dynamometer	
Start position	Athlete	Stand holding the grip dynamometer in one hand loosely at your side
Performance	Athlete	Squeeze the dynamometer as hard as possible and hold for 3 s
Measurement	Examiner	Record the result in kilograms
		Record the best of **2 trials** for each hand

Grip strength (kg):

	Excellent		Good		Average		Needs improvement	
	Dominant	Non-dominant	Dominant	Non-dominant	Dominant	Non-dominant	Dominant	Non-dominant
Girls								
14 and under	> 34	> 32	30–34	28–32	24–30	19–28	< 24	< 19
18 and under	> 39	> 27	34–39	24–27	28–34	22–24	< 28	< 22
Boys								
14 and under	> 50	> 31	42–50	27–31	34–42	24–27	< 34	< 24
18 and under	> 60	> 36	51–60	31–36	42–51	26–31	< 42	< 26

Isokinetic strength

Isokinetic strength testing provides reliable, objective information on the strength of various muscles or muscle groups. Testing is normally performed at several speeds that enable sports medicine and sports scientists to evaluate a player's strength at faster velocities.

1 A Cybex Isokinetic dynamometer has been used to perform isokinetic testing of elite junior tennis players using concentric muscular contractions in the following movement patterns:
   (a) shoulder internal/external rotation with 90° abduction;
   (b) knee extension/flexion;
   (c) trunk extension/flexion.

2 The testing protocol follows that recommended by the manufacturer (Cybex Inc., Ronkonkoma, NY).
3 Standardized warm-up, player positioning, verbal instruction and data-collection methods are followed.
4 For a complete summary of the isokinetic test protocols consult the following references:
  (a) shoulder testing (Ellenbecker 1991, 1992; Ellenbecker & Roetert 1999);
  (b) knee testing (Ellenbecker & Roetert 1995);
  (c) trunk testing (Roetert *et al.* 1996).

Isokinetic shoulder rotation strength

(Peak torque in foot pounds as a percentage of bodyweight in lbs.)

	Girls (ages 14–17)		Boys (ages 14–17)	
	Dominant	Non-dominant	Dominant	Non-dominant
External rotation ($210°\cdot s^{-1}$)	8	8	12	11
External rotation ($300°\cdot s^{-1}$)	8	7	10	10
Internal rotation ($210°\cdot s^{-1}$)	12	11	17	14
Internal rotation ($300°\cdot s^{-1}$)	11	10	15	13

Isokinetic quadriceps and hamstring strength

(Peak torque in foot pounds as a percentage of bodyweight in lbs.)

	Girls (ages 13–17)	Boys (ages 13–17)
Quads ($180°\cdot s^{-1}$)	N/A	60
Quads ($300°\cdot s^{-1}$)	45	55
Hamstrings ($210°\cdot s^{-1}$)	N/A	36
Hamstrings ($300°\cdot s^{-1}$)	30	33

Isokinetic trunk strength

(Peak torque in foot pounds as a percentage of bodyweight in lbs.)

	Girls (ages 13–17)	Boys (ages 13–17)
Flexion ($60°\cdot s^{-1}$)	100	125
Flexion ($120°\cdot s^{-1}$)	97	118
Extension ($125°\cdot s^{-1}$)	90	125
Extension ($105°\cdot s^{-1}$)	80	105

Designing a programme

The fitness-testing protocol as outlined in this chapter provides information for players and coaches to help design an appropriate individualized training programme. The tests show fitness data in the areas of flexibility, strength, power, aerobic endurance and speed and agility. You can compare your scores to those listed and evaluate where your strengths and weaknesses may be. For example, the sample player in Fig. 10.5 is a 17-year-old-male player. His test results clearly indicate very good scores in all but the strength and power categories. If over looked, this player may potentially set himself up for reduced performance and increased risk of injury. Remember, the scores given are those of high-level junior tennis players. Adult scores may vary. As with

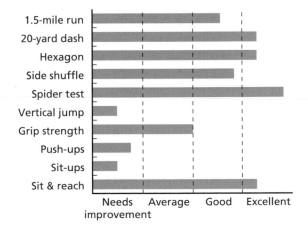

Fig. 10.5 Sample player profile.

the design of any conditioning programme, proper communication among player, coach and conditioning specialist is imperative.

References

Chandler, T.J., Kibler, W.B., Stracener, E.C., Ziegler, A.K. & Pace, B. (1992) Shoulder strength, power, and endurance in college tennis players. *American Journal of Sports Medicine* **20**, 455–458.

Ellenbecker, T.S. (1991) A total arm strength isokinetic profile of highly skilled tennis players. *Isokinetics and Exercise Science* **1**, 9–21.

Ellenbecker, T.S. (1992) Shoulder internal and external rotation strength and range of motion of highly skilled junior tennis players. *Isokinetics and Exercise Science* **2**, 1–8.

Ellenbecker, T.S. (1995) Rehabilitation of shoulder and elbow injuries in tennis players. *Clinics in Sports Medicine* **14** (1), 87–109.

Ellenbecker, T.S. & Roetert, E.P. (1995) Concentric isokinetic quadricep and hamstring strength in elite junior tennis players. *Isokinetics and Exercise Science* **5**, 3–6.

Ellenbecker, T.S. & Roetert, E.P. (1999) Testing isokinetic muscular fatigue of shoulder internal and external rotation in elite junior tennis players. *Journal of Orthopaedic and Sports Physical Therapy* **29**, 275–281.

Ellenbecker, T.S., Roetert, E.P., Piorkowski, P.A. & Schulz, D.A. (1996) Glenohumeral joint internal and external rotation range of motion in elite junior tennis players. *Journal of Orthopaedic and Sports Physical Therapy* **24** (6), 336–341.

Groppel, J.L. & Roetert. E.P. (1992) Applied physiology of tennis. *Sports Medicine* **14** (4), 260–268.

Kibler, W.B. (1990) *The Sport Preparticipation Fitness Examination*. Human Kinetics, Champaign, IL.

Priest, J.D. & Nagel, D.A. (1976) Tennis shoulder. *American Journal of Sports Medicine* **4**, 28–42.

Roetert, E.P., Piorkowski, P.A., Woods, R.W. & Brown, S.W. (1995) Establishing percentiles for junior tennis players based on physical fitness testing results. *Clinics in Sports Medicine* **14** (1), 1–21.

Roetert, E.P., McCormick, T.J., Brown, S.W. & Ellenbecker, T.S. (1996) Relationship between isokinetic and functional trunk strength in elite junior tennis players. *Isokinetics and Exercise Science* **6**, 15–20.

Chapter 11

Specific problems for the young tennis player

Introduction

The average young tennis player experiences relatively few injuries. However, if the young tennis player is participating intensely, either exclusively in tennis or in tennis as well as other sports, injuries occur with increasing frequency (Hutchinson *et al.* 1995). In addition, intensely active young tennis players can develop deleterious maladaptations in flexibility and strength in areas subject to repetitive tensile overload (Kibler & Chandler 1993a). These maladaptations have been shown to increase with years of tournament play (Kibler *et al.* 1996). They impose altered joint biomechanics (Harryman *et al.* 1990; Matsen *et al.* 1991), alter muscular force couples around the joint (Speer & Garrett 1994), may be seen as risk factors for injury causation (Herring 1990; Silliman & Hawkins 1991), and decrease maximal force production (Kibler 1995).

The young tennis player also faces problems in learning the proper biomechanical functions to perform at a high skill level, and in developing efficient physiological motor organization to generate the force necessary to hit the ball at a high level of proficiency. Inefficient biomechanics and physiology will impair ultimate performance and create conditions for increased injury risk (Kibler 1995).

This chapter will review each of those areas and discuss treatment and prevention strategies. It will also review the concept of prehabilitation, or sport-specific conditioning to allow the athlete to withstand the inherent demands imposed by the particular sport (Chandler & Kibler 1993).

Injuries

Epidemiology

Large epidemiologic studies are not available in young tennis players. Several small studies do shed light on relative incidence and location of injury. A multinational study (Kibler *et al.* 1988) showed that the incidence of injury in elite junior players was high. The incidence of injury within the past year was 68%. Overload injuries were the predominant type, with the shoulder, back and knee the most common sites. These findings were confirmed by two United States Tennis Association (USTA) studies (Hutchinson *et al.* 1995; USTA, unpublished data) and a Danish study (Winge *et al.* 1989) which documented a similar high incidence of injury, microtrauma predominance and location frequency. These studies differ slightly from those in adult players, which show a higher percentage of lower extremity injuries, but similar overall incidence and microtrauma predominance.

Causation

Based on these studies, two causative mechanisms appear to be operative to cause injuries in young tennis players. Macrotrauma-caused injuries include acute sprains, acute joint injuries, fractures, dislocations or contusions. They usually occur in the lower extremity, and result from a one-time event. Microtrauma-caused injuries include tendinitis, chronic muscle strains or joint instability. They may occur in the upper or lower extremity, and are the result of a process over time, with resultant associated tissue alterations, both locally and distantly. Young tennis players appear to respond similarly to adult players with regard to injury causation.

Special concerns

Epiphyseal and apophyseal areas of long bones are areas of concern in young tennis players. Traumatic inversion ankle injuries, or falls on the outstretched arm, may produce epiphyseal bony injuries, rather than ligament sprains. Tenderness to palpation over the epiphysis, rather than over the ligament, is the key physical diagnostic finding. Traction apophysitis, due to repetitive load on the tendon insertion on a growing bone, is very common at all tension sites. The most commonly involved areas include the Achilles tendon at the heel, quadriceps tendon at the tibial tubercle, and the wrist flexors at the humeral medial epicondyle. These injuries usually occur because the muscle–tendon unit inflexibility, either due to growth or maladaptation, and the resulting increased strain with loading damages the tendon–bone insertion.

Treatment

Treatment of injuries in young tennis players should proceed along the same lines as treatment in adults. Fractures usually heal in slightly shorter times. Overload injury treatment should include the 'complete and accurate' diagnosis of all the injuries and tissue alterations that create the clinical picture (Kibler *et al.* 1992) and rehabilitation in an orderly sequence.

Maladaptations

Inherent demands

Tennis may be considered a violent game from the standpoint of required velocities and motions in normal tennis activities. The entire body is involved in these demands. Shoulder rotation velocity approaches $1700°·s^{-1}$, shoulder horizontal adduction velocity approaches $1150°·s^{-1}$, elbow extension velocity is approximately $895°·s^{-1}$, wrist flexion $315°·s^{-1}$, and trunk rotation velocity is $350°·s^{-1}$ (Kibler 1993). Glenohumeral shoulder rotation includes an arc of $146°$ (Kibler 1993). These velocities occur very rapidly, creating large accelerations at the hip, shoulder and elbow (Kibler 1993; Kleinoder *et al.* 1995). Young athletes do not produce the same magnitude of velocities, but the attained speeds are still quite high.

These hitting activities are combined with repetitive running, starting and stopping activities that involve the legs. The average tennis point requires 8.7 changes of direction. Each change of direction creates a load of 1.5–2.7 times body weight on the plant leg, knee and ankle.

The direction changes and load applications require muscle work, both in concentric and eccentric modes. Metabolic evaluation reveals that 70% of metabolic demands in tennis are alactic anaerobic, 20% lactic anaerobic and 10% aerobic (Kibler 1993).

Skill acquisition and high-level performance in tennis requires frequent training sessions. One study revealed the young tennis players averaged 2.3 h of practice or match play 6.1 days per week (Kibler *et al.* 1988).

In summary, demands inherent in tennis are high in magnitude, high in intensity, and frequently applied. The musculoskeletal base must respond to these demands to protect itself from injury and allow skilful performance.

Musculoskeletal response

The human body adapts to the stresses applied to it during sports. Many adaptations are positive, even in young tennis players. Increased bone density, tendon collagen content, $\dot{V}o_{2max}$ and anaerobic threshold are all seen in young tennis players. However, studies have shown that adaptations in flexibility, strength and endurance may not be positive, and may be sources of injury, risk and decreased performance.

Young tennis players have been shown to have decreased back flexibility, measured by decreased sit and reach measurements, compared to age-matched controls (Kibler & Chandler 1993a; Kibler 1998). They also demonstrate trunk extensor weakness, both in absolute magnitude and in strength balance (Ellenbecker 1995).

Several studies (Kibler *et al.* 1988, 1996; Silliman & Hawkins 1991; Kibler & Chandler 1993a; Kibler 1998) have documented shoulder internal rotation and horizontal adduction inflexibility in the dominant shoulder of tennis players (Fig. 11.1). Progression with years of play has also been shown (Kibler *et al.* 1996). This appears to be associated with a true limitation of total shoulder rotation, in contrast to baseball, in which decreased internal rotation is coupled with increased external rotation.

Strength in shoulder muscles is often altered. External rotation strength, muscle work and internal rotation/external rotation ratios are altered, with external rotation being relatively weaker (Chandler *et al.* 1992; Ellenbecker 1992). This combination results in force couple imbalance of the humeral head stabilizers.

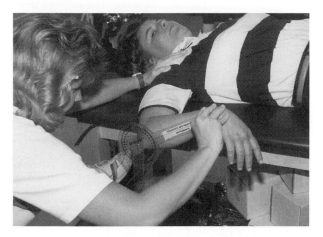

Fig. 11.1 Decreased glenohumeral range of motion. This should be measured goniometrically.

Elbow range of motion may also be altered, in both flexion/extension and pronation/supination (Kibler 1998). The clinical picture is usually a mild flexion and supination contracture.

These alterations are extremely common in even young tennis players. They are always seen at areas of repetitive tensile load. The exact genesis or function is not clear. The inflexibilities may be a body adaptation to the tensile load, so that a tight muscle may better resist the developed tension. However, most authors feel this is a capsular and/or muscle supporting tissue contracture (Harryman *et al.* 1990; Silliman & Hawkins 1991) and it causes abnormal biomechanics, such as altered lumbopelvic rhythm in trunk inflexibility (Young *et al.* 1996), increased translation in mid-ranges of glenohumeral motion (Harryman *et al.* 1990), extra load on the glenoid labrum, or lack of varus acceleration to support valgus elbow stress in glenohumeral internal rotation inflexibility (Putnam 1993).

Strength alterations may result from a plyometric-like effect to increase shoulder internal rotation strength (Warner *et al.* 1990), actual muscle damage due to repetitive load, or inhibition related decrease in tensile muscle function due to muscle spindle overload (Nichols 1994). They cause problems by destabilizing the base (the legs and trunk) that generates the force in tennis (Kibler 1995), the base (the scapula) that allows normal arm motion (Kibler & Chandler 1997), or by creating force couple

imbalances that do not control joint pertubations in normal activity (Nichols 1994; Speer & Garrett 1994).

These musculoskeletal responses should be considered maladaptations to imposed demands. They may appear at young ages in intensity training tennis players and should be identified. They can be modified with a specific conditioning programme (Kibler 1998).

Biomechanics and skill acquisition

Motor control literature reports that the best time to learn new skills is early in life. Proper organization of motor firing patterns is more easily obtained at this time. Efficiency of muscle activation will allow efficient biomechanics throughout the athlete's career, with positive implications for performance and injury risk.

However, improper learning at this time can have negative effects. The two most common means by which this can occur are training with the wrong equipment, or trying to learn skills that require more muscular force than the athlete can generate. In each situation, some less efficient biomechanical adaptation will be learned.

Rackets that are too heavy, too long or that have too large a grip create major problems as the young player tries to repetitively move the racket through the hitting zone. In addition, the extreme western grip (Fig. 11.2) places an extra strain on the young player. More motion and muscle activity in the trunk, or excessive dropping of the racket head in cocking, is often the adaptation.

Power development to hit the ball hard or with heavy topspin requires a coordinated sequential linkage of all the body segments. This linkage coordination is called the kinetic chain (Fig. 11.3) (Kibler *et al.* 1992). This also requires muscular strength, especially in the legs and trunk. Proper development of smooth coordination of the links of the kinetic chain should precede attempts at developing power shots. Many young tennis players do not have sufficient lower leg strength to hit the ball the way their older role models do. They must rely on biomechanical efficiency to hit effective shots until they have the hormonal capacity to develop strength. Inefficient adaptations include excessive trunk lean

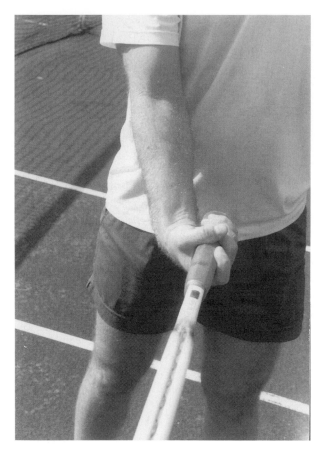

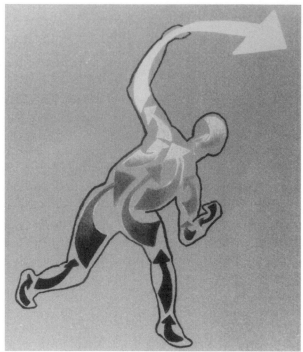

Fig. 11.3 The kinetic chain of force production. Force is produced in the legs and transferred through the trunk to the arm and racket.

Fig. 11.2 Extreme western grip places extra load on the arm due to extra forearm supination.

in the service motion, dropping or leading with the elbow in the serve and forehand, excessive wrist snap or slap in the forehand, and pulling up and away from the ball on the backhand.

Prehabilitation

Preventative conditioning should be employed to decrease problems seen in young tennis players. This technique involves understanding the demands inherent in tennis, the special demands that young tennis players face, and a pre-participation examination of the individual's flexibility, strength, power and endurance (Chandler & Kibler 1993).

Several techniques have been described to conduct the pre-participation examination (Kibler *et al*. 1989;

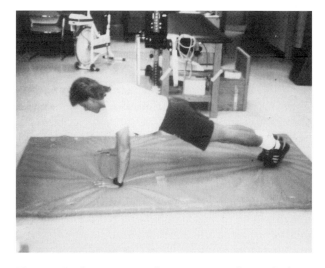

Fig. 11.4 Push-ups are a good measurement of upper body and trunk strength. Most teenage boys should be able to do 35–40 in 1 min. Teenage girls may do modified (knees on ground) push-ups and should be able to do 30 in 1 min.

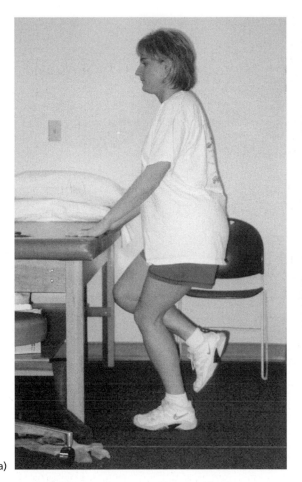

(a)

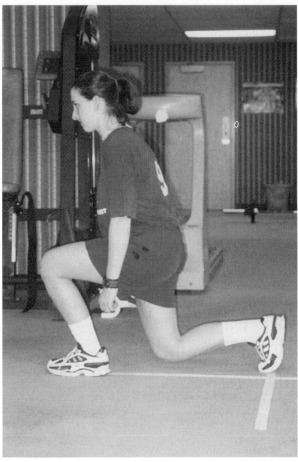

(b)

Fig. 11.5 Squats (a) and lunges (b) are good plyometric-type exercises to increase power in the legs.

Kibler & Chandler 1993b). The exact examination will depend on the facilities, but it should at least include areas of special interest in tennis players. These would include flexibility of the back, shoulder and the elbow; strength estimation such as push-ups and sit-ups (Fig. 11.4) and isokinetic evaluation of the shoulder and knee; vertical jump and medicine ball for power; and a dash or shuttle run for anaerobic power.

The exercise prescription for prehabilitation would first be based on the results of the pre-participation examination, to correct any deficits that may be discovered. In addition, tennis-specific conditioning exercises are implemented. These would include squats and lunges (Fig. 11.5) for leg strengthening, to simulate the power generation and load absorbing requirements, trunk rotations, scapular stabilizations, shoulder strengthening (Fig. 11.6), and wrist co-contractions. These exercises should integrate the entire kinetic chain, improve joint stability force couples (Fig. 11.7) (Matsen *et al.* 1991; Kibler & Chandler 1994), and improve proprioception (Fig. 11.8). Endurance exercises would emphasize simulating the metabolic demands of tennis, with relatively short duration, rapid direction change exercises such as jumping jacks, jump rope, minitrampoline and shuttle runs. Long-distance runs would be occasionally used to facilitate recovery mechanisms. The programme

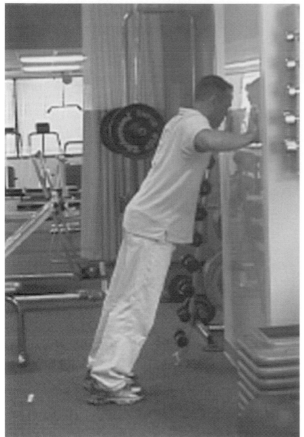

(a)

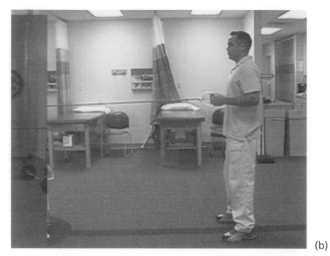

(b)

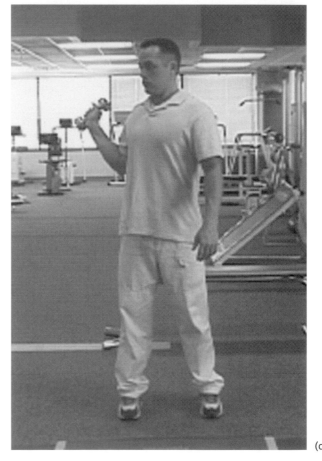

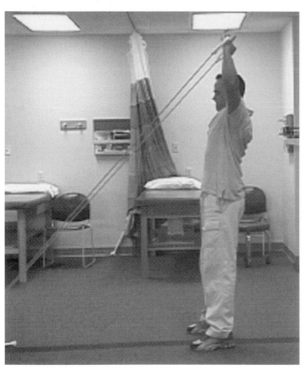

(c)

(d)

Fig. 11.6 Shoulder strengthening exercises include wall push-ups (a), tubing exercises for the scapula (b) and shoulder (c), and dumb-bells (d).

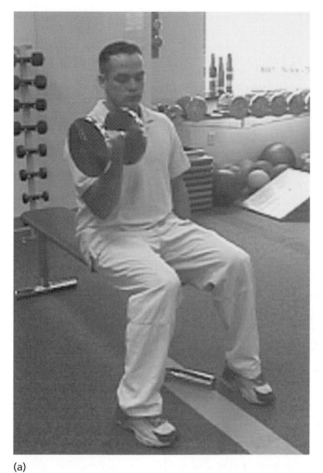

(a)

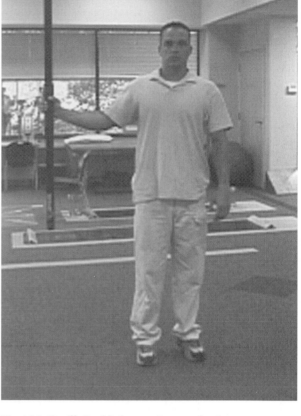

Fig. 11.8 Oscillating blade exercises emphasize proprioceptive feedback.

(b)

Fig. 11.7 Exercises should emphasize development of both the anterior (a) and posterior muscles (b) for force couple balance.

should be conducted in a periodization framework (Kibler & Chandler 1994).

Conclusions

The young tennis player presents slightly different musculoskeletal problems than the adult player. Injury site is slightly different, maladaptations are frequent and appear early in training, and skill acquisition is a major challenge, especially in the face of growth, adaptation and maladaptation. The sports medicine practitioner must understand these differences, know the demands, do serial musculoskeletal evaluations for maladaptations, and adhere to a periodized prehabilitation programme of preventative exercises to maximize performance and minimize injury risk.

References

Chandler, T.J. & Kibler, W.B. (1993) Muscle training in injury prevention. In: Renstrom, P., ed. *Sports Injuries—Basic Principles and Care*, pp. 252–261. Blackwell Scientific Publications, Oxford.

Chandler, T.J., Kibler, W.B. & Stracener, E.C. (1992) Shoulder strength, power, and endurance in college tennis players. *American Journal of Sports Medicine* **20**, 455–458.

Ellenbecker, T.S. (1992) Shoulder internal and external rotation strength in highly skilled junior tennis players. *Isokinetics and Exercise Science* **2**, 1–8.

Ellenbecker, T.S. (1995) Rehabilitation of shoulder and elbow injuries in tennis players. *Clinics in Sports Medicine* **14**, 87–105.

Harryman, D.T., Sidles, J.A., Clark, J.M. & Matsen, F.A. (1990) Translation of the humeral head on the glenoid. *Journal of Bone and Joint Surgery* **72**, 1334–1343.

Herring, S.A. (1990) Rehabilitation from muscle injury. *Medicine and Science in Sports and Exercise* **22**, 453–456.

Hutchinson, M.R., Laprade, R.F. & Burnett, Q.M. (1995) Injury surveillance at the USTA Boy's Tennis Championships: a six year study. *Medicine and Science in Sports and Exercise* **7**, 826–830.

Kibler, W.B. (1993) Evaluation of sports: demands as a diagnostic tool in shoulder disorders. In: Matsen, F.A., Fu, F.H. & Hawkins, R.T., eds. *The Shoulder: A Balance of Mobility and Stability*, pp. 379–399. AAOS, Rosemont, IL.

Kibler, W.B. (1995) Biomechanical analysis of the shoulder during tennis activities. *Clinics in Sports Medicine* **14**, 79–85.

Kibler, W.B. (1998) The role of the scapula in athletic shoulder function. *American Journal of Sports Medicine* **26**, 325–337.

Kibler, W.B. & Chandler, T.J. (1993a) Musculoskeletal adaptations and injuries associated with intense participation in youth sports. In: Cahill, B., ed. *The Effect of Intense Training on Prepubescent Athletes*, pp. 203–216. AAOS, Rosemont, IL.

Kibler, W.B. & Chandler, T.J. (1993b) Preparticipation evaluations. In: Renstrom, P., ed. *Sports Injuries—Basic Principles of Prevention and Care*, pp. 223–241. Blackwell Scientific Publications, Oxford.

Kibler, W.B. & Chandler, T.J. (1994) Sport specific conditioning. *American Journal of Sports Medicine* **22**, 424–432.

Kibler, W.B. & Chandler, T.J. (1997) Musculoskeletal considerations in overtraining. In: Kreider, R.B., Fry, A.C. & O'Toole, M.L., eds. *Overtraining in Sport*, pp. 169–191. Human Kinetics, Champaign, IL.

Kibler, W.B., McQueen, C. & Uhl, T.L. (1988) Fitness evaluations and fitness findings in competitive junior tennis players. *Clinics in Sports Medicine* **7**, 403–416.

Kibler, W.B., Chandler, T.J. & Uhl, T.L. (1989) A musculoskeletal approach to the preparticipation physical examination. *American Journal of Sports Medicine* **17**, 525–531.

Kibler, W.B., Chandler, T.J. & Pace, B.K. (1992) Principles of rehabilitation after chronic tendon injuries. *Clinics in Sports Medicine* **11**, 661–673.

Kibler, W.B., Chandler, T.J., Livingston, B.P. & Roetert, E.P. (1996) Shoulder range of motion in elite tennis players. *American Journal of Sports Medicine* **24**, 279–285.

Kleinoder, H., Neumaier, A., Loch, M. & Mester, J. (1995) Cinematographic analysis of the service movement in tennis. In: Krahl, H., Pleper, H.G., Kibler, W.B. & Renstrom, P., eds. *Tennis: Sports Medicine and Science*, pp. 16–20. Rau, Dusseldorf.

Matsen, F.A., Harryman, D.T. & Sioles, J.A. (1991) Mechanics of glenohumeral instability. *Clinics in Sports Medicine* **10**, 783–788.

Nichols, T.R. (1994) A biomechanical perspective on spinal mechanisms of coordinated muscle action. *Acta Anatomica* **15**, 1–13.

Putnam, C.A. (1993) Sequential motions of body segments in striking and throwing skills. *Journal of Biomechanics* **26**, 125–135.

Silliman, F.J. & Hawkins, R.J. (1991) Current concepts and recent advances in the athlete's shoulder. *Clinics in Sports Medicine* **10**, 693–705.

Speer, K.P. & Garrett, W.E. (1994) Muscular control of motion and stability about the pectoral girdle. In: Matsen, F.A., Fu, R.H. & Hawkins, R.J., eds. *The Shoulder: A Balance of Mobility and Stability*, pp. 159–173. AAOS, Rosemont, IL.

Warner, J.T.P., Micheli, L.J. & Arslenian, L. (1990) Patterns of flexibility, laxity, and strength in normal shoulders and shoulders with instability and impingement. *American Journal of Sports Medicine* **18**, 366–375.

Winge, S., Jorgenson, U. & Neilson, L. (1989) Epidemiologic studies in Danish championship tennis. *International Journal of Sports Medicine* **10**, 368–371.

Young, J.L., Herring, S.A., Press, J.M. & Casazza, B.A. (1996) The influence of the spine on the shoulder in the throwing athlete. *Journal of Back and Musculoskeletal Rehabilitation* **7**, 5–17.

Chapter 12

Pathophysiology of tennis injuries—an overview

Introduction

Analysis of injuries sustained in tennis competition reveals that: (i) they are very common; (ii) they occur throughout the body; (iii) they are relatively mild in disability; and (iv) they occur frequently as a result of microtrauma and infrequently from macrotrauma.

Most studies of injury patterns have been performed on elite or competitive athletes. Table 12.1 summarizes injury incidence reports from several studies—an international study (Kibler *et al.* 1988), a USTA study (Kibler & Chandler 1994) and a Belgian study (Verspeelt 1995). Table 12.2 shows injury sites from these plus an American study (Hutchinson *et al.* 1995). Table 12.3 breaks these injuries into types, either macrotrauma (sprains and fractures) or microtrauma overload. These studies, although limited due to population studied, population size and lack of a common definition of injury, are similar in their findings and probably do represent injury profiles in competitive tennis players.

Injury occurrence in competitive tennis players is quite high. Fifty to ninety per cent of players reported an injury in the 12 months prior to the questionnaire (see Table 12.1). These injuries were spread throughout the entire body, reflecting the stresses applied to all parts of the body during tennis (see Table 12.2). In general, the injuries tended towards mild disabilities. The only study that closely followed 'down time' showed that the mean time away from sport was 3.1 weeks, and no player had to give up tennis directly due to the injury (Verspeelt 1995).

Macrotrauma, such as sprains and fractures, was a causative factor in a minority of tennis injuries. These types of injury represent an event in which previously normal tissues are rendered immediately abnormal. These injuries occur as a result of an externally applied force, are unpredictable, and are difficult to prevent by conditioning activities.

The major type of injury in tennis players is due to microtrauma repetitive overload (see Table 12.3). Injuries in the upper extremity and back are almost exclusively due to overload, while lower extremity injuries are due to overload in half of the cases. Overall, microtrauma injuries account for 65–75% of all injuries seen in these studies.

Microtrauma injuries represent a process of injury in which normal tissues gradually become altered (Kibler *et al.* 1992). These alterations, most of which can be objectively measured, cause the tissues to be unable to respond adequately to sports demands. Decreased performance and overt tissue injury result from these alterations. This process may create

Table 12.1 Incidence of tennis-related injuries.

Study	Total players	Players with injury (%)	Total number of injuries
International			
English	17	11 (64.7)	14
Swedish	13	12 (92.3)	18
American	33	18 (54.5)	27
Total	63	41 (65.1)	59
USTA	34	22 (64.7)	26
Belgian	127	110 (87)	167

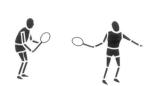

Table 12.2 Site of tennis-related injury.

	International (%)	USTA (%)	Belgian (%)	American (%)
Shoulder	7 (22)	4 (15)	21 (13)	3 (9)
Elbow	2 (6)	1 (4)	10 (9)	4 (15)
Back	4 (12.5)	2 (8)	31 (18.5)	3 (9)
Knee	4 (12.5)	5 (19)	33 (20)	7 (24)
Ankle and foot	6 (18)	7 (27)	26 (15.5)	7 (24)

Table 12.3 Types of injury by causative mechanism.

	Macrotrauma (%)	Microtrauma (%)
Overall (USTA + American)	33	67
Overall (International)	31	69
Overall (Belgian)	24	76
Individual—shoulder	6	94
Individual—back	25	75
Individual—knee	42	58
Individual—foot and ankle	48	52

adaptations in other tissues, as the athlete tries to continue to participate in sport. The incidence of these injuries may be modifiable with proper conditioning (Ekstrand & Gillquist 1983; Butler & Siegel 1990; Chandler & Kibler 1993).

This chapter will review current concepts on pathophysiology of repetitive microtrauma overload injuries, and suggest techniques for evaluation of tennis injuries based on these concepts.

Pathology in overload injuries

Pathological specimens reveal a characteristic picture of a longstanding process of injury. There are many blood vessels and a large amount of poorly organized, undifferentiated tissue, indicating a lack of organized healing to normal tissue. There are very

few inflammatory cells, indicating chronicity and lack of an ongoing attempt to heal the tissue through the normal process of tissue regeneration. This tissue has not, and cannot, respond to normal biologic signals for repair and recovery, collagen orientation, or maturation (Leadbetter 1992). This failed healing response has been termed angiofibroblastic tendinosis, reflecting the pathological picture of a degenerative lesion to a lower order of maturation (Leadbetter 1992; Nirschl 1992).

These changes probably have their genesis in the effect overload exerts on cells. Cellular effects include decreased enzyme levels, alteration in mitochondrial size, changes in RNA transcription, alterations in calcium release and uptake, and changes in myofibril attachment to the sarcomere cytoskeleton (Kibler 1995b). Recent evidence suggests that mechanical

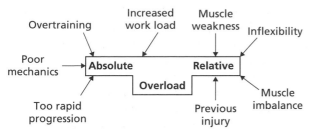

Fig. 12.1 The 'overload threshold' spectrum. Normal loads acting on subnormal tissues exert comparable tensile stresses as supranormal loads on normal tissues.

tensile load on the tissue is the most important factor in these changes (Teague & Schwane 1995). In muscle and muscle–tendon injuries, the exact mechanism is fibre and fibril strain that occurs during lengthening of an activated muscle (Lieber & Friden 1993). Implied in this description is that the load causing the lengthening and increased internal strain is important only as a relative load compared to the muscle's or tissue's ability to protect itself against the strain generated by the load, and that this 'overload threshold' is probably on a spectrum from relative to absolute overload (Fig. 12.1). Normal loads on weakened or fatigued muscles or tissues, a relative force overload, are as capable of causing excessive strain as supranormal loads acting on normal muscles or tissues, an absolute force overload.

Vascular or hormonal changes also participate in microtrauma causation. Probably all of these factors are involved to varying degrees. The net result is cellular contents that are incapable of making matrix of normal quality and quantity (Leadbetter 1992; Nirschl 1992).

These cellular alterations may be expressed on a tissue level as overt tissue injury, or non-overt tissue adaptations, such as inflexibility, weakness or inability to absorb loads. These adaptations may

not produce clinical symptoms, but do reduce performance (Chandler & Kibler 1993) and may act as risk factors for producing injuries (Ekstrand & Gillquist 1983; Knapik *et al.* 1991).

Model for injury causation

It appears that many factors may affect the process of microtrauma injury causation. A direct one-to-one cause-and-effect relationship can rarely be established between one particular anatomic or physiologic factor and a specific diagnosis.

We use a modification of Meeuwisse's model (Meeuwisse 1994) of multifactoral causation in microtrauma injuries (Fig. 12.2). Intrinsic risk factors (age, inflexibility, lack of strength, previous injury, lack of endurance) that are part of the athlete's musculoskeletal base create a predisposed athlete. This athlete then interacts with the inherent demands of the sport (biomechanical requirements, metabolic requirements, strength, agility) and other extrinsic factors (equipment, playing conditions, environment) to produce a susceptible athlete. This athlete is not normal or optimally efficient, but is functioning. An inciting event, such as more athletic exposure, more intense participation, or change in technique, may lead to overt injury and symptom production (Meeuwisse 1994). This has been termed the transitional event (Leadbetter 1992) and while it may be the moment of clinical symptoms, it is not when the clinical or anatomical problem developed. This model suggests that this process is longstanding and has many factors to be evaluated.

This model directs attention to understanding the demands inherent in tennis and evaluation of the individual tennis player's musculoskeletal base. Several studies (Elliott 1989; Giangarra *et al.* 1993; Kibler & Chandler 1994; Kibler 1995a) have analysed

Fig. 12.2 A model of multifactorial causation in microtrauma injuries. This illustrates the process on injury causation and the many factors that must be evaluated in the injury examination.

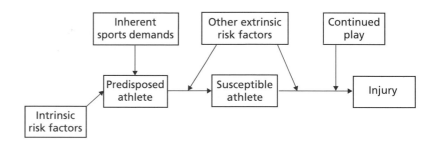

the inherent sports demands. The major findings of these studies are that tennis players face high force loads in the knee, back and arm; large motions of flexion/extension and rotation are required; and these forces and motions are frequently faced. Several studies (Chandler *et al.* 1991; Kibler & Chandler 1994; Kibler *et al.* 1996) demonstrate that intrinsic risk factors are common in tennis players. These usually are inflexibilities or alteration of muscle strength balance. This means that there are many predisposed and susceptible athletes playing tennis, and with time and intensity of competition being quite high, the incidence of injury would be predicted to be high. This prediction is borne out in the injury data.

Therefore, this model also directs attention to the importance of evaluating and conditioning the player's musculoskeletal base in light of the inherent demands, to reduce the population of predisposed athletes. This concept, called prehabilitation, has been shown to decrease inflexibility and strength deficits in a 2-year programme (Kibler & Chandler, unpublished data).

Framework for injury evaluation

In evaluation of microtrauma injuries, the clinician often has to play the game of 'victims and culprits' (MacIntyre & Lloyd-Smith 1993). The clinician must recognize all of the tissue alterations that exist as a result of the process of pathophysiology. These include local alterations in flexibility or strength, tissue injuries that produce the predominant clinical symptoms, alterations in distant areas of the kinetic chain that may be causing or affecting the local injury, and adaptations that may exist as the athlete continues to play (Kibler *et al.* 1992). By doing this type of evaluation, it often will be found that the source of clinical symptoms (the 'victim'), is not the sole source of the pathophysiological changes (the 'culprits'). We evaluate injuries based on a framework in which all

of the local and distant alterations are categorized into five complexes. These complexes appear to interact with each other in the causation of these microtrauma-moderated injuries, and are all detectable on the clinical level. These complexes also interact with each other in a negative feedback cycle, as shown in Fig. 12.3.

The five complexes are as follows.
1 *Tissue injury complex.* A group of anatomical structures that have overt pathological change.
2 *Clinical symptom complex.* Grouping of overt signs and symptoms that characterizes the injury.
3 *Tissue overload complex.* A group of anatomical structures that have clinically detectable change but are not overtly symptomatic. They are injured on the spectrum of relative to absolute overload.
4 *Functional biomechanical deficit complex.* Inflexibilities or strength imbalances that create altered athletic mechanics.
5 *Subclinical adaptation complex.* The substitute actions the athlete uses to compensate for altered mechanics to maintain performance.

The model allows description of most of the abnormalities that may exist in the 'predisposed' or 'susceptible' athlete, and emphasizes the multifactoral process that is occurring to produce the eventual clinical symptoms and altered performance. The tissue overload complex is part of the intrinsic risk factors present in the predisposed athlete, whereas the functional biomechanical deficits and subclinical adaptations characterize the susceptible athlete. The tissue injury and clinical symptom complexes are part of the overt pathology. Typically, an athlete may 'cycle' as a susceptible athlete for some time before clinical symptoms appear. Prevention of some of these injuries may be possible at this time. Appropriate pre-participation screening can detect the early development of microtrauma-induced tissue overloads and suggest correct rehabilitation before they create overt pathology.

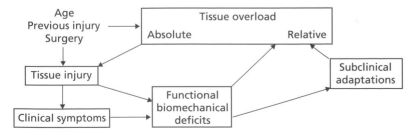

Fig. 12.3 The negative feedback vicious cycle framework for injury evaluation. This also emphasizes the process of injury causation and the type of analysis necessary for complete evaluation.

Specific injury evaluation using the negative feedback vicious cycle

All tennis injuries can be evaluated using this framework. After proper evaluation, treatment can then proceed by resolving each of the complexes. See Chapter 19 for rehabilitation principles.

Rotator cuff tendinitis (tendinopathy)

This specific injury is one of the most common injuries at all activity levels in tennis players (Fig. 12.4).
• Tissue overload—posterior capsule, shoulder external rotator muscles, scapular stabilizers.
• Tissue injury—rotator cuff impingement or tensile stretch, glenoid labrum, anterior capsule.

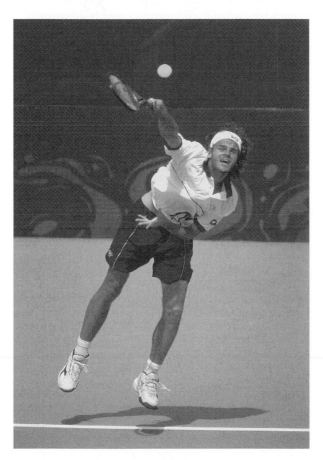

Fig. 12.4 Repeated tissue overload occurring during the explosive actions of serving and overhead shots can cause rotator cuff tendinitis. Photo © Allsport/R. Cianflone.

• Clinical symptoms—pain over anterior lateral acromion, impingement upon abduction and rotation, glenohumeral subluxation, positive 'clunk' or anterior slide test.
• Functional biomechanical deficit—functional 'lateral scapular slide', consisting of inflexibility in internal rotation, muscle strength deficits in shoulder external rotators and scapular stabilizers; in more advanced cases, superior or anterior glenohumeral translation occurs.
• Subclinical adaptations—'short arming' the throw, alteration of arm position during throwing or lifting, muscle recruitment from anterior shoulder, forearm or trunk.

Lateral epicondylitis

'Tennis elbow' is a very common problem in recreational athletes, but a rather infrequent problem in more accomplished tennis players. This injury occurs almost exclusively as a result of repetitive overload. Pathological change is seen in the extensor tendon attachments around the lateral epicondyle, especially in the extensor carpi radialis brevis.
• Tissue overload—lateral muscle mass, mainly extensor carpi radialis brevis, wrist pronators and extensors, shoulder external rotators.
• Tissue injury—same as for tissue overload, plus annular ligament and joint capsule.
• Clinical symptoms—point tender pain over extensor muscle mass, swelling in varying degree, pain on hitting backhand (usually in recreational athlete).
• Functional biomechanical deficit—extensor inflexibility and muscle weakness, decreased range of motion (ROM) in pronators and supinators, decreased shoulder external rotation strength.
• Subclinical adaptations—hitting 'behind the body', hitting with wrist movement, recruitment of triceps or alteration of position of elbow.

Medial epicondylitis

'Medial tennis elbow' is not as common as lateral epicondylitis, but is more commonly seen in advanced and competitive players. The pathology appears to be the same, with repetitive tensile microtears eventually giving rise to clinical tears

and symptoms. The overload is more frequently an absolute overload due to the large forces applied to the elbow in serving.
• Tissue overload—forearm flexor mass, biceps, pronator tests, usually absolute overload.
• Tissue injury—same as for tissue overload, ± medial collateral ligament, ulnar nerve, and/or posterior medial olecranon ('valgus overload complex').
• Clinical symptoms—point tender over flexor muscle mass, medial collateral ligament, posterior medial elbow, ± ulnar nerve symptoms.
• Functional biomechanical deficit—functional pronation contracture, consisting of elbow flexion and pronation inflexibility, tight and weak flexors, and decreased shoulder internal rotation strength, weak hip muscles.
• Subclinical adaptations—hitting 'behind the body', more overhead throwing motion, more wrist snap, more use of shoulder in throwing motion.

Low back and trunk pain

This anatomical area is the site of many tennis-related injuries. Three main types of injuries are seen. The first is located in the posterior midline, and is usually associated with the service motion or with straight-ahead activities, such as running to the net or hitting a low volley. The second is in the peripheral musculature of the quadratus lumborum or oblique abdominal muscles; it is associated with change in service motion or with groundstrokes. The third is a tear of the rectus abdominis anteriorum, which is associated with hitting overheads or many serves.
• Tissue overload—posterior back musculature, hamstrings, and hip rotators.
• Tissue injury—same as for tissue overload, with the addition of facet joints or sacroiliac joints.
• Functional biomechanical deficit—tight hamstrings, tight hip rotation and decreased trunk rotation.
• Subclinical adaptations—alteration of arm motion, excessive thoracolumbar motion, and excessive hip and leg rotation.

Leg muscle strains

Acute muscle strains or acute exacerbation of chronic muscle strains may occur in any of the leg muscles, but they seem to be most common in the adductors (groin strain), the medial head of the gastrocnemius ('tennis leg') and the hamstrings.

All of these may be acute injuries, but a substantial proportion of them are acute exacerbations of chronic injuries. The chronic injury may be mildly symptomatic or overtly asymptomatic but still capable of creating a functional biomechanical deficit. Before initiating treatment, it is important to enquire about previous injuries or prodromal symptoms and to check for anatomical deficits.

The difference between examining for acute hamstring strains and chronic hamstring strains may be seen in the evaluations. In the acute hamstring strain, the following complexes are observed.
• Tissue overload—origin/insertion of hamstring or muscle tendon junction.
• Tissue injury—medial or lateral hamstring, secondary to mechanical disruption, varying degrees of inflammation.
• Clinical symptoms—point tenderness, swelling and/or bruising, mass.
• Functional biomechanical deficit—none.
• Subclinical adaptations—none.
In the chronic hamstring strain, the following complexes are observed.
• Tissue overload—same as acute.
• Tissue injury—same as acute plus fibrosis.
• Clinical symptoms—point tender, diffuse over leg, reinjury.
• Functional biomechanical deficit—hamstring inflexibility, quadriceps/hamstring muscle imbalance, adductor inflexibility, hip extensor weakness.
• Subclinical adaptations—shortened stride, shortened kick, use of hip extensors and gastrocnemius.

Achilles tendinopathy

This injury is not very common in tennis players, but is disabling when it occurs. It usually occurs when playing surfaces are changed, such as going from hard courts indoors to soft courts outdoors in the spring. It may also occur when playing intensity increases, such as when attending a tennis camp.
• Tissue overload—gastrocnemius/soleus muscle or muscle tendon junction.
• Tissue injury—Achilles tendon, along its course or at its distal tendon bone attachment.

- Clinical symptoms—point tender, ± knot, stiffness after rest.
- Functional biomechanical deficit—inflexibility in dorsiflexion, weak plantar flexors.
- Subclinical adaptations—shortened stance, less push-off.

Ankle sprains

Just as in other sports in which running, cutting and stopping and starting are major demands, ankle sprains are the most common macrotrauma injuries in tennis players. Twisting forces, especially in plantar flexion, account for most of the injuries.

Inadequate treatment of the acute ankle sprain leads to the chronic ankle sprain syndrome, which has a more complex evaluation and which is more difficult to rehabilitate. Therefore, treatment should ensure good ligamentous stability, full flexibility, and good plantar flexion and eversion strength before return to play.

Acute ankle sprain

- Tissue overload—none.
- Tissue injury—anterior talofibular, fibulocalcaneal ligaments.
- Clinical symptoms—pain, swelling, point tender area.
- Functional biomechanical deficit—none.
- Subclinical adaptations—none.

Chronic ankle sprain

- Tissue overload—plantar flexors, evertors.
- Tissue injury—same as above, plus ankle capsule.
- Clinical symptoms—recurrent sprains, locking of joint.
- Functional biomechanical deficit—plantar flexion inflexibility and weakness.
- Subclinical adaptations—running on heels, decreased stride length.

Summary

Injuries in tennis are quite frequent, but are relatively mild. They are most commonly the result of chronic microtrauma overload. Because of these factors, emphasis should be placed on a complete understanding and assessment of the musculoskeletal factors that are associated with the clinical expression of the injury, and a good programme of prehabilitation, or preventative conditioning to decrease injury risk. This can be done by understanding the multifactorial model of injury causation that exists in microtrauma overload injuries, by looking for the conditions that create the predisposed or susceptible athlete, and evaluating for 'victims' and 'culprits' using the negative feedback vicious cycle. Effective treatment can then proceed based on this complete and accurate diagnosis.

References

Butler, D. & Siegel, A. (1990) Alterations in tissue response: conditioning effects at different ages. In: Leadbetter, W.B., Buckwalter, J.A. & Gordon, S.L., eds. *Sports Induced Inflammation*, pp. 713–731, AAOS, Rosemont, IL.

Chandler, T.J. & Kibler, W.B. (1993) Muscle training in injury prevention. In: Renstrom, P., ed. *Sports Injuries, Principles of Prevention and Care*, pp. 252–261. Blackwell Scientific Publications, London.

Chandler, T.J., Kibler, W.B., Kiser, A.M. & Wooten, B.P. (1991) Shoulder strength, power, and endurance in college tennis players. *American Journal of Sports Medicine* **20**, 455–457.

Ekstrand, J. & Gillquist, J. (1983) The avoidability of soccer injuries. *International Journal of Sports Medicine* **4**, 124–128.

Elliott, B.C. (1989) Tennis strokes and equipment. In: Vaughn, C.L., ed. *Biomechanics of Sport*, pp. 263–288. CRC Press, Boca Raton, FL.

Giangarra, C.E., Conroy, B., Jobe, F.W. & Pink, M. (1993) EMG and cinematographic analysis of elbow function in tennis players. *American Journal of Sports Medicine* **21**, 394–399.

Hutchinson, M.R., Laprade, R.F. & Burnett, Q.M. (1995) Injury surveillance at the USTA Boys' Tennis Championships: a 6 year study. *Medicine and Science in Sports and Exercise* **7**, 826–830.

Kibler, W.B. (1995a) Biomechanical analysis of the shoulder during tennis activities. *Clinics in Sports Medicine* **14**, 79–86.

Kibler, W.B. (1995b) Pathophysiology of overload injuries around the elbow. *Clinics in Sports Medicine* **14**, 447–456.

Kibler, W.B. & Chandler, T.J. (1994) Racquet sports. In: Fu, F. & Stone, R., eds. *Sports Injuries: Mechanisms, Prevention, and Treatment*, pp. 531–550. Williams & Wilkins, Baltimore, MD.

Kibler, W.B., McQueen, C. & Uhl, T.L. (1988) Fitness evaluations and fitness findings in competitive junior tennis players. *Clinics in Sports Medicine* **7**, 403–416.

Kibler, W.B., Chandler, T.J. & Pace, B.K. (1992) Principles of rehabilitation after chronic tendon injuries. *Clinics in Sports Medicine* **11**, 661–673.

Kibler, W.B., Chandler, T.J., Livingston, B. & Roetert, E.P. (1996) Shoulder rotation in elite tennis players—effect of age and tournament play. *American Journal of Sports Medicine* **24**, 279–285.

Knapik, J.J., Bauman, C.L., Jones, B.H. & Harris, J.M. (1991) Preseason strength and flexibility imbalances associated with athletic injuries in female collegiate athletes. *American Journal of Sports Medicine* **19**, 76–81.

Leadbetter, W.B. (1992) Cell-matrix response in tendon injury. *Clinics in Sports Medicine* **11**, 553–578.

Lieber, R.L. & Friden, J. (1993) Muscle damage is not a function of muscle force but active muscle strain. *Journal of Applied Physiology* **74**, 520–526.

MacIntyre, G. & Lloyd-Smith, D.R. (1993) Overuse running injuries. In: Renstrom, P., ed. *Sports Injuries, Principles of Prevention and Care*, pp. 139–160. Blackwell Scientific Publications, London.

Meeuwisse, W.H. (1994) Assessing causation in sport injury: a multi-factoral model. *Clinical Journal of Sport Medicine* **4**, 166–170.

Nirschl, R.P. (1992) Elbow tendinosis/tennis elbow. *Clinics in Sports Medicine* **11**, 851–869.

Teague, B.N. & Schwane, J.A. (1995) Effect of intermittent eccentric contraction on symptoms of muscle microinjury. *Medicine and Science in Sports and Exercise* **27**, 1378–1384.

Verspeelt, P. (1995) A review of tennis related injuries in flemish high-level tennis players. In: Krahl, H., Pieper, H.G., Kibler, W.B. & Renstrom, P., eds. *Tennis: Sports Medicine and Science*, pp. 47–51. Rau, Dusseldorf.

Chapter 13

Foot problems in tennis

Tennis is usually associated with upper extremity problems but lower extremity injuries are probably more frequent in tennis than upper extremity problems. This is not surprising, given the amount of quick starts and stops, changes in direction, and running that are required in tennis. The majority of tennis injuries are chronic and most likely due to the repetitive nature of the sport. The majority of lower leg injuries are similar to those disorders that commonly affect running athletes. However, due to the uniqueness and repetitive nature of the tennis serve and the significant amount of side-to-side movement, specific anatomical structures are placed under greater stress than they are in most other sports. This accounts for the comparatively higher incidence of problems with structures such as the plantar fascia, Achilles tendon, posterior tibial tendon and flexor hallucis tendon, which are put under increased stress during the push-off phase of the service motion.

Posterior heel pain (retrocalcaneal bursitis, Haglund's deformity, pump bump)

Incidence and injury mechanism

Heel pain is not unusual in running and jumping athletes, such as tennis players. Poor-fitting shoes can exacerbate this, with a heel counter that is too stiff and tight putting pressure on the back of the heel. As expressed in the title, heel pain has been given many names. However, the basic cause of the pain is the same; that is, an inflammation of the fluid sac (bursa) between the front of the Achilles tendon and underlying bone of the calcaneus (heel bone) (Fig. 13.1). Although inflammation of the bursa can occur without a prominence of the bone in this region,

this is uncommon. It is felt that the condition is caused by constant rubbing of the Achilles tendon against a large bony prominence of the calcaneus (Haglund's deformity).

Diagnosis and symptoms

Retrocalcaneal bursitis typically presents as a gradual onset of heel pain located at the back of the heel. The pain is often worse with weightbearing and worse when bending the foot upward (dorsiflexing). Particular types of shoe wear that put increased pressure on the heel also often exacerbate it. Usually a prominence of the heel develops (pump bump) and swelling and tenderness occur in front of the Achilles tendon on both sides of the heel. This condition can occur with tendinosis and/or partial tears of the Achilles tendon. When tears occur, the tendon is usually injured at its insertion onto the calcaneus where excess pressure is being placed on it by the bony prominence. The diagnosis is usually

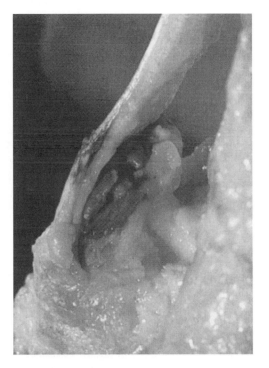

Fig. 13.1 Retrocalcaneal bursitis of the Achilles tendon—bump. (From Peterson, L. & Renström, P. (2000) *Sports Injuries: Their Prevention and Treatment*, p. 358. Martin Dunitz, London.)

apparent by physical examination, but a radiograph will confirm the presence of the bony prominence.

Treatment and rehabilitation

Initial treatment is by modification of shoe wear, instituting a soft heel counter, and relative rest. A small U-shaped pad can also be used around the tender area to relieve pressure. A small heel lift can help to move the Achilles tendon away from the bony prominence. Anti-inflammatory medicines can reduce swelling and pain. In severe cases, a couple of weeks in a walking boot, to rest the Achilles tendon and reduce inflammation, may be helpful.

In cases that do not respond to non-operative measures, surgery can be considered. Non-operative treatment should be attempted for a minimum of 4–6 months. Surgery consists of removal of the inflamed tissue and removal of the bony prominence. If the bony prominence is not removed, the condition is likely to recur. At the time of surgery the Achilles tendon insertion should be inspected and if there is any abnormal tissue it should be removed.

Impact and return to tennis

As with most overuse-type injuries, return to tennis playing is guided by pain and response to treatment. Depending on the severity of the injury and how the injury responds to shoe-wear changes and inserts, symptoms can last from a few days to several months. In those refractory cases treated surgically, time to return to tennis is variable. If the Achilles tendon had to have some debridement, return to tennis would be prolonged to 3–5 months in optimal cases.

Plantar fasciitis—sole heel pain

Incidence and injury mechanism

There are few epidemiological studies regarding the incidence of plantar fasciitis in athletes. Plantar fasciitis accounted for 9–10% of the total running disorders seen in one sports medicine clinic. In one retrospective study of lower extremity injuries in a tennis club in Northern California, 16% of the subjects indicated a history of plantar fasciitis (Feit & Berenter 1993).

Diagnosis and symptoms

Plantar fasciitis typically presents as a gradual onset of heel pain located on the bottom of the foot at the front of the heel. The pain is often worse with weight-bearing and worse when first arising in the morning. Pain can also be exacerbated by extension of the toes, which puts stretch on the plantar fascia. The cause of plantar fasciitis is not well understood, but it is thought to be related to periodic stress placed on the plantar fascia as it assists in maintaining the longitudinal arch of the foot (Fig. 13.2). During the push-off in the tennis serve the foot is brought into plantar flexion and the toes are forced into hyper-extension. This position puts the maximum stretch on the plantar fascia and probably contributes to the frequency of the injury.

Physical examination will reveal tenderness on the bottom and front part of the heel that will extend along the plantar fascia toward the front of the foot. The player will have increased pain with extension of the toes and toe raising. Hyperpronation of the foot and a tight Achilles tendon may contribute to the problem. Radiographs may show a spur on the heel but its presence is not the cause of the pain, and its removal is not necessary for a good surgical result. MRI will verify the diagnosis.

Treatment and rehabilitation

Treatment of this common disorder can be difficult, but fortunately about 75–80% of the cases resolve within 6 months using non-operative measures. Treatment protocols vary greatly but the majority rely on a stretching programme and the use of non-steroidal anti-inflammatory medicines and shoe inserts. Additionally, a period of rest, training modification and night splinting can be helpful. The basic concept of stretching and night splinting is to maintain a mild state of tension on the plantar fascia. This minimizes the change in tension during activities and avoids the repetitive microtrauma to the tissue. Unfortunately, no scientific studies support or refute this hypothesis, but some authors have reported good clinical results with both stretching and night splints.

Many types of shoe inserts have been advocated as an adjunct to therapy. These include heel cups,

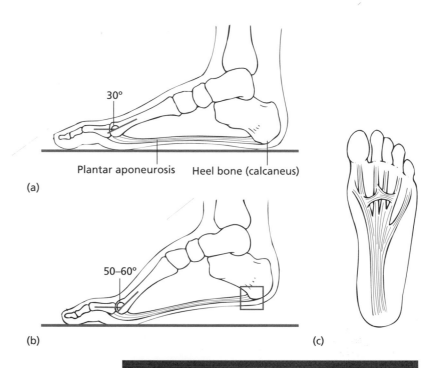

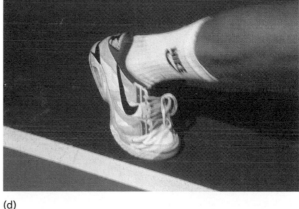

Fig. 13.2 Plantar fasciitis. (a) The foot and plantar aponeurosis (fascia) when the whole foot is loaded against the surface. (b) The plantar aponeurosis stretched during take-off. The boxed area indicates the seat of inflammation at the origin of the plantar aponeurosis from the heel bone. (c) The plantar aponeurosis seen from underneath. (From Ekblom, B. (ed.) (1994) *Handbook of Sports Medicine and Science: Football (Soccer)*, p. 177. Blackwell Scientific Publications, Oxford.) (d) When athletes push off they may experience pain.

tuli cups, heel pads, medial arch supports and heel wedges. Heel cups, tuli cups and heel pads are designed to support the fibro-fatty tissue of the fat pad beneath the heel to help cushion the heel during heel strike. This also is felt to minimize the microtrauma on the plantar fascia. Once again, little scientific evidence exists to evaluate this hypothesis, but clinical studies have shown acceptable results (Wolgin *et al.* 1994). Orthotics are designed to support the longitudinal arch and to support the heel during landing to keep the foot out of hyperpronation. Shock wave therapy on one to three occasions

shows very promising results. Steroid injections and casting are reserved for refractory cases.

In a review of 400 consecutive cases of heel pain, where patients were variably treated with steroid injections, orthoses, calf-stretching exercises, non-steroidal anti-inflammatory medications and occasional plaster immobilization, results showed that 73% improved significantly within 6 months, 20% failed to improve and 7% did not return and were lost to follow-up (Bordelon 1994).

For cases that are refractory to conservative measures, surgery to release the plantar fascia is considered.

Results of surgery are good in about 80% of the cases regardless of whether the spur is removed or not.

Impact and return to tennis

Again, as with most of the overuse-type injuries, return to tennis playing is guided by pain. Depending on the severity of the injury and how the injury responds to shoe-wear changes and inserts, symptoms can last from a few days to several months. There are tennis players that have problems from plantar fasciitis for years. In those refractory cases treated surgically, return to tennis is usually possible at about three to four months.

Flexor hallucis longus tendinopathy or rupture

Incidence and injury mechanism

Tendinopathy or partial rupture of the flexor hallucis longus tendon is most commonly reported in associ-

ation with ballet dancers. Although uncommon, with only one partial rupture of the flexor hallucis longus tendon in association with tennis reported in the literature (Trepman *et al.* 1995), we have seen this disorder in several tennis players. This is most probably due to the repetitiveness of the push-off and rotation of the foot during the tennis serve (Fig. 13.3) or pushing from side to side (Fig. 13.3). To date, however, no epidemiological studies have examined this.

Diagnosis and symptoms

Flexor hallucis longus (FHL) injury usually presents as a gradually increasing pain located 2 cm behind the bone prominence (medial malleolus) on the inside of the ankle and radiating along the course of the tendon to the big toe. Pain will be increased with active flexion and passive extension of the big toe. Sometimes, triggering of the tendon, where the toe will get caught in a fixed position, can occur if the swelling in the tendon becomes larger than the surrounding covering. The player may have tenderness and swelling on the inner side of the hindfoot. Magnetic resonance imaging (MRI) will verify the diagnosis after showing fluid inside the tendon sheath but will not always verify a rupture especially if it is a longitudinal split (Fig. 13.4).

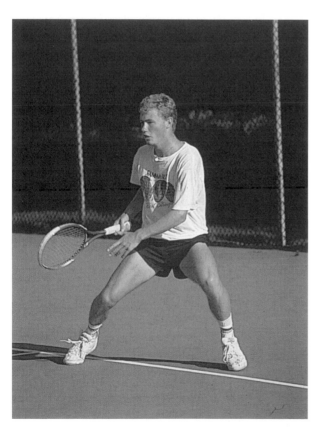

Fig. 13.3 Side-to-side motion or serving may cause hindfoot pain such as flexor hallucis longus partial tear or tendinosis.

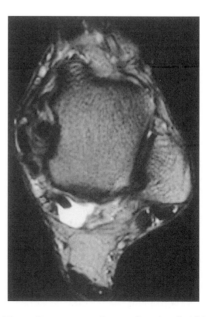

Fig. 13.4 Magnetic resonance image showing fluid in the sheath of flexor hallucis longus indicating overuse or tear.

Treatment and rehabilitation

Treatment of flexor hallucis longus injury includes anti-inflammatory medications and avoidance of activities that require forceful flexion of the big toe. Tennis players should avoid the strong push-off phase of the serve or when returning from the side. Shoes with stiffer soles can help to decrease the amount of push-off required from the FHL, by using the energy of the sole to aid in push-off. The majority of cases of fluid in the sheath will resolve within a few weeks.

With chronic tendinopathy, recovery may take up to 3 months or longer. In these cases, immobilization for 2–3 weeks in a cast or walking boot may be helpful. In all cases, modification of training can assist in recovery and prevention. In cases that are refractory to non-operative treatment, surgery may be indicated to release the surrounding tendon sheath and to remove inflamed tissue, and in case of rupture repair it or in case of tendinosis remove it.

Impact and return to tennis

Again, as with most of the overuse-type injuries, return to tennis playing is guided by pain. Depending on the severity of the injury, symptoms can last from a few days to several months. In those refractory cases treated surgically, return to tennis is usually possible at about 2–3 months. A longer rehabilitation programme to recover strength etc. is usually needed.

Stress fractures

Incidence and injury mechanism

Stress fractures in tennis players are not as common as in long-distance running sports, but they do occur. Most commonly they are the result of an abrupt change in training habits, with a sudden large increase in repetitive pounding-type activities. The most commonly involved bone in the athletic foot and ankle are the metatarsals, lateral malleolus and calcaneus. The most difficult fractures to treat, however, are the medial malleolar, base of the fifth metatarsal (Jones' fracture) and navicular stress fractures. Women have been shown to have an increased incidence of stress fracture compared to men.

Diagnosis and symptoms

Athletes typically complain of a gradual onset of pain that worsens with activity. Most commonly, they will be tender over the involved area, and may have a small amount of swelling. Diagnosis can be confirmed with plain radiographs or bone scan. In early cases, and cases with a minimal healing response, the plain radiographs will be normal. Stress fractures in the foot and ankle are particularly hard to see on plain radiographs due to the smallness of the bones and the large amount of overlap of the bones on radiograph. Therefore, a bone scan, a computed tomography (CT) scan or MRI are usually necessary to confirm the diagnosis.

Treatment and rehabilitation

Fortunately, the most common fractures, those of the lateral malleolus, and metatarsal shafts are easily treated and heal well. Treatment consists of relative rest, which means keeping activity below that which causes pain. Shoe modification and/or orthotics can help to redistribute stress in the foot to aid in healing and prevent recurrence.

Treatment of the stress fractures of the base of the fifth metatarsal (Jones' fracture) and medial malleolus is controversial, with some people advocating early surgical fixation and others advocating non-operative treatment with a non-weightbearing cast for 6 weeks or more. These fractures tend to heal slowly because, like the stress fracture of the mid-tibia, they are fractures on the tension side of the bone. So, in general, surgical fixation with screws leads to earlier return to activities. There seems to be a higher incidence of refracture with non-operative treatment.

Navicular stress fractures fortunately are not that common, but they are particularly troublesome. They are often overlooked and the diagnosis in many cases is delayed by many months. This is because of the vagueness of the symptoms and the difficulty in seeing this fracture on plain radiographs. Long delays in treatment can lead to chronic disability, because in those cases healing can be difficult to induce even with surgical fixation. Initial treatment in acute cases with no displacement of the fracture proceeds with 6 weeks of non-weightbearing casting. In cases that fail to respond to casting, or those with fracture displacement, surgery is indicated to fix the fracture with screws. Bone grafting (placing bone taken from the hip area into the fracture site) may be needed to induce healing. Surgery probably does not promote faster healing in non-displaced fractures, as for the medial malleolus and Jones' fractures. This is probably because of the more tenuous blood supply to the navicular, which is further compromised by the surgical incisions. In either case, orthotics should be worn after healing to redistribute the stresses to prevent recurrence.

Impact and return to tennis

For stress fractures of the lateral malleolus, calcaneus and metatarsal shafts, return to tennis can usually begin at 6 weeks with gradual progression of intensity.

For the medial malleolar and Jones' fractures treated non-operatively, return to tennis can usually begin at about 4 months. Those treated by surgical fixation can often begin tennis at 6–8 weeks after surgery.

Navicular stress fractures, in optimal cases, are out of tennis for 4–6 months regardless of the type of treatment, and this can be prolonged in cases that fail to respond to treatment.

Nerve entrapments and Morton's neuroma

Incidence and injury mechanism

Nerve entrapment syndromes are not common around the foot with the exception of the Morton's neuroma (interdigital neuroma) that occurs in the web space of the toes and causes pain and altered sensation to the affected toes. Any of the nerves that supply the foot can cause pain by being compressed (entrapped) by another tissue. The pain will be felt in the area that the nerve supplies and not necessarily at the site of the nerve compression. There are three main nerves to the foot: tibial nerve, deep peroneal nerve and superficial peroneal nerve. The sural nerve and saphenous nerve also supply some smaller areas of sensation to the foot, but entrapment of these nerves is rare. However, injury to these two nerves can occur from lacerations or surgical incisions. Such injuries can cause a loss of sensation to a small part of the foot as well as a painful nerve scarring (neuroma).

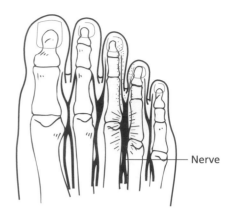

Fig. 13.5 Morton's syndrome. (From Ekblom, B. (ed.) (1994) *Handbook of Sports Medicine and Science: Football (Soccer)*, p. 177. Blackwell Scientific Publications, Oxford.)

Tibial nerve compression is probably the most common of the larger nerves to be involved in entrapment syndromes, followed by the deep peroneal nerve. The superficial peroneal nerve is rarely involved but compression can occasionally occur as the nerve exits from the fascial compartment (thick fibrous covering of the muscles) in the lower leg.

Morton's neuroma is compression of the digital nerves where they split at the web space to give sensation to the toes. This is most common at the third web space between the third and fourth toes (Fig. 13.5).

Diagnosis and symptoms

Symptoms of nerve compression will depend on where and which nerve is being compressed. Most commonly the nerve compression only affects the sensory portion of the nerve. The motor portion of the nerve is not as sensitive to compression and usually will not be involved, but in severe cases this can occur.

The tibial nerve most commonly is entrapped at the tarsal tunnel, which is a fibrous sheath behind the bony prominence on the inside of the ankle (medial malleolus) that contains the tibial nerve and some of the blood vessels to the foot. This is analogous to carpal tunnel syndrome in the wrist where the nerve is compressed by the fibrous covering that is too tight. The tibial nerve supplies sensation to the bottom of the foot and inside back portion of the heel. In tarsal tunnel syndrome, these are the painful areas. Isolated branches from the nerve can be compressed further down in the foot. In this case, a smaller portion of the area supplied by the tibial nerve—that area supplied by the particular branch that is compressed—will be affected.

The deep peroneal nerve can be entrapped at the front of the ankle joint where it courses underneath a strong fibrous structure that holds the tendons to the foot in place (extensor retinaculum). The deep peroneal nerve supplies sensation to the first web space between the big toe and second toe, so this will be the painful area. Note that the real problem is away from the painful area.

The most common nerve compression in the foot occurs in the web space between the toes (Morton's neuroma). This is caused by compression and swelling of the nerve as it branches to supply sensation to the adjacent half of the two toes. The player will have pain and sometimes numbness of this area of the toes.

Nerve conduction studies can sometimes be useful in assisting with the diagnosis, but these often do not show the problem because of the somewhat intermittent nature of the compression that depends on the local swelling around the nerve. The best diagnostic test is to inject a local anaesthetic at the site of compression and see if the pain is completely resolved.

Treatment and rehabilitation

Initial treatment is to modify shoe wear to relieve external pressure in the area of the nerve compression to reduce swelling. Anti-inflammatory medicines and/or an injection of steroids can also reduce the amount of swelling around the nerve and provide relief. In true nerve entrapment syndromes these non-operative measures have a relatively high rate of failure. If the pain is severe enough, surgery is indicated to release the offending tissue around the nerve. In the case of Morton's neuroma the area is too small for a release of surrounding tissue to be effective, so the nerve is actually cut in the area just before the swelling. This will leave half of the affected toes with permanent numbness, but the pain will be gone.

Impact and return to tennis

Return to tennis is governed by pain. Most players with this injury do not need to interrupt playing time. If the pain becomes too severe and surgery is required, return to tennis is allowed as soon as the player can tolerate it.

Sesamoid dysfunction

Incidence and injury mechanism

The sesamoids are small bones located within the flexor hallucis brevis tendon of the big toe just beneath the first metatarsophalangeal joint (Fig. 13.6). Sesamoid pain is not uncommon in running athletes. Pain can be caused by fracture, or inflammation of the sesamoid bones. Most commonly the sesamoid on the inside of the foot is affected.

Diagnosis and symptoms

Most commonly the player presents with a several-week history of gradually increasing pain located under the first metatarsophalangeal joint that worsens during weightbearing, 'pounding'-type activities and during the push-off phase of running. On examination

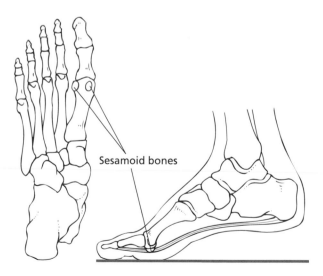

Fig. 13.6 Sesamoid bones. (From Peterson, L. & Renström, P. (2000) *Sports Injuries: Their Prevention and Treatment*, p. 421. Martin Dunitz, London.)

the patient will have localized tenderness of the affected sesamoid, and pain with active big-toe flexion and passive extension. Radiographs may be normal, or may show a fracture, irregular shape or bipartate (two parts) sesamoid. Difficulties arise in trying to differentiate these entities by plain radiographs. A bone scan can be helpful to at least show where the pathology is located.

Treatment and rehabilitation

In cases of obvious fracture, which are uncommon, a short leg walking cast, walking boot or wooden-soled shoe with taping of the toe have been used. In the usual case of inflammation, initial care consists of a moulded orthotic or pad placed just before the sesamoid to relieve pressure. The majority of cases will improve with these simple unweighting techniques, in addition to activity modification. In the refractory case, excision of the sesamoid can be considered, but complications are not infrequent, with deformities of the big toe sometimes developing.

Impact and return to tennis

Return to tennis playing is guided by pain. If the pain can be completely resolved with shoe-wear changes and orthotics, return to play can be instituted quicker. Depending on the severity of the injury, symptoms can last from a few days to several months. In those refractory cases treated surgically, return to tennis is usually possible at about 3–4 months. But, as stated above, surgical excision should be a last resort.

Hallux valgus (bunion) deformity

Incidence and injury mechanism

A bunion is a painful prominence of the large joint (metatarsophalangeal joint) of the big toe, with an angular deformity where the tip of the big toe deviates toward the smaller toes (Fig. 13.7). It is interesting to note that in societies that do not wear shoes, few bunions occur. This seems to implicate shoe wear as the main cause of bunions; this is particularly true of women's fashion shoes, with narrow pointed toes and high heels. No studies have shown an

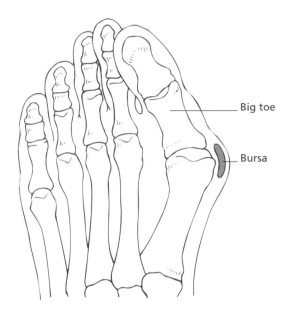

Fig. 13.7 Hallux valgus. (From Peterson, L. & Renström, P. (2000) *Sports Injuries: Their Prevention and Treatment*, p. 415. Martin Dunitz, London.)

increased incidence of bunions among athletes, so the stresses generated during push-off with the big toe do not seem to play a role in causing the problem. However, once the deformity has occurred, these stresses can exacerbate the pain and make playing difficult. Shoes with narrow toeboxes can exacerbate the problem.

Diagnosis and symptoms

The symptomatic player usually presents with swelling, redness and tenderness on the inside of the big toe joint closest to the ankle (the metatarsophalangeal joint). The player may also indicate that the big toe and second toe have begun to jam together or overlap. Radiographs taken in the weightbearing position will confirm the angulatory deformity. Sometimes the deformity will be present but will not cause pain.

Treatment and rehabilitation

Treatment is directed at relieving pain. The deformity itself is not a functional problem as long as it is not causing pain. The mainstay of treatment is convincing the player to modify his or her shoe wear to avoid pressure on the bunion. This means wearing shoes with wide toeboxes to allow space for the toes to comfortably seek their natural position. Orthotics and donut-shaped padding can sometimes be helpful in relieving stress over painful areas. Surgical treatment involves removing the bony prominence and realigning the big toe. There are various methods described to perform this. Surgical treatment is a last resort, because return to tennis following bunion surgery is unpredictable. Therefore, bunion surgery should never be carried out for cosmetic reasons; it is only indicated for where there is pain that is refractory to non-operative treatment and is interfering with the player's ability to function. Surgery may end the tennis player's competitive career. Following surgery the foot is protected with a cast or walking boot for about 3–6 weeks. A period of rehabilitation is then needed prior to vigorous activity.

Impact and return to tennis

The effect on tennis play is mainly governed by pain. If shoe-wear changes relieve the pain, the athlete can resume playing tennis immediately. In cases treated surgically, return to tennis playing in optimal cases can resume in about 3–4 months.

Hallux rigidus (stiff big toe)

Incidence and injury mechanism

Arthritic changes can occur in the metatarsophalangeal joint of the big toe, particularly in the older tennis player. Because of the stress placed on the joint during the push-off phase of the tennis serve, pain can occur in this joint (Fig. 13.8).

Diagnosis and symptoms

The symptomatic player usually presents with tenderness on the top of the big toe joint closest to the ankle (the metatarsophalangeal joint). The player will also have decreased and painful motion of the joint. Swelling is often present around the joint. Radiographs will usually show spurring on top of the joint and some narrowing of the metatarsophalangeal joint, indicative of early arthrosis is also typically

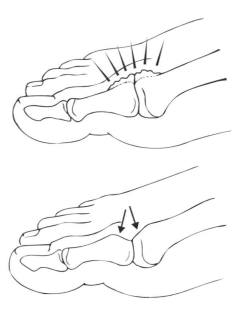

Fig. 13.8 Hallux rigidus. (From Peterson, L. & Renström, P. (2000) *Sports Injuries: Their Prevention and Treatment*, p. 418. Martin Dunitz, London.)

present. As the arthritic changes worsen, the degree of spurring and joint narrowing progress.

Treatment and rehabilitation

Initially, conservative treatment with non-steroidal anti-inflammatory medications and shoe-wear changes or stiff-soled shoes is tried. A stiff sole can decrease the amount of extension that is necessary at the big toe metatarsophalangeal joint during push off, instead using the energy of the stiff sole to assist with push-off. Most people continue to play during the early stages of this condition, modifying their activity or taking medication. If the pain becomes too severe, surgery can be considered. In cases with mainly spur formation with minimal joint cartilage changes, removal of the spurs can give relief (Fig. 13.8, bottom). However, in advanced cases with extensive joint cartilage loss, or cases in which removal of the spurs has failed, more extensive surgery may be needed such as fusion of the big toe metatarsophalangeal joint. This provides excellent pain relief but motion will no longer occur at the joint, which makes tennis playing more difficult, so this type of surgery should not be taken lightly, and should be used only as a last resort.

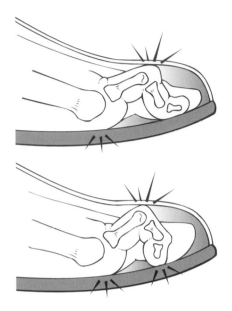

Fig. 13.9 Hammer toes. (From Peterson, L. & Renström, P. (2000) *Sports Injuries: Their Prevention and Treatment*, p. 417. Martin Dunitz, London.)

Impact and return to tennis

The effect on tennis play is mainly governed by pain. Shoe-wear changes can help alleviate some pain. Continued play may hasten arthritic changes, so there is a trade-off in terms of how much discomfort is acceptable in relation to the benefit gained from playing tennis. Once fusion is performed, tennis playing becomes more difficult, but may still be possible with a modification or reduction in playing style.

Lesser toe problems

Many problems of the lesser toes occur as the result of excessive pressure when the foot is jammed against the front of the shoe. Hammer toe can develop especially in older players (Fig. 13.9). Hard calluses, soft corns, blisters and subungual haematomas (tennis toe) are common occurrences in sports that require quick starts, stops and changes in direction. Many of these problems are caused or exacerbated by poor fitting shoes. Fortunately, most of these problems can be relieved by shoes with adequate toe box space, a snug fit in the midfoot and padding over sensitive areas (Baxter 1992; Zecher & Leach 1995). The mainstay of treatment therefore is prevention of lesser toe problems by proper shoe wear of good quality.

References

Baxter, D. (1992) The foot in running. In: Mann, R. & Coughlin, M., eds. *Surgery of the Foot and Ankle*, Vol. 2, pp. 1225–1240. Mosby, St Louis, MO.

Bordelon, R. (1994) Heel pain. In: DeLee, J. & Drez, D., eds. *Orthopaedic Sports Medicine. Practice and Principles*, Vol. 2, pp. 1806–1830. WB Saunders, Philadelphia, PA.

Feit, E. & Berenter, R. (1993) Lower extremity tennis injuries. Prevalence, etiology, and mechanism. *Journal of the American Podiatric Medical Association* **83** (9), 509–514.

Trepman, E., Mizel, M. & Newberg, A.H. (1995) Partial rupture of the flexor hallucis longus tendon in a tennis player: a case report. *Foot and Ankle International* **16** (4), 227–231.

Wolgin, M., Cook, C., Graham, C. & Mauldin, D. (1994) Conservative treatment of plantar heel pain: long-term follow-up. *Foot and Ankle International* **15**, 97–102.

Zecher, S. & Leach, R. (1995) Lower leg and foot injuries in tennis and other racquet sports. *Clinics in Sports Medicine* **14** (1), 223–239.

Chapter 14

Ankle problems in tennis

Introduction

There are two separate but related problems when considering ankle injuries. There are those problems that cause pain, and those problems that cause instability (giving way) and a feeling of unsteadiness. This chapter will break down into three main categories: (i) acute ankle injuries causing pain; (ii) chronic pain and overuse injuries; and (iii) chronic ankle instability. It is important to remember that there is much cross-over between categories. For example, an acute ankle sprain can lead to chronic ankle instability with subsequent painful giving way episodes. Thus, the breakdown is somewhat artificial but it helps to get a better understanding of the problem and treatment outcomes.

Acute ankle injuries

Acute sprain of the lateral ligaments of the ankle

Incidence

It is estimated that about one inversion injury of the ankle is suffered per 10 000 persons per day. This means that about 5000 of these injuries occur in the United Kingdom and 27 000 in the United States each day. Ankle sprains constitute 7–10% of all cases admitted to emergency departments of hospitals. This was the most common injury in cadets at the US Military Academy, with one-third of them sustaining an ankle sprain in their 4 years there (Balduini *et al.* 1987).

An ankle sprain is also the most common injury in sports. In a 1-year study in Oslo, 16% of sports injuries were acute ankle sprains. Although ankle sprains are less common in tennis than sports such as

soccer, basketball and volleyball, given the frequency with which this injury occurs in tennis it still constitutes a large number of injuries.

The large majority of ankle sprains occur in persons under 35 years of age, most commonly in the age range from 15 to 19 years. In spite of the high frequency and associated remaining disability of ankle sprains, there is great variation in the diagnostic approaches, the criteria used to define significant ligament disruption needing surgery, treatment modalities and rehabilitation techniques.

Anatomy

The ligamentous complex on the outside of the ankle is composed of three ligaments: the anterior talofibular ligament (ATFL), the calcaneofibular ligament (CFL) and the posterior talofibular ligament (PTFL) (Fig. 14.1). Most inversion sprains occur when the foot is in plantar flexion (with the toes pointed) when the most stress is on the ATFL. Consequently, this is the ligament that is most frequently torn. If the tearing force continues, the CFL will be injured next, followed by the PTFL. Isolated, complete rupture of the ATFL is present in 65% of cases of ankle sprains. A combination injury involving the ATFL and the CFL occurs in 20% of ankle sprains.

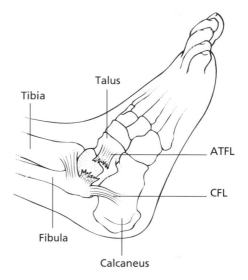

Fig. 14.1 Ankle lateral ligament tear. (From Peterson, L. & Renström, P. (2000) *Sports Injuries: Their Prevention and Treatment*, p. 367. Martin Dunitz, London.)

Diagnosis and symptoms

The most common presenting history is a player who has 'rolled' over the outside of his or her ankle. This will often occur when the athlete mis-steps or lands onto an opposing player's foot or on uneven ground. Most commonly these occurrences cause the foot to be in plantar flexion at the time of the injury.

• Immediately after the injury the player usually experiences a sudden, rather intense pain localized to the lateral side of the ankle.

• The area of maximal tenderness and swelling usually indicates which ligament has been disrupted. This area is most frequently localized over the ATFL. If the player is not seen until several hours after the injury, generalized swelling and pain make the evaluation more difficult and unreliable.

• Most players experience pain and discomfort when they try to bear weight on the injured extremity. Some players experience instability of the ankle with a feeling that the ankle 'gives way' when they try to use the leg.

• After 24–48 h, the outside of the injured ankle is usually discoloured, appearing blue and yellow due to the haematoma organization and resorption. The discolouration is often located more toward the foot than the injury itself because of the pooling affect of gravity. It is important that the entire ankle and foot are examined to be sure no other injuries have occurred.

• Standard radiographs should be taken in every patient with grade II or grade III ankle sprains (see below). They should include routine anteroposterior (AP) and lateral views as well as an anteroposterior view with the foot in 15–20° of internal rotation. In this position, which is called the mortise view, it is possible to exclude fractures.

Treatment and rehabilitation

Traditionally, ankle sprains have been classified as grade I (mild), grade II (moderate) and grade III (severe) injuries. Grade I injuries involve ligament stretch without macroscopic tearing, little swelling or tenderness, minimal or no functional loss, and no mechanical joint instability. A grade II injury is a partial macroscopic ligament tear with moderate pain, swelling and tenderness over the involved structures. There is some loss of joint motion and mild to moderate joint instability. A grade III injury is a complete ligament rupture with marked swelling, haemorrhage and tenderness. There is loss of function and marked abnormal joint motion and instability. Grading of ankle sprains, however, remains a largely subjective interpretation of the abnormal laxity observed in the ankle, and agreement between independent observers is variable.

Almost all clinicians agree that grade I and II injuries recover quickly with non-operative management and that the prognosis is excellent or good.

The treatment programme, called '*functional treatment*' includes application of the RICE principle (rest, ice, compression and elevation) immediately after the injury, a short period of protection with an elastic or inelastic tape, bandage or brace, and early motion exercises followed by early weight bearing and balance training. Applying compression is most important as it is by far the best way to decrease oedema and prevent further swelling. Ice has mainly a pain-limiting effect.

Balance training with a tilt board is commenced as soon as possible, usually after four to eight weeks (Fig. 14.2). This type of exercise should be carried out over a long period of time, usually about 3 months. Additional mobility and muscle-strengthening exercises are recommended.

Using this type of regimen, the period of disability was only 8 days in a group of US Military Academy cadets with grade I injuries and 15 days in those with grade II injuries.

Many studies have shown that early controlled mobilization (functional treatment), even for grade III injuries, provides the quickest recovery in ankle mobility and the earliest return to work and physical activity without compromising the late mechanical stability of the ankle (Renström & Kannus 1994). In addition, functional treatment is free of complications, whereas surgical treatment has some serious complications, although infrequently. Functional treatment produces no more late symptoms (giving way, pain, swelling, stiffness or muscle weakness) than surgical repair and cast or than cast alone. Furthermore, secondary surgical repair of the ruptured ankle ligaments (delayed anatomical repair) can be performed even years after the injury if necessary, with good results that are comparable to those achieved with primary repair. Therefore, even competitive athletes can initially be treated conservatively. Acute

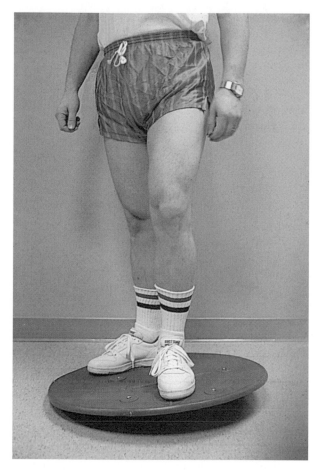

Fig. 14.2 Balance board training can be valuable.

surgery is seldom indicated. Those 10–20% of cases that may require secondary repair can be operated on in an elective phase.

In addition to functional therapy, other therapeutic modalities have been advocated to speed recovery. The most frequently used are ultrasound, temperature-contrast baths, cryotherapy (cold therapy) and electric stimulation. Unfortunately, randomized controlled studies have questioned the efficacy of these therapies. Of these different types of passive physical therapy, only cryotherapy has been proved to be effective, especially in treating pain. In regard to ankle function, tenderness, swelling and pain, non-steroidal anti-inflammatory drugs (NSAIDs) have been shown to be more effective than placebo, although the differences were not striking and seemed to disappear during extended follow-up.

Impact and return to tennis

After an ankle sprain, a player can return to tennis when he or she has full ankle range of motion, has 90% strength in the injured ankle as compared to the healthy side, and can run and cut at maximum speed without pain. During the initial return to tennis a brace should be used in order to avoid recurrent giving way. If chronic instability occurs, see p. 172.

Osteochondral and chondral fractures

Incidence and injury mechanism

Osteochondral injuries are small fractures of the cartilage surface and underlying bone, and chondral fractures are injuries sustained only by the cartilage lining that cause a flap or a small loose piece to form. These injuries can be sustained during a lateral ankle ligament sprain. Osteochondral injuries have been reported to occur in up to 4–6% and chondral lesions in 60–70% of patients who have had an ankle sprain.

Diagnosis and symptoms

The player will usually describe a history of a lateral ankle ligament sprain with the associated swelling along the outside of the ankle. Often injuries that are associated with chondral or osteochondral fractures are more violent. Most cases are initially treated as a lateral ankle ligament sprain with functional rehabilitation, unless the fracture is evident on the initial radiograph, which is usually not the case. The injury is usually identified when the player fails to respond to treatment, the player will often have persistent giving way episodes, pain on weight bearing and/or locking and catching of the ankle. A repeat radiograph at 3–4 weeks after the injury can sometimes reveal an osteochondral fracture. This occurs because the bone surrounding the fracture line begins to resorb and the fracture line becomes wider. In many cases, however, the lesion will not be evident on plain radiographs and a bone scan, computed tomography (CT) scan or magnetic resonance imaging (MRI) are necessary for diagnosis; this is particularly true when the lesion does not include bone (chondral lesions).

Treatment and rehabilitation

In cases in which the fracture has remained partially attached, results of non-operative treatment
have been good. This is achieved with protected
weightbearing with a walking boot for 4–6 weeks.
In cases in which the lesion is detached, non-
operative treatment often fails. The treatment of
choice is to remove the loose piece and roughen
the underlying bone to promote ingrowth of new
tissue. Weightbearing is restricted for 4–6 weeks
following surgery. The results of late surgery have
been variable with good outcomes in about 40–80%
of the cases. In cases in which the piece is very large,
reattaching the loose piece should be tried. The
results of this treatment have not been scientifically
verified.

Impact and return to tennis

In cases for which the lesion remains attached, and
that respond well to non-operative treatment, return
to tennis is usually possible at about 3–4 months. For
detached fragments that undergo surgery, return to
tennis is less predictable, but in optimal cases return
is possible at 3–4 months after surgery. Some patients
with chondral and osteochondral fractures will have
chronic pain.

Fractures of the ankle

Incidence and injury mechanism

Fractures of the ankle are not common among tennis
players, but they do occasionally occur. They are
much more common in jumping and contact sports.
Most fractures are caused by indirect forces rather
than a direct blow, such as when a football player
gets his foot caught in an abnormal position on the
turf during a tackle. Most fractures involve the distal
part of the bone on the outside of the ankle (lateral
malleolus); but with higher energy loads the forces
can continue around the joint to also include the
inside of the ankle (medial malleolus) and back of
the tibia (posterior malleolus). Isolated fractures of
the medial malleolus do occur but with much less
frequency.

Fractures of the small prominences of the other ankle
bones can also occur, but are fairly rare. The majority
of these are due to avulsions by the attaching ligament
or tendon. These fractures include the lateral and
posterior process of the talus, anterior process of the
calcaneus, as well as the more common avulsion of
the tip of the lateral malleolus that occurs with an
ankle sprain.

Diagnosis and symptoms

Diagnosis of acute fractures is usually quite obvious
by the amount of pain and swelling that occur at the
injury site. However, with low-energy fractures, and
particularly with the avulsion injuries, the symptoms
may mimic a common ankle sprain and the fracture
can be overlooked. Plain radiographs will usually
make the diagnosis, though special views may sometimes be necessary to see avulsion fractures at the
lateral or posterior process of the talus, or the anterior
process of the calcaneus.

Treatment and rehabilitation

Most low-energy fractures that involve only the
lateral malleolus can be treated by an ankle brace,
a walking boot or a cast for 4–6 weeks. But, if both
sides of the ankle are fractured the injury is more
unstable and usually requires surgery to fix the bones
with plates and screws. Most avulsion fractures can
be treated as a sprain with functional rehabilitation,
but with large fragments that have wide displace-
ments, surgery may be needed to reattach the fragment; this is particularly true of the lateral process
of the talus, and anterior process of the calcaneus.
Rehabilitation following casting or surgery consists
of range of motion exercises followed by strength
training.

Impact and return to tennis

Following immobilization or surgery, return to tennis
is usually possible after about 3–4 months. In severe
injury, early arthritis can sometimes develop despite
good treatment. Fortunately, however, the ankle is
fairly resistant to arthritic changes and most people
will make a full or nearly full recovery.

Posterior tibial tendon rupture

Incidence and injury mechanism

The majority of posterior tibialis tendon problems occur in middle-aged females, and complete rupture prior to this time is unusual. This is not a common injury in tennis players, but it may occur in the over-45 age group. It is included here because of the need to recognize the symptoms prior to rupture, because treatment of a complete rupture is difficult with an uncertain outcome in terms of return to vigorous activities.

It should be noted that, despite a well-described presentation and relatively consistent physical findings, tendon ruptures are frequently not recognized. In a study of 17 patients, all of whom had seen one or more physicians prior to evaluation by a foot specialist, only two cases had the proper diagnosis made before seeing the foot specialist (Mann & Thompson 1985). In addition, the average delay in diagnosis was 43 months.

The tibialis posterior is the main dynamic stabilizer of the longitudinal arch of the foot, and it is responsible for maintaining heel alignment.

Diagnosis and symptoms

The common presenting history is that of a preceding dull pain at the back (posterior) inside (medial) portion of the ankle caused by inflammation of the tendon covering. This is then followed by a minor ankle injury. Often the patient will not seek treatment immediately because of the relatively minor amount of pain. On physical examination the player will have mild tenderness just below and behind the inside portion of the ankle (medial malleolus). In the standing position the patient may display the characteristic flatfoot deformity. When viewed from behind, the patient will appear as if they have 'too many toes' due to the collapsed arch and change in the heel alignment. They will have difficulty with standing on their toes on the affected side.

Treatment and rehabilitation

Once rupture occurs, treatment is difficult. For acute ruptures in active young patients, surgical repair can be performed by direct repair, advancement of the tendon if possible or by transferring another tendon to replace the posterior tibialis. The surgical treatment will usually not restore normal foot alignment, particularly in chronic cases, but it most commonly does improve function. Surgical repair or reconstruction of the tendon is only indicated with flexible foot deformities that can be passively corrected. If there is a rigid flatfoot deformity, and conservative treatment with shoe-wear changes and orthotics has been unsuccessful, surgical fusion of the hindfoot joints can be helpful.

Impact and return to tennis

Once rupture occurs, return to tennis playing, even with good treatment, will be difficult. This is why it is important to recognize and treat the symptoms aggressively before rupture occurs.

Chronic ankle pain and overuse syndromes

Chronic ankle pain is caused by either acute injuries that do not respond to treatment, or by problems that arise from continuous overstressing of the tissues from overuse. Overuse problems can arise in the tendons in the form of tendinosis or peritendinitis, or can arise from the structures surrounding the joint, causing an arthritic or impingement type problem. Finally, in patients with persistent problems or unusual symptoms, we must consider other problems that can mimic lateral ankle ligament injuries, such as tendon ruptures, osteochondral or chondral fractures, osteochondritis dissecans, and midfoot or forefoot problems.

Posterior tibial tendinopathy

Incidence and injury mechanism

In contrast to rupture, posterior tibialis tendinosis and tenosynovitis are not uncommon in tennis players and runners, with a reported incidence of between 0.6 and 6%. Symptoms can be exacerbated by the strong push-off required during the tennis serve. Many authors stress the importance of treating posterior tibialis tendinopathy aggressively because they feel that this may be a precursor to complete rupture.

Diagnosis and symptoms

Symptoms are generally gradual in onset and increase with running activities, with the pain located just beneath and behind (posterior to) the inside of the ankle (medial malleolus) and extending along the course of the posterior tibial tendon. The player will have increased pain during push-off and when standing on his or her toes. On examination, the player will have swelling and tenderness along the tendon and will have pain when testing active function of the posterior tibialis tendon. Testing should be performed with the foot in plantar flexion to isolate the posterior tibialis tendon, and then having the patient invert the foot against resistance.

Treatment and rehabilitation

Treatment in mild cases can begin with a resting period and change in training habits. A medial longitudinal arch support can be helpful in relieving stress on the tendon and reducing symptoms. In severe or mild chronic cases that do not respond to a resting programme, cast or walking boot immobilization is recommended for a period of 2–4 weeks. If symptoms continue for longer than 4–6 months despite adequate conservative treatment, then surgery is considered. Surgery consists of opening of the tendon sheath and excising scar and inflammatory tissue. The patient is immobilized in a walking boot for 2–4 weeks after surgery. Return to sports can usually begin about 4 months after surgery. Good results following surgery have been reported in some studies but large objective studies are needed.

Impact and return to tennis

Again, as with most of the overuse-type injuries, return to tennis playing is guided by pain. Depending on the severity of the injury, symptoms can last from a few days to several months. In those refractory cases treated surgically, return to tennis is usually possible at about 4 months.

Anterior tibiotalar impingement

Incidence and injury mechanism

The term anterior tibiotalar impingement describes a bony or soft tissue build-up at the front of the ankle joint. This causes impingement of the tissue when the foot is bent upwards. The exact cause of the bony tissue build-up is unknown, but it is felt to be related to repeated microtrauma and possibly microfractures of the bone mostly on the anterior tip of the tibia that cause a bony overgrowth. Scar tissue can occur after a ligament rupture to cause soft tissue impingement on the lateral side (outside) of the joint. Sports that require jumping, sudden acceleration and deceleration, such as American football, soccer, ballet dancing and tennis have shown a propensity for this problem.

Diagnosis and symptoms

The presenting complaints are a gradually worsening pain located at the front of the ankle joint. The pain is worsened by passively bending the ankle upwards; this impinges the tissue. In prolonged cases, decreased ankle motion will occur, especially dorsiflexion (the foot bent upwards). The examination will confirm these findings, with tenderness and sometimes a palpable spur around the front of the ankle.

Treatment and rehabilitation

Treatment is initially conservative with rest, modification of activities, non-steroidal anti-inflammatory medication and bracing during activities to limit ankle motion. These treatments are designed to decrease the amount of inflammation in the soft tissues and to control symptoms. They will not remove the spur. The only method to accomplish this is surgical excision. In soft tissue impingement, arthroscopic excision of the soft tissue is effective. Return to activities can begin as soon as tolerated. Most can return to full physical activities at 3–6 weeks after soft tissue excision and 8–12 weeks after bone excision. The short-term prognosis is good, but long-term recurrence rates may be high.

Impact and return to tennis

Tennis play can continue as pain allows. Following surgically treated cases, tennis play can resume as soon as tolerated, with most being able to play tennis by about 2–3 months.

Osteochondritis dissecans of the talus

Incidence and injury mechanism

Osteochondritis dissecans describes a small area of bone beneath the joint lining that has lost its blood supply and become necrotic (i.e. dead bone) (Fig. 14.3). There is controversy as to whether osteochondritis dissecans of the talus is a separate condition from osteochondral fractures, or whether this represents a failed healing response of an old osteochondral fracture. Those that favour a separate aetiology feel this is caused by an interruption of the blood supply to a small portion of the bone that results in a small piece of dead bone. However, many, but not all, patients report a history of previous injury. It appears that those lesions that occur on the outside (lateral) have a much higher association with previous trauma than those that occur on the inside (medial).

So, in fact, most likely both scenarios are true, and they give similar long-term problems. If the small bone is well stabilized by strong scar tissue attachments, the fragment will often not cause any symptoms. However, as in osteochondral fractures, loose pieces, particularly if the opening extends through the cartilage lining the joint, will cause pain (Fig. 14.4).

Diagnosis and symptoms

The player will usually describe a chronic history of ankle pain that can be associated with recurrent giving-way episodes or locking. Some patients will have a remote history of a lateral ankle ligament sprain. Osteochondritis dissecans is more often seen on plain radiographs than its acute counterpart, osteochondral fracture. As in osteochondral fractures, however, the lesion sometimes will not be evident on plain radiographs, and a bone scan, CT scan or MRI is necessary to diagnose it.

Treatment and rehabilitation

An initial trial of non-operative treatment can be attempted. Protected weightbearing with a walking boot for 4–6 weeks is instituted to try to stabilize the

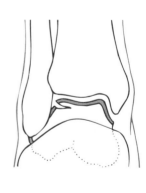
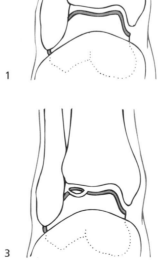
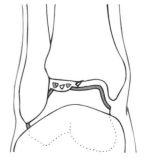

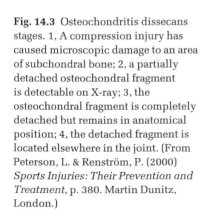

Fig. 14.3 Osteochondritis dissecans stages. 1, A compression injury has caused microscopic damage to an area of subchondral bone; 2, a partially detached osteochondral fragment is detectable on X-ray; 3, the osteochondral fragment is completely detached but remains in anatomical position; 4, the detached fragment is located elsewhere in the joint. (From Peterson, L. & Renström, P. (2000) *Sports Injuries: Their Prevention and Treatment*, p. 380. Martin Dunitz, London.)

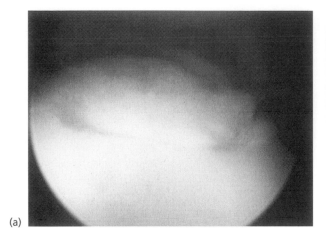
(a)

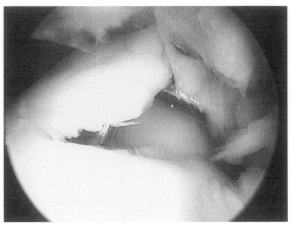
(b)

Fig. 14.4 A loose fragment of bone cartilage on the talus. (a) Fragment in place; (b) fragment opened up.

fragment so that it can heal. Results of non-operative treatment are better if the overlying cartilage is still intact. This prevents the synovial fluid from interposing between the fragment and underlying bone. If non-operative treatment fails, the treatment of choice is to remove the loose piece and roughen the underlying bone to promote ingrowth of new tissue. Weightbearing is restricted for 4–6 weeks following surgery. The results of late surgery have been variable with good outcomes in about 40–80% of the cases. In cases in which the piece is very large, some authors advocate reattaching the loose piece. The results of this treatment have not been scientifically verified.

Impact and return to tennis

In cases for which the lesion remains attached, and that respond well to non-operative treatment, return to tennis is usually possible at about 3–4 months. For detached fragments that undergo surgery, return to tennis is less predictable, but in optimal cases return is possible at 4–6 months after surgery. Some patients with osteochondritis dissecans will have chronic pain.

Chronic ankle instability

Chronic ankle problems can be caused by ankle pain or instability (giving-way episodes).

Problems related to chronic giving-way with periods of little or no pain in between episodes is most likely

the result of problems with the ligaments supporting the tibiotalar joint (ankle) or the subtalar joint (the joint in the heel between the talus and calcaneus). Sinus tarsi problems can also cause a feeling of instability. Chronic ankle instability from the tibiotalar joint is a much more common problem, but it can be difficult to differentiate between the two entities.

Chronic lateral ankle ligament instability

Incidence and injury mechanism

Chronic problems after ankle ligament injuries are very common. After either conservative or operative treatment, 10–20% of patients with a lateral ligament injury may have chronic symptoms.

Diagnosis and symptoms

Symptoms usually include persistent ankle stiffness, swelling, some pain, muscle weakness and frequent giving-way. Many of these problems are associated with ankle instability. It is important to differentiate between the two types of ankle instability: mechanical and functional. *Mechanical* instability refers to abnormal laxity of the ligamentous restraints, and *functional* instability refers to normal ligamentous restraint but abnormal function, with a feeling of giving-way and recurrent giving-way episodes. Often mechanical and functional instability occur together.

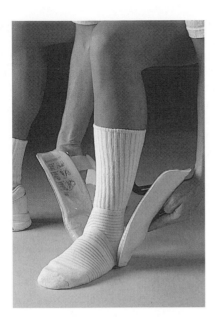

Fig. 14.5 Combined bracing and wrapping of the ankle can be effective.

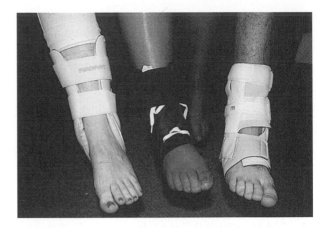

Fig. 14.6 Ankle braces can be very effective.

Treatment and rehabilitation

Strength training should be routine treatment. Balance training on a tilt board is very effective. After 10 weeks of training, a maximum effect is reached. Bracing and/or taping can help alleviate some of these problems (Figs 14.5 and 14.6). Athletes subjectively often experience a positive effect when using external supportive devices. At the beginning of a performance they provide mechanical support but the mechanical support decreases rapidly after only a few minutes of exercise. It has also been suggested that tape and braces provide increased proprioceptive feedback to assist with balancing. Finally, we must remember that the psychological effect of taping or bracing is probably high.

In cases of mechanical and/or functional instability that are refractory to bracing and external support, surgical treatment can be considered. Many surgical procedures used for treatment of chronic mechanical instability of the lateral ligaments of the ankle have been described. 'Anatomical reconstruction' (delayed repair) of the lateral ligaments, which means that the lateral ligaments are shortened and reinserted, gives good results. Postoperatively, the ankle is immobilized for 7–10 days, and then for 3–4 weeks an ankle brace (stirrup) walking boot is used for weightbearing and motion. Motion exercises are begun as soon as tolerated, followed by strength and balance training.

Impact and return to tennis

In cases of chronic lateral ankle ligament instability, tennis activities are allowed about 3 months after surgery. An ankle brace may be needed during tennis activities for 6–8 months postoperatively.

Subtalar instability

Incidence and injury mechanism

The subtalar joint is the joint between the two bones that make up the heel (the talus and calcaneus). The subtalar sprain has remained a mysterious and little-known clinical entity. The incidence is unknown, but it is widely accepted that most subtalar sprains occur in combination with lateral ankle ligament sprains. Subtalar instability is estimated to be present in about 10% of patients with chronic lateral ankle ligament instability.

Diagnosis and symptoms

Patients with chronic subtalar instability complain of giving-way episodes during activity, with a history of recurrent ankle sprains and/or pain, swelling and stiffness. This is especially prominent when walking on uneven ground. This is because the foot conforms to the ground by motion at the subtalar joint. Clinical evaluation of the subtalar joint is difficult and unreliable. Some athletes have a positive stress inversion test (former talar tilt test) and a negative anterior drawer test. Radiographs (Brodén view) can be helpful. Overall, this is an extremely difficult entity to describe and diagnose.

Treatment and rehabilitation

Treatment is initially conservative with treatment similar to that for chronic lateral ankle instability described in the previous section. This includes ankle muscle strengthening, balance training and bracing. In players that do not respond to non-operative measures, reconstruction of the ligaments between the talus and calcaneus can be performed. This can be done by shortening the local ligaments, or by using variously described tendon transfers to reconstruct the ligaments. Postoperatively, the ankle is immobilized for 7–10 days, and then for 3–4 weeks an ankle stirrup brace or a walking boot is used for weightbearing and motion. Motion exercises are begun as soon as tolerated, followed by strength and balance training.

Impact and return to tennis

Treatment and return to tennis are directed by the patient's symptoms. Ankle bracing may control symptoms and allow the player to return to tennis. In those requiring surgical treatment, tennis activities are allowed about 3 months after surgery. An ankle brace may be needed during tennis activities for 6–8 months postoperatively.

Sinus tarsi syndrome

Incidence and injury mechanism

The term sinus tarsi syndrome describes an unusual and painful condition at the outside (lateral) of the joint between the two bones that make up the heel (the talus and calcaneus). The joint is referred to as the subtalar joint. The sinus tarsi is an area within the joint that contains ligaments, synovial tissue (joint lining tissue which can secrete fluid) and blood vessels. There is no actual contact between the two bones, or their cartilage lining within the sinus tarsi. Thus, the weightbearing forces are transmitted through the subtalar joint by the cartilage lining of the bones around the sinus tarsi. It is not well understood why people develop pain from the sinus tarsi area. Most likely this is due to injury to the ligaments within the sinus tarsi causing local swelling and irritation.

Diagnosis and symptoms

About 70% of patients will recall a traumatic origin for their pain. This is usually a lateral ankle ligament sprain caused by 'rolling over' the outside of the ankle. This injury, if severe enough, can continue through the sinus tarsi to disrupt the strong ligamentous attachment from the talus to the calcaneus. The player will initially be treated for a lateral ankle ligament sprain, and pain along the bony prominence at the outside of the ankle (lateral malleolus) will improve. The player will present several weeks after the original injury with pain and tenderness over the outside of the heel of the foot at the sinus tarsi. This pain becomes more prominent as the other ligaments heal. Pain will be exacerbated by walking on uneven ground, as the subtalar joint must move to allow the foot to conform to the ground. Diagnosis of sinus tarsi syndrome is difficult because of the many conditions that can cause pain near this region. An injection of local anaesthetic and steroid into the sinus tarsi can serve both as a diagnostic tool and as treatment for this condition. MRI may secure the diagnosis by showing increased amount of fluid (Fig. 14.7).

Treatment and rehabilitation

Treatment is initially conservative with rest, modification of activities, non-steroidal anti-inflammatory medication and bracing during activities to limit ankle motion. These treatments may be tried independently, or in conjunction with a steroid injection. The number of injections should be limited to one a week in 2–4 weeks, however, because of the potential harmful effects of the steroids on the surrounding tissue. The injections can be aided by doing them under the guidance of a CT scan or fluoroscope. Ankle

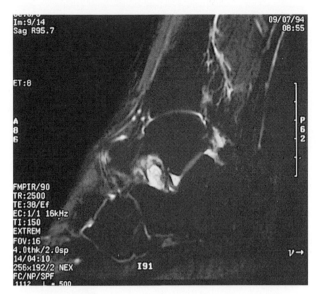

Fig. 14.7 Magnetic resonance image showing increased amount of synovial fluid in the sinus tarsi.

muscle-strengthening and balance-training exercises are also instituted at this time.

Most patients will improve with these conservative measures, but it is not unusual to have pain for many months, or to develop chronic pain with this condition. In refractory cases excision of the inflamed tissue may provide relief. In those cases with chronic pain a fusion of the subtalar joint may be needed to gain relief.

Impact and return to tennis

Treatment and return to tennis are directed by the patient's pain. Continuing participation will not cause structural damage but may exacerbate the inflammation and pain. In those chronic situations that require fusion, return to tennis playing will be difficult.

Recommended reading

Balduini, F.C., Vegso, J.J., Torg, J.S. & Torg, E. (1987) Management and rehabilitation of ligamentous injuries to the ankle. *American Journal of Sports Medicine* **4**, 364–380.

Lysholm, J. & Wiklander, J. (1987) Injuries in runners. *American Journal of Sports Medicine* **15**, 168–171.

Mann, R. & Thompson, F. (1985) Rupture of the posterior tibial tendon causing flat foot: surgical treatment. *Journal of Bone and Joint Surgery* **67A**, 556–561.

Renström, P. & Kannus, P. (1994) Injuries of the foot and ankle. In: DeLee, J. & Drez, D., eds. *Orthopaedic Sports Medicine: Practice and Principles*, Vol. 2, pp. 1705–1767. WB Saunders, Philadelphia, PA.

Chapter 15

Lower leg and Achilles
tendon problems in tennis

Epidemiology

Lower extremity injuries account for the majority of injuries in most sports. Tennis is often associated with upper extremity problems. However, some epidemiological tennis studies have shown lower extremity injuries to be nearly equal to or exceeding upper extremity problems. This is not surprising, given the amount of quick starts and stops, changes in direction, and running that are required in tennis. In addition, these same studies have indicated that most tennis injuries are chronic and most likely due to the repetitive nature of the sport. Unfortunately, epidemiological studies on tennis injuries do not comment extensively on the lower extremity problems, but in our experience the majority of lower leg injuries are similar to those disorders that commonly affect running athletes. However, due to the uniqueness and repetitive nature of the tennis serve and the significant amount of side-to-side movement, specific anatomical structures are placed under greater stress than they are in most other sports. This accounts for the comparatively higher incidence of problems with structures such as the plantar fascia, Achilles tendon, posterior tibial tendon and flexor hallucis tendon, which are put under increased stress during the push-off phase of the service motion.

Biomechanics

It is generally agreed upon that most of the power during the tennis serve is generated from the lower extremity and trunk. This power is then transferred to the upper extremity and racket to propel the ball forward. Studies on ground reaction forces created during tennis serves indicate that upward thrust dominates, but the forces are relatively low in magnitude. However, very few biomechanical studies consider lower extremity forces, preferring to concentrate on upper extremity motion instead.

Studies on rearfoot stresses during side-to-side movements in tennis players found that stresses were dependent on the type of landing technique used. During competition, first ground contact occurs mainly on the forefoot (55%). While this relationship is maintained for professionals during practice, the relationship is typically reversed for the non-professionals, with the heel making contact with the ground first 58% of the time during practice. This change in technique may be a contributor to injury mechanisms.

Playing surface and shoes

The playing surface has also been reported to change the injury patterns in tennis. Lower injury rates have been reported on clay surfaces (Nigg & Segesser 1988). It is speculated that the lower coefficient of surface friction contributed to lower injury rates. But a lower limit of friction appears to exist, below which injury rates increase, as one report has shown that 21% of tennis injuries were related to slipping on wet courts.

In relation to this is the subject of shoe wear, as not only the surface, but also the shoe, will contribute to the coefficient of friction and the player's ability to start, stop, and change direction quickly. Probably the most common problem with shoe wear in athletes, as it is with the general public, is that of poor-fitting shoes. Shoes that are too small will contribute to bunions, bunionettes, corns, calluses and nail problems, particularly when the toe box is narrow. Shoes that are too loose will contribute to blistering. Well-cushioned heels have been shown to decrease the injury rate in military recruits and aerobic dancing. This is felt to be a result of the better shock absorption of the well-padded heel. Shoes that have too much flexibility in the sole will contribute to forefoot hyper-dorsiflexion (foot is bent upwards) injuries, such as hallux rigidus (stiffness of the big toe base joint) (Fig. 15.1). The modern tennis shoe has a high heel counter that helps to prevent rearfoot angulation, thereby relieving stress on the Achilles tendon, posterior tibialis tendon and plantar fascia.

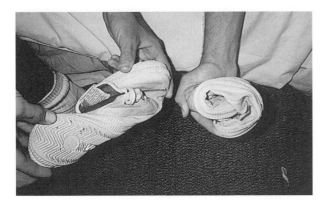

Fig. 15.1 Shoes with too much sole flexibility can cause forefoot problems.

Chronic lower leg pain

There are a variety of causes of chronic leg pain in the tennis player. These include: medial tibial stress syndrome ('shin splints'), chronic compartment syndrome, tibial and fibular stress fractures, muscle strains and tendonitis or tendinosis. These are often difficult to diagnose and can sometimes occur at the same time. Careful history and physical examination, sometimes combined with special tests, such as a bone scan or magnetic resonance imaging (MRI), can help to sort this out.

Medial tibial stress syndrome ('shin splints')

The term 'shin splints' refers to exertional lower leg pain. This is most likely caused by a stress reaction in the bone. Some believe the cause is a chronic inflammation of the fibrous tissue that covers the muscle or bone. Most commonly this occurs on the inside part of the back of the lower leg. Studies in runners have indicated that 10–15% of all injuries are due to medial tibial stress syndrome, accounting for as much as 60% of all lower leg injuries. In tennis players this problem occurs when the player goes to hardcourt from the more forgiving claycourt. The player needs to gradually adjust to the new surface over a period of at least 1 week.

Diagnosis and symptoms

Medial tibial stress syndrome is an exercise-induced pain that occurs in the lower leg. The pain is not associated with an increase in the muscle compartment pressure (this is known as chronic or exertional compartment syndrome and is described in the next section). The pain is relieved by rest, much the same as an exertional compartment syndrome. A bone scan can sometimes show a diffuse reaction from the periosteum (outer layer) of the bone, usually on the inside and back border of the tibia, but the bone scan can often be normal or an uptake can be seen on the delayed phase. Some authors have proposed an association with abnormal pronation of the foot, but this relationship is not scientifically verified.

Treatment and rehabilitation

Treatment is based on a period of rest to relieve symptoms and/or avoiding pain-causing activities. This is followed by a gradual return to activities with a strengthening programme. Stretching, moist heat, orthotics, taping and anti-inflammatory medications also have been used as an adjunct. Initial return to barefoot running on grass following a rest period has been proposed, but no objective studies have verified this.

The role of surgical intervention in cases that do not respond to non-operative treatment is controversial. For cases in which the athletes have not responded to a compliant period of rehabilitation and are ready to end their sporting career because of the pain, surgery may be indicated. The majority of authors have shown acceptable results from opening the thick covering around the muscles (incision of the fascia—fasciotomy). Surgery for this condition should not be taken lightly, as many patients may continue to have some problems, but most will improve and return to play tennis at some level.

Impact and return to tennis

Return to tennis is allowed as soon as the pain resolves and the player can tolerate the activity. This can range from a few days to many months, with some individuals never completely eliminating the symptoms. If the pain becomes intolerable, the options are to give up the inciting activities or try surgical treatment.

Stress fractures

Stress fractures in tennis players are not common but they do occur. Most commonly they are the result of an abrupt change in training habits, with a sudden large increase in repetitive pounding-type activities. The tibia is the most commonly involved bone in the athlete, accounting for 49% of all stress fractures. The fibula is also commonly involved especially in runners. Women have been shown to have a much-increased incidence of stress fracture compared to men.

Diagnosis and symptoms

Stress fractures of the tibia have three typical areas of development: adjacent to the knee, the middle one-third and close to the ankle. Athletes typically complain of a gradual onset of pain that is worsened with activity. Most commonly, they will be point tender over the involved area, and may have a small amount of swelling. Diagnosis can be confirmed with plain radiographs or bone scan. In early cases and cases with a minimal healing response the plain radiographs will be normal, in 50% of the cases a bone scan is diagnostic.

Treatment and rehabilitation

Near the knee and ankle, the fractures usually develop on the compression side of the bone (i.e. inside–back or posteromedially). In this case, the fractures typically respond with an exuberant healing response and will do quite well with a period of rest, followed by a gradual return to activity that is dictated by continued pain relief. Average rest time is 4 weeks, with a return to full sports in about 3 months. However, a recent study showed that functional bracing with a long brace reduced the return to full sports participation to an average of 21 days as compared to a group without the brace that returned at an average of 77 days (Swenson *et al.* 1997).

In contrast, the fractures in the mid-tibia form on the tension side of the bone (i.e. front or anterior). These tend to heal very slowly and have sometimes gone on to complete fracture. Treatment options for this difficult problem include non-weightbearing casting for 3–6 months, drilling, or excision and bone grafting. The average time to return to activities with these treatments is 8 months to 1 year. Recently, some have advocated surgical placement of a rod down the middle of the tibia. This can allow the athlete to return to activity in as little as 6 weeks (Andrish 1994). Experiments in Sweden with high-energy shock wave treatment, i.e. a bone crush injury technique, seem to give even better results.

Impact and return to tennis

For the compression-type stress fractures located near the joints, tennis playing usually can be resumed at about 3 months, but this is predicated by a gradual return to pain-free activity. For the mid-shaft tension side stress fractures, non-operative treatment usually sidelines the athlete for a minimum of 1 year. In contrast, with placement of the rod down the middle of the tibia, or using the shock wave technique, return to tennis can probably be accomplished in about 3–5 months.

Exertional compartment syndrome

The muscles in the lower leg are contained within four well-defined 'compartments' (Fig. 15.2) made up of fibrous tissue called fascia that surrounds the muscles. Elevated pressures within the tight fibrous borders of the four lower leg muscle compartments can cause pain. Exercise causes swelling of the muscles by increasing the circulation and in the long term hypertrophy. The compartment's surrounding walls can be tight and inelastic, and there will then not be enough space for the larger muscle volume. The pressure in the space can become abnormally elevated and cause pain. The most common location is the anterior compartment (80%) and in the posterior medial compartment (20%).

Diagnosis and symptoms

Exertional compartment syndrome presents as pain, cramping and aching in the lower leg that is brought on by exercise. The exercise causes increased pressure within the muscle compartments. Pain is relieved with rest as the compartment pressures normalize.

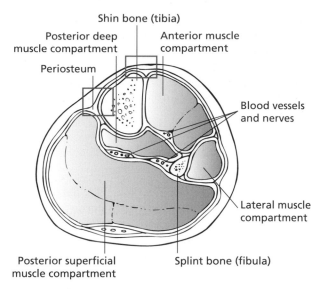

Posterior deep muscle compartment

Shin bone (tibia)

Periosteum

Anterior muscle compartment

Blood vessels and nerves

Lateral muscle compartment

Posterior superficial muscle compartment

Splint bone (fibula)

Fig. 15.2 Compartments in the lower leg which can be subjected to compartment syndrome. The squares indicate common sites of tenderness at the anchor points of muscle compartments to the periosteum of the shin bone. (From Ekblom, B. (ed.) (1994) *Handbook of Sports Medicine and Science: Football (Soccer)*, p. 183. Blackwell Scientific Publications, Oxford.)

Pain in both legs is not uncommon. Intermittent numbness and tingling can occur if the pressures get high enough in the compartments carrying the nerves.

This syndrome is distinguished from 'shin splints' by the presence of elevated compartment pressure measurements. The compartment pressures are measured by introducing needles attached to special pressure measuring devices into the compartments. Compartment pressure cut-offs to determine the presence of exertional compartment syndrome are somewhat arbitrary and based largely on retrospective data. Currently, the most commonly used technique is to measure pressures in the compartments at pre-exercise, and at 1 and 5–10 min postexercise. Pressures of >15 mmHg pre-exercise, or >30 mmHg at 1 min postexercise, or >15 mmHg at 5–10 min postexercise are felt to be diagnostic of exertional compartment syndrome (Pedowitz *et al.* 1990). It is important to be sure that the exercise period recreates the athlete's usual symptoms to have an accurate measurement.

Treatment and rehabilitation

Treatment is largely based on the athlete's desires. If the athlete wishes to restrict his or her activities to control symptoms, this is certainly acceptable. A trial of non-operative treatment is usually attempted prior to compartment pressure measurements, with a period of rest. The resting period includes avoidance of pain-causing activities. Aerobic conditioning can be maintained by biking or swimming. The rest period is followed by gradual return to activities, anti-inflammatory medication, and shoe modification.

In cases that do not respond to relative rest and in which compartment syndrome measurements confirm the diagnosis, surgical opening of the compartment by cutting the fibrous covering (fascia) is indicated. The skin is sutured shut but the fibrous covering is left open to allow the muscles to have a larger space in which to expand. The entire length of the affected compartments must be opened to be effective. Acceptable results regarding pain relief and return to activities are obtainable when patients are selected carefully.

Impact and return to tennis

Return to tennis is largely based on patient symptoms and pain tolerance. In true exertional compartment syndrome, non-operative treatment often fails. Following surgery, return to full tennis activity is usually achievable in 2–4 months in well-selected cases.

Tendon and muscle strains

Due to the repetitive nature of the sport, especially the push-off phase of the tennis serve, and the amount of time spent running and hopping, it is no surprise that tendon and muscle strain disorders account for a large percentage of tennis injuries. These include the gastrocnemius–soleus complex and Achilles tendon injuries, and posterior tibialis and flexor hallucis longus tendon disorders.

Calf muscle strain (medial gastrocnemius and soleus strain)—'tennis leg'

Perhaps no injury is associated with tennis more than 'tennis leg', which is an acute strain of the

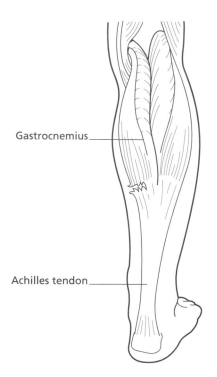

Gastrocnemius

Achilles tendon

Fig. 15.3 Calf muscle injuries, so-called tennis leg. (From Peterson, L. & Renström, P. (2000) *Sports Injuries: Their Prevention and Treatment*, p. 344. Martin Dunitz, London.)

medial gastrocnemius muscle (Fig. 15.3). A strain of the soleus muscle can also occur, but is less common. As is typical of most muscle strains, the injury occurs just adjacent to the muscle–tendon junction. The gastrocnemius–soleus complex and Achilles tendon are particularly vulnerable in tennis because of the amount of time spent landing on the forefoot. The situation may be exacerbated in non-professional players because of a change in landing habits displayed during competition as compared to practice. More landing occurs on the forefoot during competition. If the foot is suddenly pushed upward while the knee is extended during landing, injury to the gastrocnemius–soleus complex or Achilles tendon can occur.

Diagnosis and symptoms

Most commonly, gastrocnemius strains affect the medial (inside) portion of the muscle about one-third of the way down the lower leg. The rupture is located in the muscle–tendon junction. The soleus muscle can be injured closer to the knee. The injured athlete complains of a sudden sharp pain along the inside of the calf. This results in pain or an inability to push off from the foot, and pain when attempting to stand on his or her toes. There is an obvious tenderness over the affected area.

Treatment and rehabilitation

Treatment is based on reducing swelling and symptoms, with a graduated functional rehabilitation programme. Crutches may be used in the acute period to assist with pain relief, but they can be discarded as soon as the player can tolerate full weight bearing. A small heel lift may also be beneficial in the acute stages to reduce symptoms, but this should be removed as soon as possible to allow for normal function. A graduated stretching and strengthening programme that is tailored to the player's symptoms can begin within 3–5 days. Prognosis for these injuries is excellent, but patients can have residual aching that may last for several months.

Impact and return to tennis

Return to tennis can occur anywhere from several days to 4–8 weeks depending on the severity of the injury. This is mainly guided by pain, with a gradual return to full activity.

Complete Achilles tendon ruptures

Incidence and injury mechanism

The main function of the Achilles tendon is to generate forceful plantar flexion of the foot (i.e. pointing of the toes) to push off during running and jumping. The Achilles tendon is part of the soleus and gastrocnemius complex. The Achilles tendon is an extremely strong tendon. Peak Achilles tendon forces in running subjects have been estimated to be about 12.5 times bodyweight. However, the rate of force application may be more important than the magnitude of the force applied as a cause for tissue damage.

Achilles tendon ruptures are not uncommon in tennis, and the incidence seems to be rising in association with a more active middle-aged population

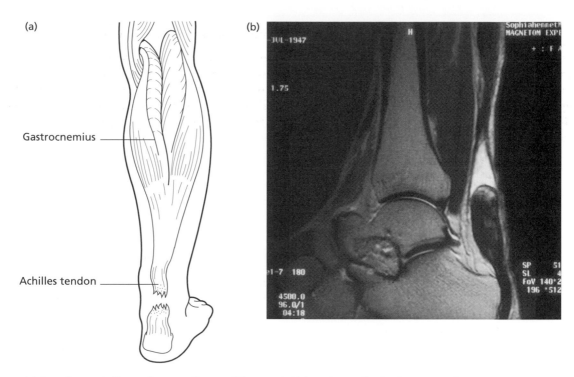

Fig. 15.4 (a) Complete Achilles tendon tear. (From Ekblom, B. (ed.) (1994) *Handbook of Sports Medicine and Science: Football (Soccer)*, p. 181. Blackwell Scientific Publications, Oxford.) (b) Magnetic resonance image of Achilles tendon tear.

(Fig. 15.4). In many studies, basketball and racket sports account for half of the injuries. The tendon is particularly vulnerable when the foot is forcefully bent upward while the gastrocnemius–soleus complex is contracting. The situation is further exacerbated when the knee simultaneously straightens. This is particularly true when landing following a tennis serve or stroke.

The tendon is more vulnerable during middle age as the normal tendon tissue starts to break down (degeneration). This process begins at about the age of 30–35 years. The region between 2 and 6 cm above the calcaneal insertion is the most common area of rupture. The relatively poor blood supply to the area may contribute to this.

Diagnosis and symptoms

Most ruptures occur without previous symptoms. Athletes complain of a sudden pain in the posterior calf. Often, the player will state that he or she felt like someone kicked him or her in the back of the leg

but no one was there. The rupture is also usually accompanied by an audible 'pop' that the player will sometimes say sounded like a gunshot. There is some immediate pain, but it is usually not too severe. The rupture causes a defect in the tendon between 2 and 6 cm above the insertion on the heel. If, however, significant swelling occurs, the defect may not be felt. The player will be unable to stand on his or her toes, but many patients will still be able to generate some active motion of the foot, although it will be weakened. Thompson's squeeze test will confirm the diagnosis. This test is performed by squeezing the calf muscle and examining the foot for the expected plantar flexion response (i.e. downward pointing of the toes). It is best performed with the player kneeling on a chair, or lying on his or her stomach. The absence of plantar flexion confirms an Achilles tendon rupture.

Treatment and rehabilitation

Treatment of Achilles tendon ruptures has remained controversial. Conservative treatment with a cast or walking boot is possible and may be successful with initiation of the treatment within 48 h after the injury. However, the disturbing problem with casting is the high risk for re-rupture and the prolonged weakness that occurs. The non-operatively treated group has a re-rupture rate of about 5–15%. More recently, several studies have advocated a non-operative functional rehabilitation programme that emphasizes relatively early motion (Thermann *et al.* 1995). The typical protocol consists of a walking cast for 3–6 weeks followed by a progressive rehabilitation programme with decreasing heel lifts. Early results of this technique have shown outcomes in non-athletes that are similar to surgical treatment in terms of strength and return to function, and this technique has a lower complication rate. However, caution should be used until better prospectively randomized trials are available.

As compared to the standard non-operative treatment, patients with surgical repair have significantly lower rates of re-rupture, higher rates of resuming sports activities at the same level, lesser degrees of calf atrophy and fewer complaints 1 year after injury (Cetti *et al.* 1993). These results could be explained by the immobilization that occurs with non-operative treatment. Immobilization will lead to an inability to maintain tension in the tendon and to major atrophy (less volume) of the calf muscle. This causes poor repair of the tendon structure. The most important factor with surgical repair is that it allows earlier rehabilitation so tension can be placed on the tendon. This tension will allow proper orientation of the tendon microstructure, which will result in good strength. Thereby the risk of re-rupture will decrease and an early return to sports is possible. With surgical repair, early mobilization, allowing the foot to move from 0° to 20° of flexion after 7–10 days, is possible. There is, however, a higher complication rate with surgery including delayed healing, skin slough and infection. Most of these problems usually heal quickly.

Impact and return to tennis

Following a complete Achilles tendon rupture treated by surgical repair, return to full tennis playing is possible usually at about 4–6 months. Return after non-operative treatment varies considerably; with return to full tennis activity sometimes possible after 8–12 months.

Partial Achilles tendon ruptures

Partial ruptures of the Achilles tendon are not uncommon in tennis, although epidemiological studies are limited in this area. One problem with evaluating this injury is differentiating a partial tear from an Achilles tendinosis or peritendinitis. In fact, partial tears can result in a chronic tendinosis. As discussed in the section on acute complete Achilles tendon ruptures, the tendon is particularly vulnerable when the foot is forcefully bent upward (dorsiflexed) while the gastrocnemius–soleus complex is contracting.

Diagnosis and symptoms

Partial tear of the Achilles tendon is characterized by a history of sudden pain, with localized tenderness and swelling. The area of partial rupture is most often in the area of poor blood supply to the Achilles tendon at about 2–6 cm above the tendon insertion onto the heel. In the case of partial ruptures no palpable defect in the tendon is felt. Instead there is a tear in the tendon microstructure that initiates the problem. The player will have pain when standing on his or her toes, but most players will still be able to do this. Thompson's squeeze test (as discussed in the previous section) will show a normal response of the foot. That is, when squeezing the calf muscle the foot will exhibit the normal plantar flexion response (i.e. downward pointing of the toes).

Treatment and rehabilitation

Treatment of partial Achilles tendon tears is begun with a conservative programme. If the tear is substantial a walking boot could be used for 2–4 weeks. Otherwise a small heel wedge can be used in the initial period to relieve pain but the player should wean out of this as soon as possible. A physical therapy programme can begin as soon as possible. The treatment protocol is identical to that outlined for Achilles tendinosis in the next section. Briefly, this includes a structured programme of stretching and eccentric muscle strengthening, with the use of orthotics, shoe inserts and correction of training errors as needed. These injuries often do not heal well. The reason for this is unknown, but it may be related to the poor blood supply to the area of injury.

The indication for surgical treatment of partial Achilles tendon tears is the same as for Achilles tendinosis (it may be that the tendinosis is a result of chronic partial tears), that is, persistent pain and loss of physical performance, with symptoms typically lasting longer than 6 months. Following surgery on the Achilles tendon, about 70–80% of athletes make a successful comeback. Return to sports, such as tennis and running, is usually delayed for 4–8 months after surgery.

Impact and return to tennis

Return to tennis playing is guided by pain. Depending on the severity of the injury, symptoms can last from a few days to several months, with some players never completely recovering. In those cases treated surgically, return to tennis is usually possible at about 6 months, but there is no guarantee that the surgery will correct the problem.

Chronic Achilles tendinopathy

Tendinitis has been the clinical term applied to virtually all painful tendon structures. Unfortunately, this is a misleading term, since the majority of these injuries do not have an inflammatory response. The characteristic pattern has instead been a degeneration (microruptures, splitting and disorientation of the fibres) of the tendon microstructure. So, despite the common use of the term 'tendinitis', the more appropriate description of the majority of injuries is tendinopathy. A localized lesion is called tendinosis. Tendinosis is most likely a reflection of the failed adaptation of the tendon to the physical load of recurrent microtrauma. Degenerative changes precede spontaneous rupture of tendons in most players.

Many feel that tendon degeneration can be exacerbated by malalignment syndromes such as excessive pronation, which place more stress on the tendon. The inside of the Achilles tendon is placed under increased tension when the foot is placed in hyperpronation. Achilles overuse injury with tendon swelling can also be caused by a non-healing partial tear (Fig. 15.5).

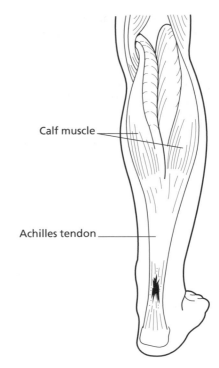

Calf muscle

Achilles tendon

Fig. 15.5 Tendinosis—partial tear in Achilles tendon. (From Ekblom, B. (ed.) (1994) *Handbook of Sports Medicine and Science: Football (Soccer)*, p. 182. Blackwell Scientific Publications, Oxford.)

Diagnosis and symptoms

Typical presenting complaints with chronic Achilles tendinopathy are a gradual onset of pain and stiffness in the Achilles tendon that most commonly occurs between 2 and 6 cm above the insertion into the heel. If the player can recall a more sudden onset, the chronic problems are often caused by a non-healed partial tear. The pain typically increases with activity and is relieved by rest to a varying degree, depending on the amount of involvement. Often the patient will develop a tender nodule along the tendon and pain will be increased with passive motion and toe standing or walking. With the development of magnetic resonance imaging (MRI), the ability to evaluate tendon overuse injuries has improved dramatically. MRI not only gives a correct diagnosis, but it also evaluates the extent and size of the injury (Fig. 15.6). Ultrasound evaluation is also valuable in expert hands.

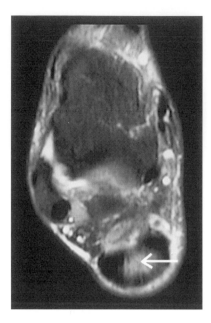

Fig. 15.6 Magnetic resonance image of Achilles tendinosis. The arrow denotes the tendinosis change in the tendon.

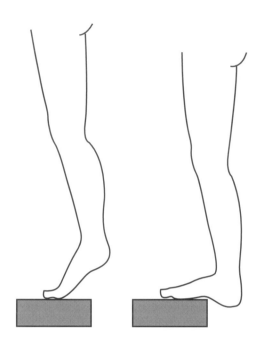

Fig. 15.7 Concentric contraction (left) and eccentric action (right) of the calf muscles.

Treatment and rehabilitation

Treatment of Achilles tendinosis should be directed at treating the cause of the injury. Orthotics to correct malalignments are often helpful, and shoes with a good heel support and a heel wedge may prevent excessive pronation. Correction of training errors is a key component in a successful programme.

The treatment of tendon overuse injuries is related to and depends on the healing process. A properly carried out exercise programme is the key to success. Tendon strength is a direct function of its microstructure. The microstructure responds favourably to tension and motion. It is therefore important to stimulate protective motion as early as possible. Eccentric training, activating the muscle while the muscle is elongating, provides the maximum achievement of load. Eccentric exercises can be very effective for this condition, but supervision is needed (Fig. 15.7). Two to three months of well-planned eccentric exercises have been so efficient that planned surgery has in many cases been avoided. Stretching is used extensively in the treatment of overuse injuries. Function and activity level in chronic tendon injuries are mostly dictated by the athlete's pain. The player should listen to the tendon: 'the tendon talks'. If the

programme is carried out correctly, there should be little or no pain, perhaps with the exception of during the last set of 10 repetitions. As the tendon strengthens, the pain should diminish. Team work with a trainer and/or a physical therapist is recommended. With these principles non-operative treatment is effective in most cases.

The indication for surgical treatment of chronic Achilles tendinopathy is persistent pain and loss of physical performance, with symptoms typically lasting longer than 6 months. In competitive athletes fewer than 10% of overuse injuries require surgery. The goal of surgery is to remove any offending tissue and relieve any external pressure on the tendon. This gives the desired effects on the tendon of inducing vascular ingrowth and creating new and better organized scar tissue. Following surgery on the Achilles tendon, about 70–80% of athletes make a successful comeback. Return to sports, such as tennis and running, is usually delayed for 4–8 months after surgery. Twenty per cent, however, need repeat surgery, and about 3–5% are forced to abandon their sports careers because of these injuries (Kvist 1991).

Impact and return to tennis

As with most of the overuse-type injuries, return to tennis playing is guided by pain. Depending on the severity of the injury, symptoms can last from a few days to several months, with some players never completely recovering. In those cases treated surgically, return to tennis is usually possible at about 4–6 months, but, as with most overuse injuries, there is no guarantee that the surgery will correct the problem.

References

Andrish, J. (1994) The leg. In: DeLee, J. & Drez, D., eds. *Orthopaedic Sports Medicine: Practice and Principles*, Vol. 2, pp. 1603–1631. WB Saunders, Philadelphia, PA.

Cetti, R., Christensen, S., Ejsted, R., Jensen, N. & Jorgensen, U. (1993) Operative versus nonoperative of Achilles tendon rupture. *American Journal of Sports Medicine* **21**, 791–804.

Kvist, M. (1991) Achilles tendon injuries in athletes. *Sports Medicine* **18**, 173–201.

Nigg, B. & Segesser, B. (1988) The influence of playing surfaces on the load on the locomotor system and on football and tennis injuries. *Sports Medicine* **5** (6), 375–385.

Pedowitz, R., Hargens, A., Mubarak, S. & Gershuni, D. (1990) Modified criteria for the objective diagnosis of chronic compartment syndrome of the leg. *American Journal of Sports Medicine* **18** (1), 35–40.

Swenson, E., DeHaven, K., Sebastianelli, W. *et al.* (1997) The effect of a pneumatic leg brace on return to play in athletes with tibial stress fractures. *American Journal of Sports Medicine* **25** (3), 322–328.

Thermann, H., Zwipp, H. & Tscherne, H. (1995) Functional treatment concept of acute rupture of the Achilles tendon. *Unfallchirurg* **98** (1), 21–32.

Recommended reading

Fyfe, I. & Stanish, W. (1992) The use of eccentric training and stretching in the treatment and prevention of tendon injuries. *Clinical Journal of Sport Medicine* **11**, 601–624.

Kannus, P. & Jozsa, L. (1990) Histopathological changes preceding spontaneous rupture of a tendon. *Journal of Bone and Joint Surgery* **73A**, 1507–1525.

Leadbetter, W. (1992) Cell matrix response in tendon injuries. *Clinics in Sports Medicine* **11**, 553–578.

Chapter 16

Knee injuries in tennis

Introduction

Knee problems are relatively common in tennis players because of the required amount of cutting, twisting, sprinting, jumping, and starting and stopping. The knee joint acts as an important link in transferring energy during tennis activities such as serving, volleying and hitting groundstrokes. The knee is required to generate force and absorb impact to allow tennis specific motions to be performed with maximum efficiency.

Statistics show that approximately 19% of all tennis injuries occur in the knee. The knee is the fourth most common anatomical site of injury, ranked behind the shoulder, back and ankle. The majority of the injuries are acute traumatic injuries (70%) with the remaining knee injuries being attributed to overuse syndromes.

The playing surface has been shown to change the injury pattern in tennis. Lower injury rates have been reported for clay surfaces. It is speculated that courts with lower coefficients of friction contribute to lower injury rates, e.g. a player can slide on a clay court. The foot is more likely to be stuck to the ground on rubber or hard courts with high friction. When the athlete tries to twist or turn, the knee may rotate with the foot fixed to the surface and a ligament or meniscus tear can occur. However, there also appears to be a lower limit for the coefficient of friction, below which injury rates increase. This is primarily due to the increased number of falls on a wet slippery surface.

The tennis surface can also be one of a number of extrinsic contributing factors in overuse injuries of the knee. Hard surfaces are fatiguing to the legs and may produce overuse problems. Forgiving surfaces such as clay, where the player can slide, are less likely to result in internal knee problems, but the sliding can be stressful for the kneecap. Other extrinsic factors—those factors related to the environment—include training errors, improper shoes and unsuitable environmental conditions. Intrinsic factors—factors related to the individual—can also play a role in overuse syndromes. These include such things as kneecap malalignment and muscle imbalance.

Tennis shoes can be an important part of injury prevention. The tennis shoe must be able to provide impact resistance and provide a high degree of support without hindering the tennis player's mobility. Most competitive players have different shoes for each surface.

Knee injuries within the joint

The most common intra-articular—within the joint—knee injuries include meniscal, chondral and ligamentous lesions. Fat-pad syndrome and plica synovialis syndrome are also occasionally experienced by tennis players.

Meniscus tear

The menisci are the two small C-shaped cushioning structures made of cartilage that lie between the two main bones that make up the knee joint (femur and tibia). This is usually what laypeople speak of when they refer to a 'cartilage tear'. The menisci provide shock absorption to protect the knee from developing breakdown of the articular cartilage—the cartilage that lines the ends of the bones (Fig. 16.1). The menisci transmit 50–100% of the load across the knee joint. Forces across the knee can range from two to four times bodyweight. Because of the stress on the menisci, it is not surprising that injuries to the menisci are common in middle-aged and elderly players.

Meniscus tears can occur by an acute trauma, but they can, and often do, occur without a specific traumatic event. The acute tears most commonly occur with a twisting or rotational movement. In the older tennis players, meniscal injuries usually occur because the structure is gradually starting to break down (degeneration) as a result of the ageing process.

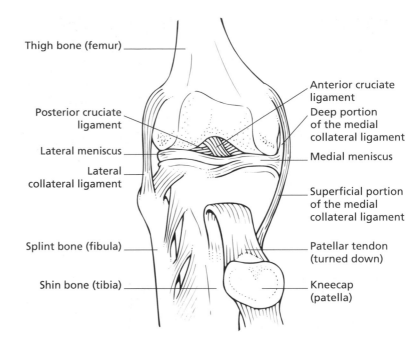

Thigh bone (femur)

Anterior cruciate ligament

Posterior cruciate ligament

Deep portion of the medial collateral ligament

Lateral meniscus

Medial meniscus

Lateral collateral ligament

Superficial portion of the medial collateral ligament

Splint bone (fibula)

Patellar tendon (turned down)

Shin bone (tibia)

Kneecap (patella)

Fig. 16.1 Anatomy of the knee. (From Ekblom, B. (ed.) (1994) *Handbook of Sports Medicine and Science: Football (Soccer)*, p. 184. Blackwell Scientific Publications, Oxford.)

Diagnosis and symptoms

For acute tears, a sudden pain will occur following a twisting or turning event. Degenerative tears will have a more gradual onset of symptoms, but an acute tear can occur to an already weakened degenerative meniscus (Fig. 16.2). Following the tear some minor swelling will occur in the knee, and running or other pounding actions may cause the knee to ache. For large tears, locking of the knee may occur due to the loose fragment impinging in the joint and preventing the knee from fully straightening.

Typical findings include tenderness over the joint lines in 75–85% of the cases. There is often discomfort with extremes of range of motion especially flexion and rotation. The diagnosis is usually apparent by the combination of the patient history and the physical examination. In difficult or unusual cases magnetic resonance imaging (MRI) can verify the diagnosis with excellent accuracy (Fig. 16.3). Arthroscopy can both verify and treat the lesion (Fig. 16.4).

Treatment and rehabilitation

Many meniscus tears cause no or minor symptoms. Therefore, the usual initial treatment for a torn

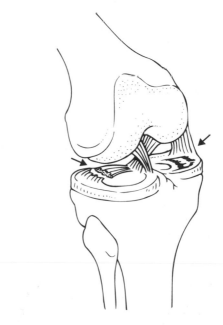

Fig. 16.2 Different types of meniscus tear. Right, Longitudinal rupture; left, transverse rupture. (From Ekblom, B. (ed.) (1994) *Handbook of Sports Medicine and Science: Football (Soccer)*, p. 187. Blackwell Scientific Publications, Oxford.)

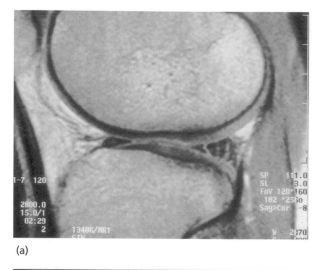

(a)

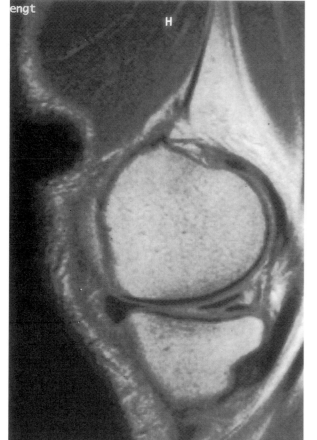

(b)

Fig. 16.3 Magnetic resonance image of meniscus tear. (a) Vertical tear; (b) horizontal tear.

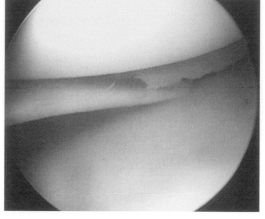

(a)

(b)

Fig. 16.4 Meniscus tear: (a) before and (b) after arthroscopic surgery.

meniscus is to begin physical therapy to strengthen the quadriceps and hamstrings, control the swelling and give the injury a chance to settle down on its own. This is usually performed for about 4–6 weeks. In the event that the athlete does not respond to conservative measures, arthroscopic surgery can be performed to treat the tear. The exception to this treatment is when a meniscal tear is causing locking of the knee. In this case the athlete should have arthroscopic surgery to address the meniscal tear to avoid long-term loss of motion and secondary joint injury.

Most meniscal tears require that a portion of the meniscus be removed. In a few cases, almost always in young patients, the meniscus can be preserved and repaired. This is indicated when the tear is peripheral, i.e. at the outer edge of the meniscus close to the capsule. After repair, the rehabilitation time is much longer than after simple partial excision.

There is nothing special about the rehabilitation programmes. It involves control of the swelling, and regaining range of motion, leg strength and endurance.

Impact and return to tennis

The rehabilitation time and return to tennis after an excision of a partial tear depend on the location and extent of the meniscus injury. If the tear is small, return to preinjury level will be approximately 2–4 weeks postsurgery. A return to tennis after 1–3 months is most common. After meniscal repair the return to tennis is delayed to 3–5 months.

Degenerative joint disease and chondral lesions

Damage to the intra-articular surface—the cartilage that lines the bones within the joint—is common in older athletes. These chondral lesions are commonly located on the undersurface of the patella (kneecap) and on the femur (thigh bone), particularly on the inside portion of the joint (medial side). Damage and/or removal of a meniscus cartilage can predispose the knee to chondral lesions. Small, localized lesions can also be secondary to osteochondritis dissecans; this disorder is discussed in more detail in the following section.

In the older athletes, early signs of osteoarthrosis or arthritis—degenerative joint disease—is a common pattern. In athletes with pre-existing degenerative changes it is common for the joint to become irritated and symptomatic due to repetitive microtrauma of tennis.

Diagnosis and symptoms

Damage to the joint surfaces causes aching and pain with motion. Many athletes will complain of start-up pain following a prolonged period of sitting. Intermittent swelling is a frequent sign of chondral lesions.

Major degenerative joint disease is verified on conventional radiographs, particularly when the radiographs are taken in the weightbearing position. The radiographs will show a decrease in the distance between the femur and tibia, indicating a thinning of the joint lining, which looks like a space on the radiograph. Localized minor chondral lesions are best diagnosed by arthroscopy. MRI can sometimes show chondral lesions, but the accuracy to date is not very good. However, new MRI techniques are emerging that look more promising.

Treatment and rehabilitation

Treatment of chondral injuries is very difficult, with unpredictable results. Traditional conservative treatment should be done as long as possible. This includes avoiding pain-causing situations and improving the thigh muscle strength and endurance.

Small full-thickness cartilage lesions that cause persistent pain and swelling can be treated with drilling or picking of the area to increase blood flow and induce a healing response to the damaged region. For lesions that do not respond to this some new techniques have been tried. The first technique involves covering of the defect by transplanting a piece of the bone lining (periosteum). The periosteum is taken from the bone just below the knee (tibia) and sutured over the defect. The second technique is similar, except that cartilage cells that are grown in the laboratory are injected underneath the covering to assist in regrowth. This technique requires a previous operation to harvest cartilage cells that can then be grown in cultures in the laboratory. This is very expensive, in addition to the need for a second operation. The third technique removes small, cylindrical pieces of cartilage with its underlying bone from areas of less weightbearing and transplants them to the defective area. This technique leaves small gaps between the transplanted cylinders that must fill in with new cartilage and it removes normal cartilage from other areas of the knee.

The results of these techniques are difficult to predict, but it does appear that in the short term many patients improve. For all of the techniques, however, it is unknown how well the repaired tissue will hold up under vigorous stress, such as tennis playing.

If a tennis player has generalized degenerative joint disease (Fig. 16.5), the above surgeries are generally not useful. The best treatment in this case is education about the condition, and activity

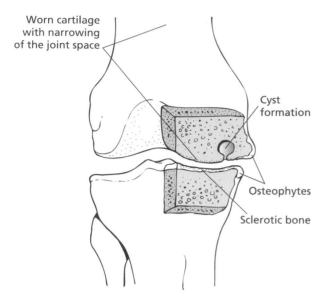

Fig. 16.5 Degenerative knee. (From Eriksson, B. (1988) *Medicine in Sports*. Prisma, Stockholm.)

modification. Switching to doubles play may prolong the athlete's tennis playing career. Tennis players with degenerative joint disease should participate in muscle-strengthening exercises. If pain is persistent and chronic swelling is present, an arthroscopy with debridement may be useful, but the long-term results of such treatment are generally not good. In the long term, when the problem begins to affect activities of daily living and/or sleep, total joint replacement is indicated. Total joint replacement will not return an athlete to vigorous sport because the mechanical joint cannot withstand the stress. Sometimes the player can enjoy some careful doubles tennis.

Impact and return to tennis

Chondral injuries represent a difficult problem. Treatment options in present-day medicine are not very good and offer unpredictable results. Those with chondral lesions should continue to play but they should be aware of the risk of accelerating the degenerative changes. The risk of how rapidly the degenerative changes will progress is unpredictable. An individual decision must therefore be made by assessing symptoms, possible risks, and psychological and cardiovascular benefit of continuing to participate in tennis, and at what level.

Osteochondritis dissecans and loose bodies

Osteochondritis dissecans (loose piece of bone and cartilage) is a disorder thought to be caused by an interruption of blood supply to a portion of the bone underlying the articular cartilage. The small bone and cartilage fragment (osteochondral fragment) comes loose from its underlying bed and begins to cause pain (Fig. 16.6). Some osteochondral fragments may remain stable enough that they do not cause any pain. The exact incidence of osteochondritis dissecans is unknown. Tennis players with this disease are usually young and symptoms are often vague and poorly localized.

Diagnosis and symptoms

The player may complain of pain, stiffness and swelling. If there is locking, catching and giving-way, a loose body should be considered. Sometimes the osteochondral fragment can fall out of its bed into the joint to form a loose body. The most common source

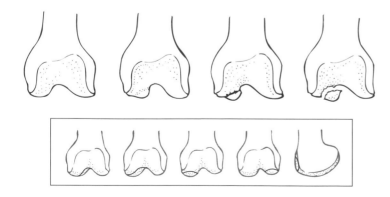

Fig. 16.6 Osteochondritis dissecans in the knee. (From Peterson, L. & Renström, P. (2000) *Sports Injuries: Their Prevention and Treatment*, p. 307. Martin Dunitz, London.)

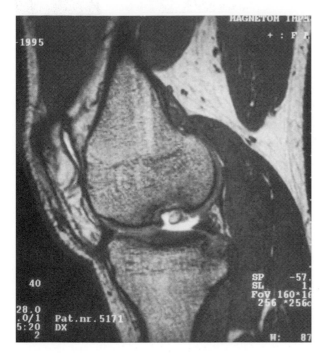

Fig. 16.7 Magnetic resonance image of osteochondritis dissecans. (From Peterson, L. & Renström, P. (2000) *Sports Injuries: Their Prevention and Treatment*, p. 307. Martin Dunitz, London.)

of loose bodies in the knee joint is osteochondritis dissecans. When the injury becomes worse the symptoms may be continuous.

The diagnosis can usually be made with regular radiographs. The medial femoral condyle (the inside portion of the femur) is involved in approximately 75–85% of cases. MRI (Fig. 16.7) and computed tomography (CT) scanning will secure the diagnosis and can sometimes aid the assessment of the fragment's stability.

Treatment and rehabilitation

The method of treatment depends on the age of the patient and the size and viability of the fragment. As long as the fragment is still within its bed, very young individuals can be treated initially with decreasing activity. In patients who continue to be symptomatic, arthroscopy should be performed to evaluate the lesion and fix it to the underlying bed if necessary. Very young patients have a good prognosis, and most will heal without surgical treatment.

Adults are treated more aggressively with an attempt to get the fragment to heal. This is usually done by securing the fragment to the underlying bed by surgical fixation. Following fixation, immediate range of motion exercises are instituted but a player is kept non-weightbearing for up to 8 weeks.

For fragments that are unable to be replaced, removal is usually the best option. If the player continues to be symptomatic following removal, one of the techniques described in the previous section can be tried to attempt to restore the articular surface.

Impact and return to tennis

The times of return to tennis vary, depending on the age of the player and the size, nature and location of the lesion. Return to play usually is not possible for 4–6 months for large lesions, or for loose lesions that require surgical fixation. Large lesions can cause chronic problems. Small loose fragments that are easily excised by arthroscopy may cause minimal morbidity and allow an early return to tennis.

Synovial plica syndrome

A thick fold in the synovial lining of the joint called a plica can be formed in the knee (Fig. 16.8). This can occasionally cause pain around the kneecap (patella). The most common area of plica formation is on the inside of the knee adjacent to the patella. Most plica are asymptomatic.

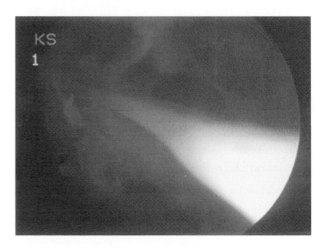

Fig. 16.8 Synovial plica.

Diagnosis and symptoms

A plica can occasionally cause pain or catching when it rides over the inside portion of the articular surface of the femur during bending and straightening of the knee. Inflammation of the joint lining (synovitis) and articular cartilage damage may also cause similar symptoms.

Treatment and rehabilitation

Most plica do not cause symptoms. This is usually a diagnosis of exclusion. If plica are symptomatic they can first be treated by muscle strengthening and flexibility training. If symptoms persist, this syndrome is treated successfully with arthroscopic debridement.

Impact and return to tennis

Plica rarely cause long-term problems. Even in those that are persistent and require surgical debridement, return to tennis can proceed at a pace determined by the individual player's symptoms. Usually, this can be accomplished within 3 weeks.

Fat-pad syndrome

The fat pad lies beneath the patellar tendon and serves as a cushion to the tendon. The fat pad can be injured and develop scar tissue within it following repetitive trauma. The fat pad becomes firm and pinches within the joint when the knee is straightened.

Diagnosis and treatment

This is a difficult entity to diagnose. Players will have pain in the front of the knee with active or passive straightening of the knee. Fat-pad syndrome is often a diagnosis of exclusion.

Treatment and rehabilitation

Fat-pad syndrome can be treated by arthroscopic debridement. However, it can sometimes return due to the traumatic effects of the debridement itself. Institution of early range of motion can lessen the recurrence rate.

Impact and return to tennis

Following debridement, players can return to tennis as soon as possible. This is usually possible within about 3 weeks.

Knee ligament injuries

The most commonly injured ligaments are the medial collateral ligament (MCL) and the anterior cruciate ligament (ACL). These injuries usually occur from twisting and cutting manoeuvres.

Medial collateral ligament injury

The MCL stabilizes the knee against side stress placed on the inside of the knee (Fig. 16.9). It is the most commonly injured knee ligament in tennis. The injury usually occurs during a twisting situation when the knee is forced into a knock-kneed position with external rotation.

Diagnosis and symptoms

The player will have pain and tenderness on the inside of the knee over the ligament. The player will also have pain when testing the ligament by manually putting stress on it by gently forcing the knee into the knock-kneed position with the knee slightly bent. This injury will generally not cause a large amount of swelling in the joint because the ligament is outside the joint. If a large amount of swelling is present within the joint, other injuries should be sought.

Treatment and rehabilitation

Benign injuries are classified as grade I and involve tearing only a few fibres of the ligament. Grade II injuries are partial tears with some stretching of the ligament, but with the ligament still intact. Grade I and II injuries are treated with early mobilization without protection. MCL grade III injuries are more severe and often are combined with other ligament injuries. Isolated grade III injuries are treated conservatively with protection in a brace for about 4–6 weeks. If a grade III injury is combined with an ACL injury, treatment is usually still by functional rehabilitation with a protective brace

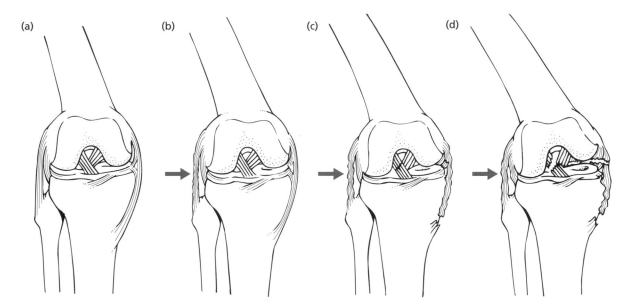

Fig. 16.9 Knee ligament injuries. (a) Normal knee; (b) deep medial collateral ligament injury; (c) complete medial collateral ligament injury; (d) with ACL injury. (From Peterson, L. & Renström, P. (2000) *Sports Injuries: Their Prevention and Treatment*, p. 275. Martin Dunitz, London.)

for 4–6 weeks. This is then followed by treatment of the ACL injury.

Impact and return to tennis

For grade I and II injuries, return to tennis is most commonly possible in 3–6 weeks after a strength training rehabilitation programme. Often return to tennis can begin even earlier for grade I injuries. Return to tennis for isolated grade III injuries is often possible after 2–3 months. If an ACL tear is also present, return to tennis is usually not possible until 6–9 months, after treatment of the ACL.

Anterior cruciate ligament injuries

The ACL is the front ligament of two ligaments that lie within the joint (Fig. 16.9). Its main function is to prevent the leg bone (tibia) from moving forward in relation to the thigh bone (femur). In fact, the ACL absorbs 86% of the total strain in this direction. The ACL is vital to allow participation in cutting, twisting and turning activities, such as vigorous tennis. This is the reason surgery is usually performed in young tennis players.

Diagnosis and symptoms

The diagnosis is made from the history that is characterized by feeling a pop and experiencing acute intensive pain. The trauma is usually from a cutting motion to one side, followed by a quick twisting motion to the other side. Landing after a serve can cause a rotational trauma and an ACL tear. In cases with this history and acute swelling within the joint, an ACL tear is noted 70% of the time. The diagnosis is verified by the Lachman test, where the examiner tries to move the tibia forward while stabilizing the femur. An ACL tear is verified when the tibia moves forward more than the normal side and the ligament fails to provide a distinct stopping point during the test.

Treatment and rehabilitation

In the young active tennis player, the treatment of a complete ACL tear is usually surgical. The non-surgical treatment of complete ACL tears in young active players may often lead to recurrent giving-way episodes that can cause tears in the meniscus. In players that continue to have recurrent giving-way, the risk for developing arthritis in the knee is greatly

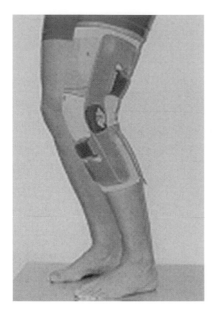

Fig. 16.10 Knee brace that can be effective and not cumbersome.

increased. In elderly and recreational tennis players, it is possible to treat ACL injuries with a functional rehabilitation programme and brace. If there are continuous problems then delayed surgery is possible. Recreational tennis can often be played without a fully functioning ACL if the quadriceps and hamstring muscles are well trained.

Indications for ACL surgery are participation in high-risk activities such as aggressive tennis. If there is a combined ligament injury the indication for surgery increases. Age plays a secondary role to activity level.

Surgery is carried out as a delayed procedure mostly 2–10 weeks after the injury. Currently, ACL reconstruction using autogenous grafts such as patellar tendon or quadrupled hamstring tendons are recommended.

Many tennis players use functional knee braces. These braces are not efficient in aggressive sports activities; however, they may be helpful in less demanding tennis (Fig. 16.10). The mechanism by which these braces may help is still unknown.

Impact and return to tennis

With current technique and rehabilitation, time for return to tennis is about 4–6 months. Return to competitive tennis 6 months after surgery is possible in about 80% of players.

Posterior cruciate ligament and lateral collateral ligament injuries

These injuries are rare in tennis. Isolated injuries of the posterior cruciate ligament (PCL) are often treated conservatively with aggressive quadriceps strength training. The prognosis for early return to tennis with proper rehabilitation is good.

Complete tears of the lateral collateral ligament (LCL) combined with injury to other lateral structures are notorious for providing treatment difficulties and poor outcomes. The best option is to address these injuries within the first week by surgical repair. Fortunately, these injuries are extremely rare in tennis players.

Extensor mechanism problems

Patellofemoral pain syndromes

Patellofemoral pain (pain around the kneecap) syndromes are common in young tennis players. About 16% of tennis players will experience patellofemoral pain. In players under the age of 14, the incidence is 7% in boys and 11% in girls.

The causes of patellofemoral pain are varied. Traumatic injuries, such as patellar fracture or traumatic injury to the articular cartilage from a direct fall or blow can occur. Patellofemoral pain can also be caused by chronic problems, such as breakdown of the articular cartilage, which can be associated with malalignment and/or instability. Malalignment refers to anatomical irregularities that can cause the patella to sit incorrectly within its associated femoral groove. Patellofemoral instability is the inability of the patella to consistently stay correctly within the groove of the femur where it is supposed to track. Conditions that cause excessive pressure on the tissues that connect to the outside of the patella predispose to these pain syndromes. To make this complex syndrome easier to grasp and understand, classification systems have been developed. Patellofemoral problems can clinically be divided into subluxation, tilt, subluxation and tilt, and chondromalacia. It is important to differentiate between these problems because surgical treatment options are slightly different. The wrong treatment can lead to worsening of the problem and increased pain.

Subluxation of the patella

Subluxation of the patella is defined as a partial dislocation of the patella (kneecap) from the femoral groove (Fig. 16.11). This can be a result of previous trauma that damages the soft tissues that hold the patella in place, or it can be a result of anatomical variations in the individual (malalignment). Patellar subluxation may lead to areas of high pressure on portions of the articular cartilage with risk of damage and early arthritis.

Diagnosis and symptoms

Patients with subluxation alone may complain more of giving-way than of pain. Sometimes there will be a feeling of sharp pain followed by giving-way. There is often aching after activity. Pain is often non-specific but mostly located in the front of the knee. The pain increases with knee bending and squatting. Repeated gliding on clay courts may exacerbate the pain.

It is important to assess the alignment patterns by careful clinical examination. When the patellar tendon attaches to the tibia in a more lateral position than normal there is a large angle (Q angle) formed from the groove where the patella tracks to the insertion point. The normal Q should be less than about 17° in women and less than about 15° in men with the knee flexed in 30°. An increased Q angle can increase the likelihood that the patella will subluxate laterally. Other lower extremity malalignments that can contribute to subluxation are increased femoral anteversion, excessive external tibia torsion, and exaggerated pronation. The clinical examination should be performed both in the standing and in seated position. Examining the knee while the athlete actively flexes and extends the knee can aid in finding causative factors.

Some special radiographs, such as the Merchant view, can assist in the diagnosis. This test shows how the patella sits in the femoral groove. More information is provided if the test is carried out with quadriceps contractions. CT scan tracking studies allow precise reproducible imaging of patellofemoral relationships at different angles and reveal normal alignment, excessive lateral tilt, and subluxation of the patella.

Treatment and rehabilitation

All of the disorders that cause patellofemoral pain are initially treated with quadriceps strengthening, endurance, balance and flexibility training. The main goal of the exercises is to strenghten the activity of the vastus medialis portion of the quadriceps muscle. This muscle pulls the patella in a medial direction to limit lateral subluxation or dislocation. Electrical stimulation of the vastus medialis may be helpful in regaining strength and neural recruitment. Activity modification and functional training are also very important. Bracing to prevent the patella from moving laterally may be helpful, especially in cases of patellar subluxation or dislocation. Some patients experience relief with patellar taping. The purpose of patellar taping is to attempt to move the patella into better alignment, thereby reducing pain and facilitating an exercise programme.

Surgery is needed in a few of these cases. In those patients a high Q angle and subluxation or dislocation, moving the insertion site of the patellar tendon medially to reduce the Q angle (tibia tubercle transfer) leads to improvement in the majority of the patients.

Impact and return to tennis

Return to tennis can proceed on a symptomatic basis with the conservative programme. Most patients will be able to resume some level of tennis with bracing or taping while participating in the rehabilitation programme. For those athletes requiring surgery, return to tennis is usually possible 4–5 months after surgery.

Increased lateral tilt of the patella

Increased lateral tilt of the patella means that the outside (lateral) border of the patella sits lower within the groove than the inside (medial) border (Fig. 16.11). This can result in increased pressure on the lateral patellar articular surface that can cause degeneration and damage on the articular cartilage of the lateral patellar surface or femoral groove. There may also be degeneration on the medial side of the patellar surface due to the absence of contact pressure necessary for healthy articular cartilage. Chronic lateral tilt may develop adaptive shortening of the soft

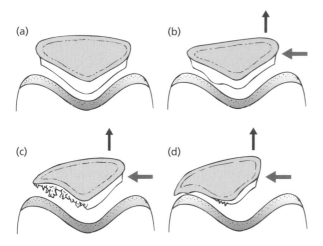

Fig. 16.11 Patellar tracking. (a) Normal; (b) lateral tracking causing some damage on the lateral angle; (c) subluxation and some lateral tilt, causing further damage; (d) subluxation and severe lateral tilt. (From Peterson, L. & Renström, P. (2000) *Sports Injuries: Their Prevention and Treatment*, p. 303. Martin Dunitz, London.)

tissues that attach to the lateral border of the patella (lateral retinacular tissues) and concomitant reactive lengthening of the medial retinacular structures. With knee flexion the tension on the lateral structures will increase and may cause compression of small nerves. This is called excessive lateral pressure syndrome.

Diagnosis and symptoms

Athletes with this problem will complain of pain in the front of the knee that will be worse with squatting and deep knee bending activities. Players with only lateral tilt will have a normal Q angle, but will have tight lateral retinacular structures. These patients will have abnormal tightness when trying to move the patella in a medial direction or when trying to tilt the lateral border of the patella up. Some patients may have tenderness over the lateral retinaculum.

Treatment and rehabilitation

The treatment of lateral tilt, in addition to the conservative programme mentioned in the previous section on patellar subluxation, includes stretching of the lateral retinacular tissues and the iliotibial band. As with all the conservative programmes, strength training of the quadriceps muscles, especially the vastus medialis obliques, is most important. Occasionally surgery is needed in refractory cases. Surgical treatment of this problem is by cutting of the lateral structures (lateral retinacular release). Care must be taken not to extend the release into the quadriceps tendon or medial instability can occur. For cases with no subluxation, tibial tubercle transfer should not be performed, as this can also cause medial instability.

If there is a combination of patellar tilt and subluxation there is a risk for both degradation of the lateral facet and instability of the patella. In this case, a tibial tubercle transfer would be indicated, as described in the section on subluxation of the patella.

Impact and return to tennis

As with most patellar pain syndromes, tennis play can usually continue at some level while rehabilitation is undertaken. In those cases that do not respond to conservative therapy and go on to surgical lateral retinacular release, return to tennis is usually possible at about 4–6 weeks.

Chondromalacia patella (patellar cartilage degeneration)

There are two major causes for injury to the articular joint surface of the patellofemoral joint. One cause is blunt trauma to the patella (i.e. falling directly on the patella). This trauma causes cartilage matrix breakdown. The second cause is chronic malalignment, which causes abnormal tracking of the patella in the femoral groove. Lastly, some degeneration of the patella cannot be associated with a specific cause. Damage of the patellar cartilage without trauma can occur with normal alignment, but it is more common with abnormal alignment. The grading of the damaged patellar cartilages is seen in Fig. 16.12.

Symptoms and diagnosis

Pain may result from abnormally stressed peripatellar structures or from abnormal articular loading. A grinding sound or feeling may occur during motion. As is the case with all patellofemoral disorders, athletes with this problem will complain of pain in

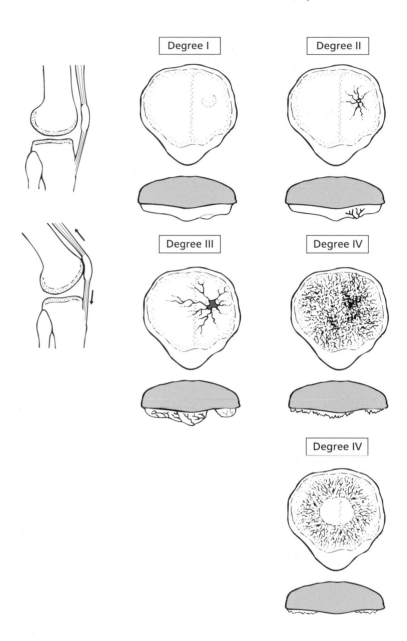

Fig. 16.12 Patellar cartilage damage. (From Peterson, L. & Renström, P. (2000) *Sports Injuries: Their Prevention and Treatment*, p. 318. Martin Dunitz, London.)

the front of the knee that will be worse with squatting and deep knee bending activities.

Treatment and rehabilitation

The treatment is most commonly symptomatic, but should be directed toward the cause of the problem. Avoidance of abuse and muscle strengthening are the two most important factors in managing this difficult problem. The programme is outlined in the previous sections. If malalignment is present, surgery to move the patellar tendon insertion to a more natural position may help. This usually involves elevating and moving the tibial tubercle to the inside (anterior and medial).

Impact and return to tennis

Return to tennis must be gradual and depends on the extent of the injury and the amount of intervention that is necessary. In most cases, tennis play can continue while the athlete is undergoing treatment. Play may need to be reduced to a less strenuous level, with a gradual build-up to the previous level of play.

Patellar dislocation

Rotational stress to the knee while weightbearing may cause the patella to dislocate. This is more frequent in players with predisposing malalignment such as increased Q angle or valgus position of the lower leg.

Symptoms and diagnosis

The patella will sit to the outside of the femoral groove after an acute dislocation. For this to occur the structures on the inside of the knee that hold the patella in the groove must be torn. The patella can quite easily be put back in position by straightening the leg. This usually requires no direct manipulation of the patella itself. This can occur because the patella sits above the level of the femoral groove when the knee is fully straightened.

Treatment and rehabilitation

Treatment is most often by a short period of immobilization to control pain, followed by a functional rehabilitation programme. A brace to hold the patella in position is often useful during the rehabilitation programme. It is important during the initial period to avoid rotational exercises of the knee. The healing time is usually about 6–8 weeks, but rehabilitation should continue at least 4–6 months. Surgery is sometimes required.

Impact and return to tennis

Return to tennis is usually possible between 2 and 4 months. For several months following the injury, a patellofemoral brace to hold the patella in the femoral groove may be of value during tennis playing.

Quadriceps tendinopathy and tears

This condition is caused by overuse of the quadriceps muscle group either by repeated jumping or by heavy extension exercises such as weightlifting. This is a common condition during preseason training that occurs often after an athlete begins to train heavily following a long period of inactivity. Complete quadriceps tears can occur in elderly recreational players during sudden eccentric motions such as landing after a smash. Fortunately, complete tears are not very common.

Symptoms and diagnosis

The athlete will experience pain at the top of the patella, particularly when performing squatting, knee extension activities or stair climbing. The athlete will also have tenderness at the top of the patella where the quadriceps muscle inserts into the patella. Acute complete tears will only occur following an obvious injury. If an acute complete tear has occurred a defect will be felt in the tendon at the top of the patella and a MRI evaluation will secure the diagnosis (Fig. 16.13).

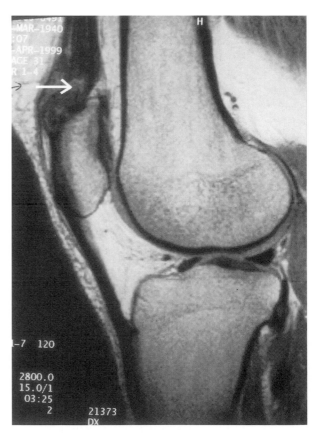

Fig. 16.13 Magnetic resonance image of complete quadriceps tendon tear (arrow).

Treatment and rehabilitation

As with most of the patellofemoral problems, most of the problems with quadriceps tendinosis will resolve with physical therapy to stretch the quadriceps and hamstring muscles, followed by a gradual strengthening programme. The player should avoid activities that exacerbate the pain. In prolonged cases that last more than 6–9 months, and are diminishing performance, surgery can be considered to remove the degenerative portion of the tendon that is causing the pain.

Complete tears require urgent surgical repair to reattach the tendon. This should be performed within the first 7–10 days to avoid muscle contraction.

Impact and return to tennis

Most players can continue playing tennis during the rehabilitation for quadriceps tendinosis, but they may need to lower their level of competition to avoid the pain. As with all the patellofemoral pain syndromes this is an individualized programme that depends on the athlete's pain level.

If surgery is required to remove the degenerative tissue, return to light tennis activity can usually begin at about 2–3 months, with a gradually increasing level of activity. Full return to tennis may take up to 4–6 months, however. Following surgical repair of a complete quadriceps tendon rupture, return to tennis is usually not possible until about 6 months after the repair.

Patellar tendinopathy

Patellar tendinopathy is a problem caused by similar mechanisms to that which cause quadriceps tendinopathy, and in fact patellar tendinopathy is probably more common. Instead of the pain being localized to the quadriceps tendon at the top of the patella, the pain is localized to just below the patella at the insertion of the patellar tendon. Tennis requires repetitive flexion/extension manoeuvres during serving and overhead smashes, gliding out to the corners and running towards the net to return drop shots. These tennis actions include forceful concentric and eccentric quadriceps muscle action involving the patellar tendon. A change in direction involves decelerating eccentric action of the extensor

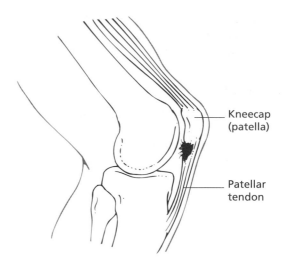

Fig. 16.14 Patellar tendon partial tear or tendinopathy. (From Ekblom, B. (ed.) (1994) *Handbook of Sports Medicine and Science: Football (Soccer)*, p. 185. Blackwell Scientific Publications, Oxford.)

mechanism, which is followed by an explosive concentric quadriceps activity to move backward. Repetitive motions cause extensor mechanism problems.

Symptoms and diagnosis

The tennis player often experiences pain with vigorous quadriceps activity such as jumping and landing after smashes. Clinical findings include pain, tenderness and sometimes swelling at the lower pole of the patella. Occasionally there is an osseous fragmentation of the patella. A small partial rupture can occur in the posterior portion of the tendon at the insertion to the patella (Fig. 16.14). A very distinct tenderness can then be palpated over that area, and an MRI will confirm the extent.

Treatment and rehabilitation

Conservative therapy with stretching, strengthening and eccentric activities is successful in 80% of the players. A physical therapist should help plan all individual programmes. Some people will obtain some relief from braces or straps that put pressure on the patellar tendon (Fig. 16.15). The exact mechanism of action of the strap is not well understood, but some people do get some benefit.

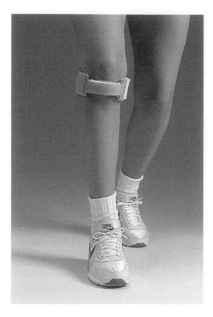

Fig. 16.15 Patellar tendon strap.

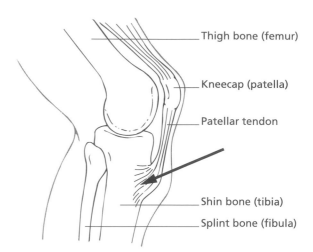

Thigh bone (femur)

Kneecap (patella)

Patellar tendon

Shin bone (tibia)

Splint bone (fibula)

Fig. 16.16 Osgood–Schlatter's disease. The lesion is indicated by an arrow. (From Ekblom, B. (ed.) (1994) *Handbook of Sports Medicine and Science: Football (Soccer)*, p. 186. Blackwell Scientific Publications, Oxford.)

If the condition becomes chronic, with decreased function and pain lasting longer than 6–9 months, surgery can be considered. Surgery consists of removal of the degenerative portion of the tendon that causes the pain. MRI and ultrasound are helpful in confirming the location and size of the lesion of the tendon.

Impact and return to tennis

For mild cases of patellar tendinopathy, tennis play can usually continue during treatment, but the player may need to play at a lower level during the rehabilitation period. Return to tennis after surgery of a partial tear of the patellar tendon can take a long time. The average time to return to play is between 4 and 6 months.

Osgood–Schlatter's disease

Pain located at the insertion site for patellar tendon into the tibia can occur in junior tennis players. In growing individuals, the soft tissues such as tendon and muscles are stronger than the bone. Excessive tensile forces may cause stress and result in fragmentation at the insertion site (Fig. 16.16).

Symptoms and diagnosis

Young teenage athletes with this condition will complain of pain and swelling over the patellar tendon insertion on the tibia. Knee radiographs will verify the fragmentation. There is distinct tenderness over the swollen tubercle on palpation. Young tennis players localize the problems to this area during squatting, deep knee bending, and jumping.

Treatment and rehabilitation

The disease often is untreated with spontaneous healing. The player should avoid abuse of the knee and thereby painful situations. At the end of adolescence, the condition disappears.

Impact and return to tennis

The cornerstone of treatment of this condition is rest and avoidance of painful activities. The player can continue activities that do not cause pain. Return to full tennis is usually possible at about 6 weeks, but the athlete should adjust his or her training programme to avoid overuse of the knee so that the condition does not return.

Fig. 16.17 Bursitis around the knee. (a) Acute bleeding in anterior patellar bursa; (b) untreated bleeding, adhesions and loose bodies; (c) residual condition with adhesions, scar tissue and loose bodies. (From Peterson, L. & Renström, P. (2000) *Sports Injuries: Their Prevention and Treatment*, p. 325. Martin Dunitz, London.)

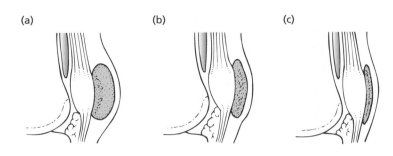

(a)   (b)   (c)

Knee bursitis

The knee is surrounded by a number of bursae. The most common types of bursitis are the pre-patellar bursitis, pes anserinus bursitis and semimembranosis bursitis (Fig. 16.17). There can occasionally be a biceps femoris bursitis. A bursitis inside the iliotibial band over the lateral femoral condyle is called 'runner's knee' and may occur in tennis players.

Pre-patellar bursitis

Pre-patellar bursitis is common in contact sports but is only occasionally seen in tennis. The usual mechanism of injury is a direct fall against the ground. This causes bleeding within the bursa. Occasionally, the haemorrhagic bursitis can lead to adhesions and chronic fluid within the bursa.

Diagnosis and symptoms

Diagnosis of pre-patellar bursitis is quite evident by the fluid-filled sac on the front of the patella. In the acute traumatic cases this is usually mildly tender. In cases where there is marked tenderness and surrounding redness, an infected bursa must be suspected. In this case aspiration of the bursa should be performed to evaluate for bacteria.

Treatment and rehabilitation

In straightforward non-infected cases, aspiration is usually not necessary because the fluid will usually recur. Aspiration can be performed for a very large bursa to relieve pain, and aspiration is mandatory if infection is suspected. Compression for 4–6 days will help to minimize the swelling, while the body reabsorbs the fluid.

In chronic cases, an injection of corticosteroid can sometimes induce healing, but surgery may be necessary to remove the bursa.

Impact and return to tennis

Tennis play can continue with a pre-patellar bursitis, but the player should avoid landing on the knee. If surgery is necessary, return to tennis is usually possible within 2–4 weeks.

Pes anserinus bursitis

Pes anserinus bursitis is an inflammation of the bursa between the insertion sites of three tendons on the inside front portion of the tibia just below the knee joint: the semitendinosus, sartorius and gracilis tendons. This injury is not common but can occur in tennis when the player glides from one side to the other on clay. Biomechanical abnormalities such as increased knee valgus, external rotation of the tibia or excessive tightness of the hamstrings have been implicated as potential causes of pes anserinus bursitis.

Diagnosis and symptoms

The player will usually complain of pain at the pes anserine area while running. The diagnosis is confirmed by the distinct tenderness over the pes anserinus bursa.

Treatment and rehabilitation

Sometimes an orthotic insert can help in cases of foot malalignment. A cortisone injection is indicated if conservative treatment fails.

Impact and return to tennis

This is usually a self-limited process. Sometimes a period of rest will be needed to induce the healing process. In most cases, however, tennis play can continue as much as the pain will allow.

The semimembranosis bursa

The semimembranosis bursa is located beneath the semimembranosis tendon as it crosses the tibial plateau at the back inside portion of the knee joint. The semimembranosis bursa can sometimes be inflamed and cause a sensation of pain or pressure in the back of the knee.

Diagnosis and symptoms

The diagnosis is made by localized pain on resisted flexion of the knee and direct tenderness over the semimembranosis tendon insertion on the posterior aspect of the tibia.

Treatment and rehabilitation

Conservative treatment including stretching and muscle exercises, particularly of the hamstring muscles, is indicated to decrease inflammation. In some prolonged cases an injection of corticosteroid can help to reduce the swelling.

Impact and return to tennis

As with most of the bursal inflammations, players with inflammation of the semimembranosis bursa can continue playing as much as their pain will allow.

Runner's knee (iliotibial friction syndrome)

Runner's knee is an overuse injury caused by excessive friction between the lateral femoral epicondyle and the iliotibial band. It is usually associated with extrinsic factors such as running downhill or on the side of a sloped track or road. Shoes that are worn out on one side of the sole can be a factor. Malalignment, such as increased pronation with secondary increased internal rotation of the tibia, can also be the cause of this condition. This injury is unusual in tennis but may occur during preseason preparation.

Diagnosis and symptoms

The player will complain of pain during activity, with pain and tenderness located on the outside portion of the knee on the elevated portion—the epicondyle—just above the joint line. Often the player will complain of more pain during the rest period after the activity is over. He or she may also describe 'knee stiffness' located in the same outside portion of the knee following prolonged sitting.

Treatment and rehabilitation

The treatment is designed for care of poor biomechanics, such as giving orthotics to neutralize hyperpronation. Stretching of the iliotibial band and the lateral thigh muscles is an important component. A localized cortisone injection can cure the condition. If conservative therapy does not help, there are good results with surgery that include a small incision of the iliotibial band. This can be done under local anaesthesia on an outpatient basis.

Impact and return to tennis

Tennis play can continue as much as the pain will allow. A short period of rest may be necessary to induce the healing process. In cases that require surgery, return to tennis is usually possible in about 2–4 weeks.

Prevention of knee injuries

Most knee injuries in tennis are due to overuse. These can be prevented by eliminating deficiencies in player equipment, technique and environment. Maintaining proper fitness is a key component in preventing injuries. Many athletes do not warm up properly and do not participate in a structured stretching programme. Most players go directly to the court and start to hit with no warm up. If tightness of the quadriceps mechanism and the hamstring muscles is present, this may result in an overload of forces at the knee. Repeated stretching can help reduce the potential for injury.

If a player develops knee pain, it is important to obtain a correct diagnosis and to begin effective treatment. If swelling within the knee joint itself is present, abuse of the knee must be avoided and modification in exercise intensity must be undertaken to avoid permanent injury. Once the problems are corrected, tennis play can resume.

Recommended reading

Fulkerson, J. (1991) Operative management of patellofemoral pain. *Annales Chirurgiae et Gynaecologiae* **80**, 224–229.

Fyfe, I. & Stanish, W. (1992) The use of eccentric training and stretching in the treatment and prevention of tennis injuries. *Clinics in Sports Medicine* **11** (3), 601–624.

Nigg, B. (1993) Excessive loads and sports injury mechanism. In: Renström, P., ed. *Sports Injuries: Basic Principles of Prevention and Care, IOC-FIMS Encyclopedia of Sports Medicine IV*, pp. 107–115. Blackwell Scientific Publications, Oxford.

Nirshl, R.P. & Sobel, N.P. (1994) Injuries in tennis. In: Renström, P., ed. *Clinical Practice of Sports Injury: Prevention and Care, IOC-FIMS Encyclopedia V*, pp. 460–474. Blackwell Scientific Publications, Oxford.

Chapter 17

Spine injuries in tennis

Functional anatomy of the spine

The spine, being the axis organ of the body, apparently has contrasting functions. On the one hand, it is a 'column' anchored in the pelvis that supports the head and stabilizes the body. The firm stiffness of the different bony segments is ensured by a number of muscles and ligaments. The second primary characteristic of the spine is the flexibility and is an essential requirement for all involuntary and voluntary movements. This flexibility is based on the large number of single elements—the vertebrae—whose own minor single movements sum up to the large degree of movement of the spine as a whole by means of changes in muscle contractions. The bony casing of the spinal cord, protected in the bony spinal canal, is considered the third important function.

The 'healthy' spine has typical curves within the lordotic (convex to the front) cervical and lumbar spine and the kyphotic (convex to the back) thoracic spine and sacrum in the sagittal level. As a result, the lateral view shows an apparent dynamic or elastic-like double S-shape. The curves are a result, on the one hand, of the particular shape of the individual vertebra and, on the other hand, of the tilted position of the vertebrae to one another. Sideward movements in the frontal level may occur but are of no significance as long as they are not combined with functional disorders.

The individual components of the spine—the single vertebrae—are generally shaped in the same manner regardless of which height they are located at. They can anatomically be divided into two main parts: the weight-bearing cylindrically shaped vertebral body in the front and the vertebral arch with its spinous and transverse processes as well as the superior and inferior articular processes in the back surrounding the myelon. Consequently, there are three jointed connections in

the functional unit of the spine—two adjacent vertebrae with an intervertebral disc between the two (Fig. 17.1). The two adjacent vertebrae with the intervertebral disc build the front-sided anterior column and have a static function, whereas the four articular facets of the adjacent vertebrae build the back-sided posterior column and have a primarily dynamic function. Together, the front-sided and back-sided columns build the column system of the spine and form the three-joint-complex. Junghanns (1986) describes the unit consisting of an intervertebral disc, the ligamentous structures (anterior and posterior longitudinal ligament, yellow ligament), the paired intervertebral joints and the costovertebral joints located at the level of the dorsal spine as a 'movement segment'.

The high level of strain that the functional unit can take and therefore that the spine as a whole can take is a result of the static and dynamic joining of the vertebrae to one another. Being a static element, a strongly developed ligament system connects the vertebrae in a tense manner. The most important ligaments are the anterior and posterior longitudinal ligaments that stretch over the front and back of the vertebrae, the Lig. flavum that forms the boundary of the spinal canal in dorsal direction as well as various ligaments between the spinous processes, the transverse processes and the articular processes. The active dynamic stabilization is achieved through the paraspinal back muscles, which also carry out static functions. In addition, contributing considerably to the stabilization of the spine, and of particular importance are the flexors and extensors of the spine, many of which achieve their power transmission to the body through the thoracolumbar fascia (Young 1996) (Table 17.1).

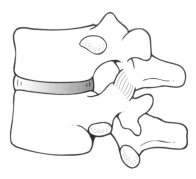

Fig. 17.1 The functional unit of the spine: two adjacent vertebrae with an intervertebral disc. (From Kapandji 1974.)

Table 17.1 The spine flexors and extensors.

Flexors/rotators	Extensors/rotators
M. rectus abdominis	M. latissimus dorsi
Mm. obliqus ext. et int.	long and short spinal
M. transvs. abdominis	extensors/rotators
M. psoas	M. gluteus maximus

The interaction between the passive elements (the ligaments) and the active elements (the muscles) allows for slight swayings within the physiological framework but at the same time helps avoid injuries caused by instability under the condition that an appropriate state of training has been reached.

Another important element of the spine is the intervertebral disc. It consists of a jelly centre, the nucleus pulposus, and a fibrous ring, the anulus fibrosus, surrounding it. The jelly centre functions as a ball bearing and is movable depending on the strain put on the disc. Aside from the main directions of movement of the spine—ventral and dorsal floxion, sidewards inclination and rotation—there are also minimal sagittal, axial and transversal shiftings possible that, when seen as the sum of several spine segments, cause a functionally relevant degree of movement. The healthy elastic intervertebral disc can hold out extreme degrees of strain. This strain increases from cranial to caudal and, corresponding to this, the greatest thickness of the intervertebral discs can be found in the lumbar spine region. The height decreases slightly when under strong strain and then reaches the original height during the period of no strain. According to Kapandji (1974), the length of the spine of an average adult therefore decreases approximately 2 cm towards the evening due to the reduction of the height of the intervertebral discs, which is caused by compression. The elasticity of the intervertebral disc is reduced with advancing age and a regeneration fails to appear so that a higher risk of tearing and therefore of slipped discs is then present.

The spine is involved in nearly every movement of the body. It is always complex segments of the spine that are affected, never single segments. The individual movements of the functional unit of two adjacent vertebrae are not of significance (1–2° per facet joint (Young 1996)) when considering the mobility of the entire spine. The degree of mobility of complex segments of the spine is of prime importance whereby low levels of mobility of the individual functional units are compensated for. The movement in major directions is possible in all three movable parts of the spine—cervical spine (seven vertebrae), thoracic spine (12 vertebrae), lumbar spine (five vertebrae). There is a difference, however, in the degree of mobility. Thus, the cervical spine has the largest amplitude in movement while the thoracic spine has a close to balanced degree of mobility in all directions. Due to the vertical sagittal positioning of the joint facets, the lumbar spine has the major focus of mobility in ventral flexion and dorsal extension with only a slight capability of rotation (Table 17.2). The spine lumbar segments L4/L5 and L5/S1 thereby allow for 80–90% of the possible amount of flexion/extension.

Table 17.2 Extent of mobility of the spine in degrees (Kapandji 1974).

	Flexion	Extension	Sideward inclination/side	Rotation/side
Cervical spine	40°	75°	35–45°	45–50°
Thoracic spine	45°	25°	20°	35°
Lumbar spine	60°	35°	20°	5°
Complete spine	110°	140°	75–85°	90–95°

The first 60° of the ventral flexion are carried out by the lumbar spine segments, and the next 25° by the hip joints (Young 1996). During dorsal extension a dorsal rotation of the pelvis initially takes place. This is followed by the extension through the M. erector spinae and the gluteal muscles. Only this combined movement—lumbopelvic rhythm—allows for the final degree of movement to occur. Sideward inclination is distributed more or less evenly among the three movable segments of the spine. Rotation decreases considerably from cranial to caudal because the articular facets are increasingly positioned in a turned position at the sagittal level in this direction and thus virtually prevent a rotation (Fig. 17.2).

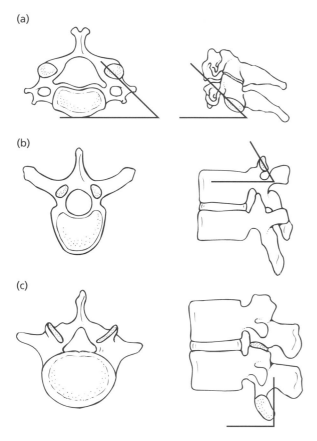

(a)

(b)

(c)

Fig. 17.2 The position of the articular facet surfaces from cranial (left) and lateral (right) in the individual segments of the spine (a, cervical spine, b thoracic spine, c lumbar spine); there is an increasing straightening up of the articular facets from the cervical spine to the lumbar spine in the frontal level and an increasing rotation in the sagittal level (according to Alexander 1985).

The connection of the lumbar spine, usually consisting of five vertebrae, and the fourth spine section, the sacral bone, is referred to as the lumbosacral connection. In this area, the capability of sidewards inclination and rotation between the fourth and fifth lumbar vertebra and the first sacral vertebra is restricted not only through the sagittal positioning of the vertebral joints but also considerably through strong iliolumbar ligaments connecting the mobile elements of the lower spine to the pelvis. The first 'mobile' vertebra is the third lumbar vertebra with a cranial positioning in this area. It has a distinctively strong vertebral arch since, on the one hand, the M. longissimus extending in caudal direction is attached here, and, on the other hand, the fibres of the M. spinalis extending in cranial direction also begin here. In comparison to this, the segment level L4–S1 is referred to as the 'static' connection to the pelvic girdle due to the firm fixing of the ligaments (Kapandji 1974). On the other hand, Magora (1976) refers to the segment of movement L5/S1 as the most 'dynamic' part of the lumbar spine which, being the 'centre of movement' in this area, receives the biomechanical strains of everyday life. Burri and Rüter (1980) confirm this opinion with regards to the flexion/extension movement and the capability of rotation but disagree, however, with the comments on sidewards inclination, which reaches a maximum in the segments L3/L4 in the lumbar spine area (Table 17.3). The biomechanical strain and overstrain, caused by the weight of the trunk, even increasing by sports-related maximum of mobility of the lower lumbar spine connected with the static pelvis, affects a relatively small weight-carrying anatomical region—the lumbosacroiliac zone.

The spine is set wedge-shaped into the pelvic girdle through the sacral bone consisting of five sacral vertebrae that are fused together. Both articular connections to the pelvic girdle—the sacroiliac joints—are firmly braced through strong ligaments as taut joints with little mobility. It is here that the position of the body is transmitted from the spine through the sacroiliac joints to the pelvic girdle and then follows to the lower extremities. The closeness of the sacroiliac joints to the psoas muscle and to the N. obturatorius may cause differential diagnostic difficulties in some cases.

Table 17.3 The extent to which the individual segments are movable within the lumbar spine in degrees (Burri & Rüter 1980).

	Flexion/extension	Sidewards inclination	Rotation
L1/L2	12	6	2
L2/L3	14	6	2
L3/L4	15	8	2
L4/L5	17	6	2
L5/S1	20	3	5

The thoracic spine consists of 12 vertebrae whose joint surfaces are turned out in ventral and dorsal direction and thus enable rotation as opposed to the lumbar spine. The thoracic vertebrae are connected to the ribs, which complete the bony thorax in a jointy manner. A special role with regard to anatomy and function is taken on by the 12th thoracic vertebra whose caudal articular facets are adapted to the lumbar spinal column.

The cervical spine is set up into two functional components. The upper cervical spine, consisting of the first two cervical vertebrae—atlas and axis— supports the head and differs anatomically and functionally from the lower cervical spine which is similar to the rest of the spinal column.

Biomechanical strain on the spinal column in tennis

Although back pain is a common symptom among recreational athletes as well as among tennis professionals, the pathophysiology, biomechanics and clinical findings of existing injuries are not clearly defined (Hainline 1995). Furthermore, it is questionable whether sports-related strain in tennis is solely responsible for pathological changes of the spinal column or whether anatomical–pathological disorders in form and function that already exist cause the pain that can be typically found in the sport of tennis.

The lumbar spine is prone to injury due to the maximal sidewards inclination, rotation and hyperextension that occurs in tennis through existing shear forces when serving and hitting an overhead smash (Elliott 1988; Hainline 1995). The hyperextension, rotation and lateral flexion take place so as to attain an optimal initial preflexing of the body and hitting arm (arched flexing). This is followed by a powerful dynamic movement in the corresponding opposite direction towards the hitting point (Fig. 17.3).

The normal forehand groundstroke requires an axial rotation of the vertebral column of about 90° so that the hitting arm can be swung back far enough behind the body. The reference lines usually chosen to determine the degree of rotation are the shoulder area on one hand and the pelvis area on the other hand. The actual hitting phase which follows is characterized by a powerful rotation of the body and shoulder in the opposite direction (Hainline 1995). A stroke straining much further is the two-handed backhand that also leads to a rotation of the spine. As is the case with the serve and smash, an extreme strain is placed on the lumbar spine, which is more or less 'non-rotatable'. The one-handed backhand requires less rotation in the hitting phase, as does the forehand because the shoulder on the 'hitting side' is already facing the net when hitting a backhand. The required rotation of the body by the backwards–forwards swing is considerably larger for the two-handed backhand (Fig. 17.4) since the non-dominant shoulder must be rotated further so as to turn the body towards the net. The lumbar spine is exposed to an extreme biomechanical phase of strain in particular by the stretched backhand because the pelvis is in a more or less locked position (Hainline 1995).

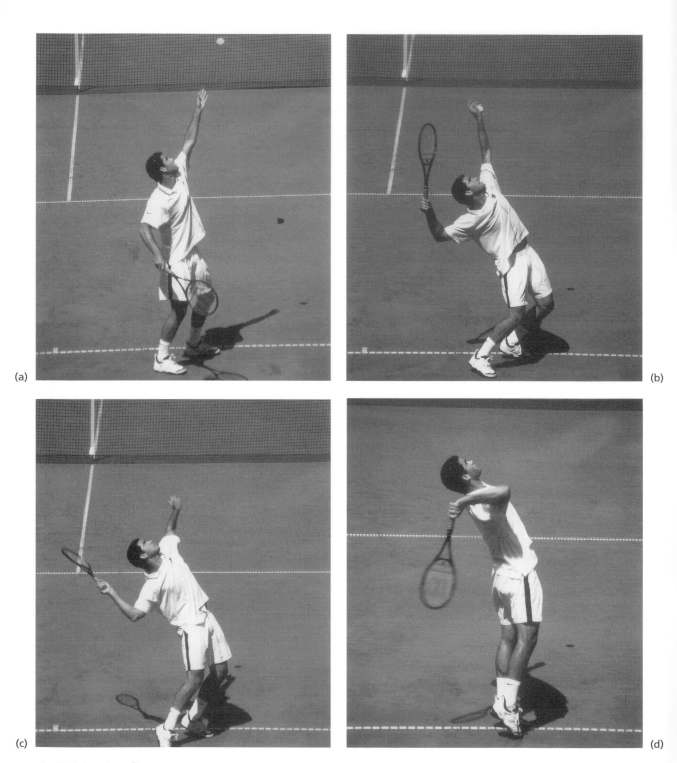

(a)

(b)

(c)

(d)

Fig. 17.3 (*continued*)

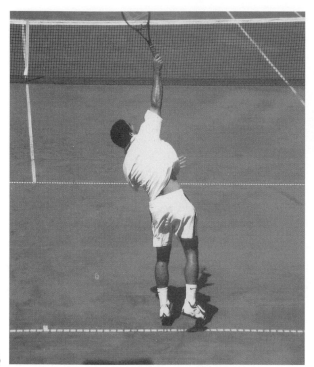

(e)

Fig. 17.3 (*continued*) The various phases of the serve in tennis. The extreme positioning into which the body is moved during reclination/flexion, sidewards inclination and rotation can be clearly seen.

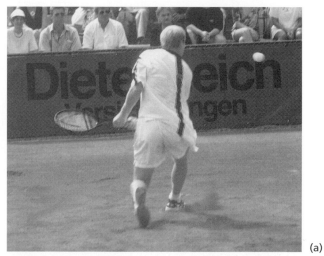

(a)

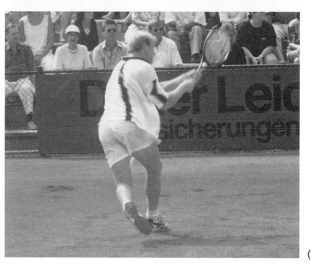

(b)

Fig. 17.4 The two-handed backhand with a body rotation of almost 180° towards the backhand side with respect to the shoulder–pelvis area.

The spine is exposed to an extreme level of strain through tennis-specific movements due to the weight of the body itself, external power and a high level of acceleration (Alexander 1985). It must be noted here that the spine is affected by all powers placed on the upper extremities (hitting arm) and all powers placed on the lower extremities (pushing off from the ground and stopping). The spine is exposed to two different forms of strain: (i) the static strain through compression and shear forces in stationary positions (e.g. weightlifter); and (ii) the dynamic strain characterized by the variation of the strain and inertia forces where there is a disproportion of the stopping and starting movements in tennis which leads to an abrupt change of acceleration of the lower extremities and a related reaction of the trunk, so that the lumbosacral region gets stressed.

The lumbosacral connection is considered to be a weakness in the biomechanics of the spine. The vertical force that is passed on through the lumbar spine is split into two directions in this segment. The first force vector extends vertically to the top surface of the first sacral vertebra in dorsocaudal direction and results in a compression of this part of the spine. The second power vector extends in a right angle to the first one, parallel to the top surface of S1 in ventrocaudal direction and therefore results in a shear force component (Le Veau 1977) (Fig. 17.5).

The strain put on the lumbosacral connecting area is influenced by three factors: the weight of the body, the lumbosacral angle and the level of training of the back

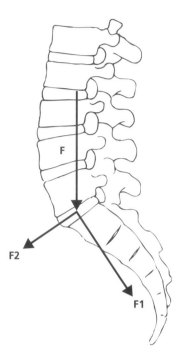

Fig. 17.5 The dividing of the powers at the lumbosacral connection: the power (F) parallel to the body axis and affecting the top plate S1 is divided here into a compression power (F1, perpendicular to the top plate in dorsocaudal direction) and into a shear force component (F2, parallel to the top plate S1 in ventrocaudal direction). A greater lumbosacral angle (standard: 124–164°; average 144° (Junghanns 1986)) leads to an enlargement of the shear force component and thus to a greater strain upon the ligaments with a higher risk of developing lumbosacral instabilities in the form of spondylolisthesis L5/S1.

muscles (Alexander 1985). In addition to the static strain upon the connection L5/S1, there are other dynamic forces in tennis that have to be absorbed by the spine: the force of the ball onto the racket, the arm and then onto the spine, the acceleration forces and the interaction of muscle contraction and ligament stretching. These forces occur to different extents in various phases in tennis (hitting phase, running phase and stopping phase).

The serve is considered to be the most important single factor in tennis with respect to lumbar spine injuries and is described as the most risky stroke. Kinematic and kinetic studies conducted by Elliott (1988) were not able to reveal a direct explanation for this. However, it seems that a rhythmic series of movements is essential for the prevention of injuries

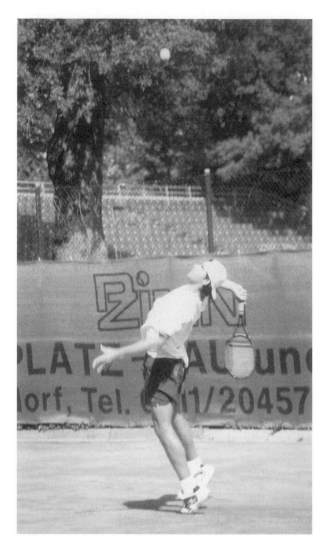

Fig. 17.6 The ball toss when serving. The extremely high toss can be seen here. A flexed hip due to a shortened hip flexor is shown which is characteristic for a muscular imbalance. In extreme cases, this can lead to the end of tennis as seen from a sports medicine point of view. While bending backwards as required the hip cannot be stretched and this has to be compensated for by an excessive reclination of the lumbar spine.

during the serve. Therefore, every change and interruption of the rhythm leads to an avoidable and incorrect strain upon the lumbar spine.

The ball toss for the serve plays an important role in the prevention of excessive hyperextension and lateral flexion. The correct ball toss enables an optimal

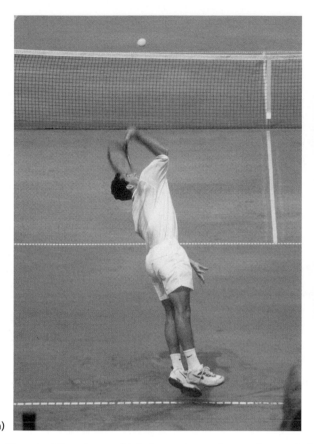
(a)

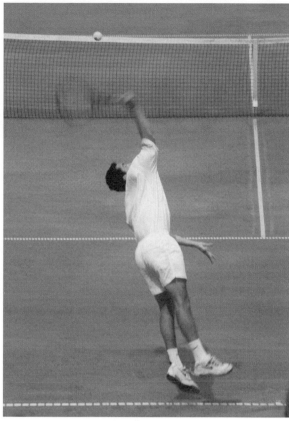
(b)

Fig. 17.7 The point at which the maximum degree of power is developed just before the ball is hit.

rhythmic swing and thus reduces the chance of injuries (Elliott 1988). Hitting the ball at its highest point is a particularly important factor in order to maintain the rhythm. This is due to the fact that a ball thrown at the height of the racket surface gives the player eight times more time to hit the ball as compared to a ball thrown 120 cm higher (Beerman & Sher 1981). Because the time available for the first two phases of the serve is considerably reduced here, the ball is usually thrown higher and is then not hit until it is on its way back down. Therefore, many of the top tennis players hit the ball just after the highest point has been reached which is at the beginning of the phase in which the ball falls back down (Plaggenhoef 1970). Other players even have an extremely high ball toss in their serving technique (Fig. 17.6).

Other top athletes, however, prefer tossing the ball with considerably more power and hit the ball in a clearly more accelerated phase. The possible duration of contact with the rapidly falling ball is significantly shortened in this technique and a precise rhythmic movement is even more important so as to reduce the chance of injuries. Nigg (1986) describes the degree of power in addition to rhythmic movements as critical variables for the aetiology of pain and injury during the serve. The serve requires the highest amount of power as opposed to all other strokes in tennis (Yoshizawa *et al.* 1987). The maximum muscle activity is not being reached at the exact moment the ball is hit but during the upward motion of the serve before the hitting point. The serving arm is behind the body and the spine is laterally flexed, hyperextended and rotated to a maximum (Miyashita *et al.* 1980; Van Gheluwe & Hebbelinck 1986) (Fig. 17.7).

Electromyographical studies revealed a greater and longer muscle activity during the serve among poorer players than was the case among top athletes (Elliott 1988).

Epidemiology of spine injuries among tennis players

Spine injuries and damages caused by overstraining are common among athletes. This is naturally the case for sports in which the spine is considerably involved. These are primarily 'contact sports' (soccer, American football, handball, rugby), power sports involving strength (weightlifting and wrestling) and sports with a high share of flexion, extension and rotation movements of the spine and in particular of the lumbar spine (swimming, gymnastics, javelin as well as the racket sports squash, badminton and tennis). Acute injuries occur in large numbers among 'contact sports' and power sports involving strength whereas 'asymmetrical' sports have a higher number of injuries due to overstraining. Of course, training intensity, duration and frequency all play an important role in the development of injuries resulting from overstraining. Acute injuries are more likely among recreational players in racket sports.

Harvey and Tanner (1991) discovered that pulled ligaments/muscles and sprains in the lumbar spine region are the most common cause of backaches that occur in 5–8% of all sports injuries. They expressed the opinion that a number of predisposed factors, which do not seem to be related to the specific type of sport, lead to the development of these symptoms (Harvey & Tanner 1991). These factors include a growth thrust, an abrupt increase in the intensity and frequency of training, poor techniques, insufficient equipment and differences in individual leg lengths. In addition, anatomical standard variations or already existing pathological changes of the spine can also contribute to the development of acute injuries and in particular to overstraining reactions.

The occurrence of spine injuries in tennis is described differently in various studies. The mentioning of the back area as the affected part of the body ranges from 'quite often' (Chard & Lachmann 1987) and 'often' (Hainline 1995) to 'most often' (Hutchinson et al. 1995). Exact numbers of how often acute spine injuries and damages through overstraining occur among tennis players under consideration of the training condition can rarely be found in literature whereby only the lumbar area is looked at in these studies.

Krahl (1995) treated 164 WTA and ATP tennis professionals from 1989 to 1992 while giving assistance during the largest tennis tournaments (Australian Open 1990, French Open 1990 and 1992, Wimbledon 1991, US Open 1989–91, ATP Masters 1990–92). It was noted that back injuries or damages through overstraining were the most common injuries in 16.4% (n = 27) of the cases (Krahl 1995). These numbers are similar to those of Chard and Lachmann (1987) who found that 20% of all tennis players have back problems. Marks et al. (1988) treated 143 tennis professionals of which 43 had lower back pain. Thirty eight per cent of these players had to give up in a tournament due to these pains.

The experience gained through the medical services of the ATP tour should be mentioned here. The information was obtained through analysis of medical check-ups of 299 tennis professionals (Krahl et al. 1997). Two hundred and ninety players with completely documented orthopaedic examinations were looked at and pathological results requiring further diagnostics, therapy or preventive measures were localized most often in the shoulder area (n = 58, 24.1%). Relevant medical results in the spine area were found among 43 players (17.8%) whereby the lumbar spine was affected in over 60% of the cases (Fig. 17.8).

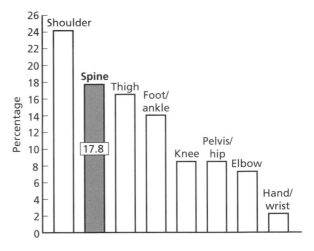

Fig. 17.8 Data of the ATP-Tour Medical Service Committee: 290 preventive check-ups with 241 orthopaedic pathological findings related to their anatomical regions (Krahl et al. 1997).

Young players that are still growing seem to be especially prone to spine injuries although the statistics in literature about sports medicine vary greatly. Hutchinson *et al.* (1995) gave assistance to the United States Association National Boys' Tennis Championship over a 6-year period and discovered that 304 of 1440 young male tennis players (21.1%) had acute or recurring injuries whereby back injuries ranked in first place. Kibler *et al.* (1988) were able to find out in their group that nine out of 97 young competitive tennis players also had back problems. Swärd *et al.* (1990a, b, 1992) noted that 50% of 30 young Swedish top athletes had lower back pain. A radiological correlate was found in 50% of the athletes with these symptoms. One hundred and fifteen of 127 injured young Flemish top tennis players had signs of overstraining whereby the torso was affected in 26 cases (22.6%) (localized second most often following the knee). Acute injuries were noted in 32 cases whereby the torso was affected in five of these cases (15.6%) (localized third most often following the thigh and ankle areas) (Verspeelt *et al.* 1995).

Larsen (1991) discovered five injuries per 1000 practice hours among 160 players of a typical Danish tennis club. In this study, damages through overstraining were predominant as compared to acute injuries (2/3 : 1/3) (Larsen 1991). Overstraining damages were found by Winge *et al.* (1989) among 67% of 104 top tennis players. According to Swärd *et al.* (1990b), 50–85% of the top athletes have back problems with a radiological confirmation of pathological changes in 36–55% of the cases.

Back pain is equally divided among sex and age groups (Larsen 1991). On the other hand, Swärd *et al.* (1990b) were able to show that the symptoms were stronger and more frequent among males. Chard and Lachmann (1987) agree with this report (males 66%, females 58%) and found out that 59% of the injured were older players (>25 years of age).

As mentioned above, there are no epidemiological studies available on the incidence of cervical and thoracic spine injuries in tennis. Merely some thought has been given to a differential diagnostic classification of pathological changes of the cervical spine and of the shoulder–arm syndrome with primary symptoms being pain and paraesthesia as well as of the epicondylitis humeri radialis (Wanivenhaus 1986; Waldis 1989; Murtagh 1990).

Pathological changes of the 'tennis spine'

Sports injuries of the spine affect three different anatomical structures—soft tissue, the intervertebral disc and the bone (Tall & DeVault 1993). Injuries concerning soft structures are most common (pulled muscles, stretched ligaments, etc.). These are usually acute injuries, which normally have a spontaneous healing process and require a symptom-orientated therapy.

Progressive degenerative development is the centre of focus with respect to intervertebral disc problems (Tall & DeVault 1993). There should be a distinction made between a degenerative reduction in the height of the intervertebral disc connected with a loss of elasticity (osteochondrosis) and a damaged disc which can lead to an initial protruding of the disc (protrusion) or even to a slipped disc in the spinal canal (prolapse) (Fig. 17.9). Thus, a tearing of the outer fibrous bounds of the disc (anulus fibrosus) often occurs by repeated lateral flexion and rotations and finally results in a protrusion or prolapse. Chard and Lachmann (1987) noted lumbar spine injuries among tennis players in 16% whereby a clinical indication of a disc prolapse was given in almost half of the cases (43%).

An increasingly degenerative diminishing of the height of the intervertebral disc results in stronger pressure put onto the small vertebra joints especially by means of extreme tennis-related rotation of the lumbar spine which is actually more or less 'unrotatable' in a functional–anatomical sense. This strain can lead to a progradient facet arthritis and can thus cause a stenosis of the spinal canal with compression of the spinal nerves and cord in a later state (Fig. 17.10).

On the other hand, the diminishing height of the intervertebral disc causes an increasing destabilization of the corresponding segment of movement and therefore leads to the danger of degenerative vertebral slipping (pseudo-spondylolisthesis).

In the bony parts of the vertebral column, repeated microtraumatizations due to extreme hyperlordosis of the lumbar spine result in degenerative changes of the border plates of the vertebra (spondylosis) which, due to the increased formation of posterior bony spurs (spondylophytes), causes a narrowing of the spinal canal that can, at an early stage, be symptomatic only during hyperextension. Furthermore, traumatic

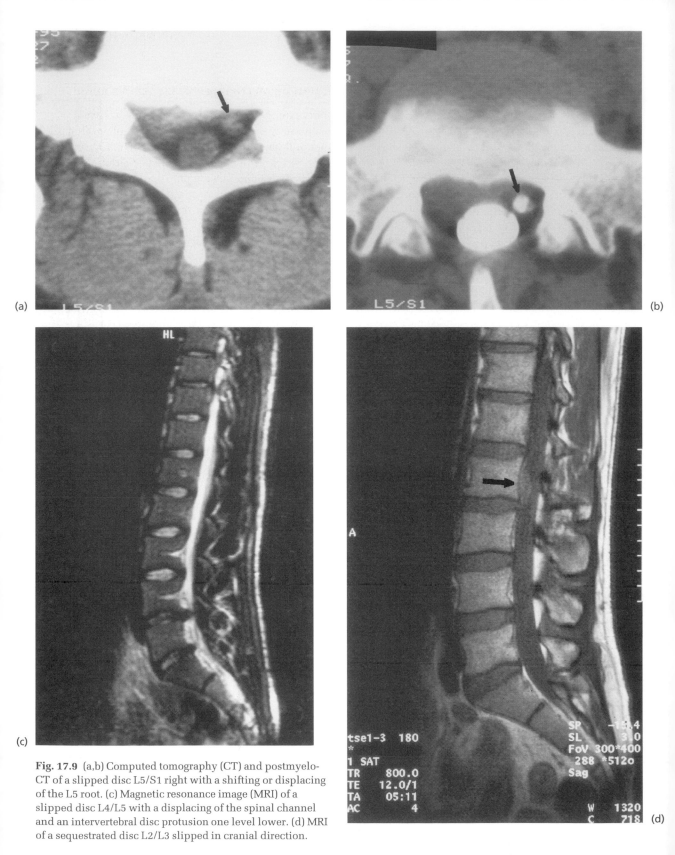

Fig. 17.9 (a,b) Computed tomography (CT) and postmyelo-CT of a slipped disc L5/S1 right with a shifting or displacing of the L5 root. (c) Magnetic resonance image (MRI) of a slipped disc L4/L5 with a displacing of the spinal channel and an intervertebral disc protusion one level lower. (d) MRI of a sequestrated disc L2/L3 slipped in cranial direction.

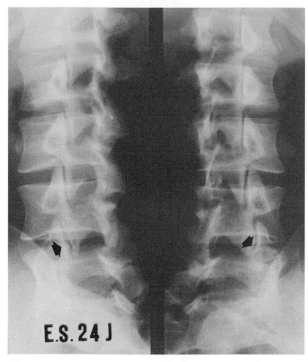

(a)

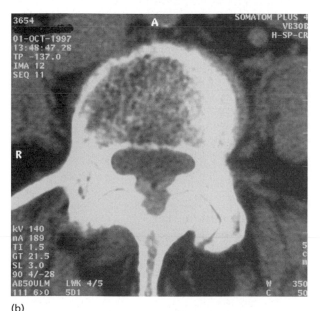

(b)

Fig. 17.10 (a) Radiograph of the beginning of a facet arthritis (see arrow). (b) Computed tomography of an extremely advanced hypertrophical facet arthritis that has resulted in a spinal stenosis.

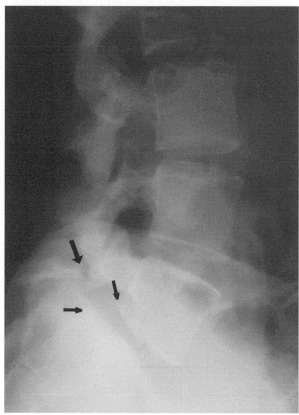

Fig. 17.11 Radiograph of a spondylolysis (large arrow) with a resulting spondylolisthesis (small arrows at the vertebrae back edges which are shifted against one another).

fractures or stress fractures resulting from chronic overstraining are found in the interarticular portion area of the vertebral arch with respect to pathological instability (spondylolysis) (Fig. 17.11) (Swärd 1992). In rare cases, acute compression fractures and dislocations may occur. However, these two types of injuries primarily affect the cervical and thoracic spine areas, and occur most often in 'contact sports' (Tall & DeVault 1993).

The type of injury in the lumbar spine area depends on the direction, the power and the target area of the occurring forces (Alexander 1985). Pulled muscles, distortions, disc injuries and vertebral arch fractures are common injuries. The injuries of the interarticular area between the superior and inferior articular process may cause spondylolysis, which can lead to vertebral slipping (spondylolisthesis) by insufficient stabilization of the segments. The lower part of the

Table 17.4 The differential diagnostic results among 27 tennis professionals with lumbar spine problems (Krahl *et al.* 1995).

Facet syndrome	6
Disc degeneration	5
Sacroiliacal locking	4
Lumbosacral malformation	4
Muscle spasm	3
Spondylosis	3
Spondylolisthesis	2

lumbar spine (L5/S1 > L4/5) is especially at risk because in this area the vertebral arches are not as well developed. Thus, a fracture of the interarticular part can be noted here quite often (Kapandji 1974; Magora 1976).

The most common diagnosis among 27 WTA and ATP tennis professionals that were treated by Krahl (Krahl *et al.* 1995) was the facet syndrome with more or less characteristic pseudoradicular symptoms (a combined back and lower extremity pain that cannot be related to a pathological process of a single spinal nerve root) (Table 17.4).

Several pathological changes of the spine can be observed in large numbers among athletes with the described mechanisms of strain. Swärd (1992) noted abnormal vertebra configurations, Schmorl's nodes (juvenile disc herniation into the bordering vertebra), changes of vertebral ring apophysis followed by spondylosis, which is found in 50% of the cases among athletes with back pain, and scoliosis (fixed lateral bending of the spine with similar rotation of the vertebra), which can be recorded in 76.7% of those athletes with asymmetrical strains upon the shoulder and body (tennis, javelin). Swärd (1992) interpreted this mild secondary scoliosis during ventral flexion and the simultaneously existing asymmetrical muscle development to be a 'physiological adaptation' of the vertebral column to an asymmetrical capacity to absorb and transfer power. The mobility of the vertebral column was 7 cm greater among these athletes. However, a correlation to back pain could not be proven.

In contrast to this, Swärd *et al.* (1990b) were able to find a close correlation between height reductions of intervertebral spaces, Schmorl's nodes, abnormal vertebral ring apophyses and changed vertebral configurations and back pain among 142 top athletes of which 30 were tennis players already between 14 and 25 years of age. They were also able to observe to a significant degree that at least two of these pathological changes occurred simultaneously among these athletes (Swärd *et al.* 1990b).

Ottolenghi *et al.* (1985) were able to note that there was a higher number of incidences in which changes in the interarticular part of the vertebral arch (posterior apophyses) took place within the lumbar region. These changes could be the pathophysiological basis for the development of spondylolysis along with the risk of spondylolisthesis and early arthritic changes.

Prevention, therapy and rehabilitation of spine injuries in tennis players

The therapy and prevention of back injuries in tennis should be directed towards the stress situation placed on the lumbar spine which is unique to this sport with respect to rotation, hyperextension and lateral flexion. The quick and repeated strains lead to a tiring of the vertebral column stabilizers and overcome the viscoelastic protective mechanisms of the intervertebral discs and ligament structures (Silver *et al.* 1985; Haher *et al.* 1993). Therefore, an optimal muscle and proprioceptive safeguarding of this specific situation of strain should be strived for.

Consequently, therapy and especially prevention must be orientated towards recurrent microtraumas and not primarily towards the prevention of extreme individual macrotraumas. Secondary changes, such as facet arthritis, spinal stenosis and instabilities with resulting spondylolysis and spondylolisthesis can only be effectively avoided in this manner.

Prevention, therapy and rehabilitation of back injuries among tennis players calls for an understanding of pathophysiology, pathobiomechanics and knowledge of predisposing factors, which is of great importance for well-aimed actions in the case of an injury.

Prevention and rehabilitation of spine injuries in tennis players

Instruction for the athlete is of special importance for the prevention of back injuries as well as for the rehabilitation following the acute treatment of every spine injury. The athlete should learn how to avoid straining movements with respect to the risk of injury of the lumbar spine (Nachemson 1985). Fitness training of the athlete generally aims at an optimizing through flexibility, power and stamina which means an effective minimizing of asymmetrical strains and injuries combined with a simultaneous increase in stamina (Groppel & Roetert 1992).

From this knowledge it can be concluded that players as well as coaches should include flexion and extension exercises to stretch muscles, tendons and ligaments and therefore to increase the flexibility of the lumbar spine. Isometric strengthening of the abdominal muscles should also be included in daily practice as well as in a rehabilitation phase following a back injury so as to balance out muscle imbalances, because abdominal muscles are often neglected in strength training as opposed to the back extensors that are usually strong but too short (Alexander 1985; Hainline 1995).

The lumbar stabilizing as a means of minimizing the static and kinetic strains upon the spine requires a maximum control of the torso and lumbar spine and can be learnt in the next stage of rehabilitation (e.g. ball exercises). This stage includes the mutual rhythmic movements of the lumbosacral region and of the shoulder and pelvis area. This helps relieve the strain on the intervertebral disc concerned, which underlines the particular importance of the lumbar stabilizing here (degeneration, hernia) (Hainline 1995).

A study group at Alfried Krupp Hospital in Essen developed a physiotherapeutic exercise programme that is available to ATP players in form of a pamphlet. Within the ATP Medical Services Committee, Michaelis *et al.* (1997) completed a corresponding training programme, which concentrates on strengthening the back and abdominal muscles, stabilizing the torso as well as on coordination training (Fig. 17.12). This training plan should be integrated into the daily plan of the players and aims at maintaining a balanced training level of the antagonistic abdominal and back muscles through strengthening of the hypotrophic or atrophic muscle groups and stretching of the antagonists that have a tendency towards shortening.

The lumbar stabilization should depend on the type of sport and should include modifications of the individual strokes whereby an intensive cooperation between the athlete and the trainer on the one hand and the physiotherapist and the physician on the other hand is necessary. Not only sport-related but also stroke-related peaks of strains should be counteracted upon in practice (e.g. by players with extreme components of hyperflexion, rotation and lateral flexion in their serve). The balancing out of muscular imbalances and the increasing of flexibility in the lumbar area are especially important for the serve (Copley 1980). A distinctive contribution to the prevention of damages to the spine, especially when serving, is made through proper development of technique. Thus, an optimal ball toss and a rhythmic movement during the serve takes considerable strain off of the lumbar spine. Furthermore, the switch from the two-handed to the one-handed backhand should be considered by the player and the coach to avoid excessive trunk rotation.

Due to the same pathogenesis, the treatment or prevention of degenerative joint diseases (facet arthritis, spinal stenosis) corresponds to that of the intervertebral disc illness. Avoiding hyperextension and rotation so as to take strain from already damaged vertebral joints should be the main aim in physiotherapy.

In conclusion, emphasis should be placed on a sufficient warm-up phase with stretching and a corresponding 'warm-down' following a game or practice (Elliott 1988).

Therapy of acute and chronic back injuries in tennis players

In all cases, the primary therapy consists of a phase of relief of strain/break from sports as well as a reduction or elimination of pain. The therapy of lumbar injuries described above is applied to different degrees for different types of injuries. An acute, uncomplicated pulling within the lumbar area calls for a body position that relieves of strain and for a pain therapy (e.g. local ice application). This also includes the manual easing of reflex muscle spasms and stretching (Cailliet 1981). Ultrasound and special massage techniques are additional possibilities of therapy with the same objective. In the case of an extreme indication, a spine manipulation may also be included in the treatment of uncomplicated spine injuries. Oral application of

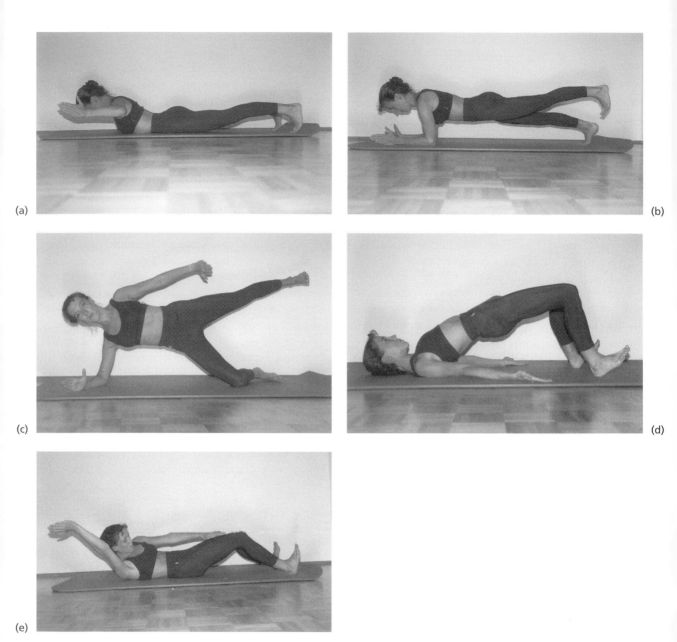

Fig. 17.12 Physiotherapeutical exercises for stabilizing the spinal column by means of strengthening the stomach and back muscles. (a) Arms in U-position, feet on toes. Lift the upper body up to tip of breast bone; shoulder blades are pulled towards spine and gluteal region, knees straight. (b) The 'push-up position'. Elbows underneath the shoulders, watch the straight configuration of your body, breathe regularly. Alternate lifting of one leg, try to walk or to walk into splits and back. (c) Side position. Lift yourself up on your forearm and yours knees until thighs, trunk and head are in line. Extend the upper arm alongside the body. Out of this position lift up the upper leg in slight hyperextension and internal rotation of the hip and try small movements up and down with this leg. (d) Bridging. 'Bridging' means stabilizing hips and trunk, stretching of the hip flexors when lifting thighs and trunk into line. (e) Abdominal muscles. On your back, slight knee flexion; push your heels into the ground. Pull your hands alternating to your right/left knee. Lift your body just until the shoulder blades lift off the ground. Do the exercises slowly and breathe regularly.

Table 17.5 The use of surgical methods when treating a slipped disc depending on the stage of the illness (Mayer & Brock 1993). (From Krämer 1996.)

Stage	I	II	IIIa	IIIb
Disc pathology	Compact, annulus fibrosus intact	Opened, annulus fibrosus mainly intact	Subligamentar sequester	Extraligamentar sequester
Conservative	++	++	+	
Nucleotomy	+	++		
Chemonucleolysis		++	+	
Microdiscectomy			+	++

+, Possible; ++, recommended.

systemic non-steroidal anti-inflammatory drugs is only necessary short term if at all. The exercises described above for increasing flexibility and strengthening the lumbar region follow once the pain is gone or has been reduced.

The acute treatment of an intervertebral injury or illness requires a prolongation of the relief of strain phase, which can be a special position in bed with 90° bending of hips and knees if needed. Non-steroidal anti-inflammatory drugs can be used here over a longer period of time to reduce pain. In addition, the systemic and epidural application of glucocorticoids can be considered (Green 1975; Benzon 1986). The following physiotherapy does not only aim at increasing the abdominal and torso flexibility and their strengthening but also focuses on relieving the strain on the intervertebral disc through stabilization. It is especially important for the player to learn how to avoid incorrect movements and imperfect stroke techniques (Hainline 1995). A decisive indicator of when to start practice again is the pain itself, which should be completely eliminated. Surgical measures to relieve nerve tissue should only be considered in exceptional cases where players have neurological failures as a result of nerve root compressions or within a cauda equina syndrome (Hainline 1995). Pain symptoms without neurological failures resistant to conservative therapy may sometimes require surgical intervention in individual cases.

There are a number of surgical techniques available for slipped disc operations: chemical liquefaction and drainage of the nucleus pulposus (chemonucleolysis, a method that has lost clinical relevance in recent years), mechanical removal of the disc (percutaneous endoscopic or conventional nucleotomy, microdiscectomy), thermic removal of the disc (percutaneous laser discectomy). The decision of whether an operation is needed at all and the surgical method both depend on the stage that the intervertebral disc prolapse has reached (Table 17.5).

Following details given by the patient and a thorough clinical examination, the so-called picture-giving methods are of great importance for the indication and operation planning: conventional radiographs (lateral and anteroposterior view), computed tomography (CT) scan with three-dimensional reconstruction (Fig. 17.13), magnetic resonance imaging (MRI), myelography (radiograph after application of contrast medium into the spinal canal), discography (radiograph after application of contrast medium into the disc), postmyelography CT scan and postdiscography CT scan. The radiograph methods in particular should not be used without criticism but should be closely orientated to the given symptoms and to the examination results.

To avoid the above, preventive measures are particularly of great importance in professional tennis as well. Therefore, a player can only profit from the ATP tour if he or she undergoes a medical check-up in which reproducible examination steps are given. These cover of course the orthopaedic examination of the vertebral column whereby the results show that

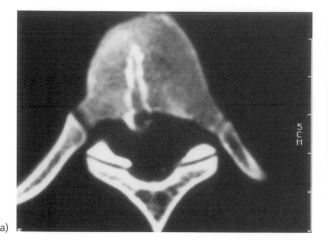

(a)

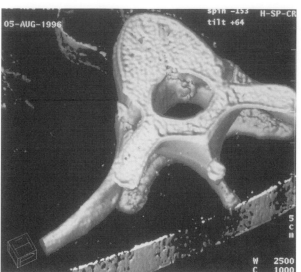

(b)

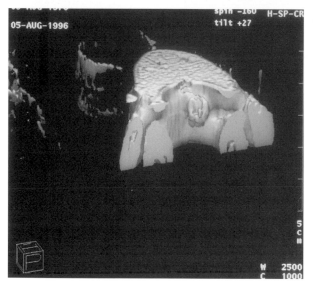

(c)

Fig. 17.13 Computed tomography (CT) (a) and a three-dimensional CT reconstruction (b,c) of a thoracic slipped disc.

every seventh player requires treatment, even though some of them might not have any pain at the time of examination. As a result, longer 'sport-free' periods due to injuries occur frequently. Preventive exercises on a regular basis are even more important among players without any symptoms. This is of benefit to the player's health and competitiveness and as a result also to his or her career on a long-term basis.

Preventive medical check-up in tennis players

Regarding the spine, not every juvenile tennis player has the physical requirement for a career at a high level lasting for years. Medical check-ups allow for

the early discovery, if possible at a young age, of 'elimination factors', which affect the suitability for the sport of tennis over many years in a negative manner. According to Krahl (1995), the illnesses include the following once they have reached a certain stage: congenital (Fig. 17.14) or acquired malformation of the spine that lead to an important loss of function, structural disorders of the vertebra that lead to pain and an important loss of mobility like the acute juvenile kyphosis (Scheuermann's disease), stiffness of spine sections like scoliosis and kyphosis, degenerative diseases (osteochondrosis, spondylosis and facet joint arthritis) and muscle imbalances.

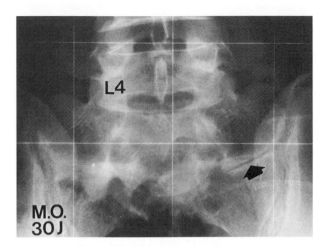

Fig. 17.14 Example of a congenital malformation: the sacralization of L5 causes a restriction in movement in this area which has to be compensated for by the other segments. This can result in a permanent overstraining of these other segments with chronic pain symptoms.

In conclusion, it can be said that prevention, therapy and rehabilitation of spine injuries and diseases is to be seen as a task for all persons involved in the sport of tennis. The physiotherapist and the physician play the major role in the therapy and rehabilitation whereas the coach and the player do so in the prevention.

References

Alexander, M.J.L. (1985) Biomechanical aspects of lumbar spine injuries in athletes: a review. *Canadian Journal of Applied Sport Sciences* **10**, 1–20.

Beerman, J. & Sher, L. (1981) Improve tennis service through mathematics. *Journal of Health, Physical Education and Recreation* **55**, 15–19.

Benzon, H.T. (1986) Epidural steroid injections for low back pain and lumbosacral radiculopathy. *Pain* **24**, 277–279.

Burri, C. & Rüter, A. (1980) *Verletzungen der Wirbelsäule*. Springer-Verlag, Heidelberg.

Cailliet, R. (1981) *Low Back Pain Syndrome*. FA Davis, Philadelphia, PA.

Chard, M.D. & Lachmann, S.M. (1987) Racquet sports—patterns of injury presenting to a sports injury clinic. *British Journal of Sports Medicine* **21**, 150–153.

Copley, B.B. (1980) A morphological and physiological study of tennis players with special reference to the effects of training. *South African Journal of Research in Sports, Physical Education and Recreation* **3**, 33–44.

Elliott, B.C. (1988) Biomechanics of the serve in tennis—a biomedical perspective. *Sports Medicine* **6**, 285–294.

Green, L.N. (1975) Dexamethasone in the management of symptoms due to herniated lumbar disc. *Journal of Neurology, Neurosurgery and Psychiatry* **38**, 1211–1218.

Groppel, J.L. & Roetert, E.P. (1992) Applied physiology of tennis. *Sports Medicine* **14**, 260–268.

Haher, T., O'Brien, M. & Kauffman, C. (1993) Biomechanics of the spine in sports. *Clinics in Sports Medicine* **12**, 449–454.

Hainline, B. (1995) Racquet sports: Low back pain injury. *Clinics in Sports Medicine* **14**, 241–265.

Harvey, J. & Tanner, S. (1991) Low back pain in young athletes. A practical approach. *Sports Medicine* **12**, 394–406.

Hutchinson, M.R., Laprade, R.F., Burnett, Q.M. II, Moss, R. & Terpstra, J. (1995) Injury surveillance at the USTA Boys' Tennis Championships: a 6-year study. *Medicine and Science in Sports and Exercise* **27**, 826–830.

Junghanns, H. (1986) *Die Wirbelsäule unter den Einflüssen des täglichen Lebens, der Freizeit, des Sports*. Hippokrates Verlag, Stuttgart.

Kapandji, I.A. (1974) *Funktionelle Anatomie der Gelenke. Band 3: Rumpf und Wirbelsäule*. Enke-Verlag, Stuttgart.

Kibler, W.B., McQueen, C. & Uhl, J. (1988) Fitness evaluations and fitness findings in competitive junior tennis players. *Sports Medicine* **7**, 403.

Krahl, H. (1995) Lumbar spine problems of professional tennis players. In: Krahl, H., Pieper, H.-G., Kibler, W.B. & Renström, P.A., eds. *Tennis: Sports Medicine and Science*, pp. 120–124. Rau-Verlag, Dusseldorf.

Krahl, H., Altchek, D., Settles, P. *et al.* (1997) Medical care of athletes in tennis world wide—concept of the ATP Tour Medical Service Committee. Presented at Fourth IOC World Congress on Sports Sciences, Monte Carlo, Monaco, October 24.

Krämer, R.J. (1996) *Bandscheibenbedingte Erkrankungen*. Thieme-Verlag, Stuttgart.

Larsen, J. (1991) Tennisskader—skadehyppighed og—monster. *Ugeskrift for Laeger* **153**, 3398–3399.

Le Veau, B.F. (1977) *Williams and Lissner's Biomechanics of Human Motion*. WB Saunders, Philadelphia, PA.

Magora, A. (1976) Conservative treatment in spondylolisthesis. *Clinical Orthopaedics and Related Research* **117**, 74–79.

Marks, H.R., Haas, S.S. & Wiesel, S.W. (1988) Low back pain in competitive tennis players. *Clinics in Sports Medicine* **7**, 277–287.

Mayer, H.M. & Brock, M. (1993) Percutaneous endoscopic discectomy: surgical technique and preliminary results compared to microsurgical discectomy. *Journal of Neurosurgery* **78**, 216–225.

Michaelis, P., Michaelis, U. & Krahl, H. (1997) ATP-Tour: rehabilitative and preventive lower back and spine exercise. In: *Manual of the ATP-Tour*. Medical Services Committee.

Miyashita, M., Tsunoda, T., Sakurai, S., Nishizono, H. & Mizuno, T. (1980) Muscular activities in the tennis serve and overhead throwing. *Scandinavian Journal of Sports Science* **2**, 52–58.

Murtagh, J. (1990) The painful arm. *Australian Family Physician* **19**, 1423–1426.

Nachemson, A.L. (1985) Advance in low back pain. *Clinical Orthopaedics and Related Research* **200**, 266–273.

Nigg, B.M. (1986) Biomechanical aspects of running. In: Nigg, B.M., ed. *Biomechanics of Running Shoes*, pp. 1–26. Human Kinetics, Champaign, IL.

Ottolenghi, G., Alessi, G.C., Oggero, P. & Buccelli, R. (1985) Alterazioni del rachide lombosacrale da micropolitraumatismi sportivi. *Minerva Medica* **76**, 2203–2212.

Plaggenhoef, S. (1970) *Fundamentals of Tennis*. Prentice Hall, Englewood Cliffs, NJ.

Silver, J., Silver, D. & Godfrey, J. (1985) Injuries of the spine sustained during gymnastic activities. *British Medical Journal (Clinical Research)* **293**, 861–868.

Swärd, L. (1992) The thoracolumbar spine in young elite athletes. Current concepts on the effects of physical training. *Sports Medicine* **13**, 357–364.

Swärd, L., Eriksson, B. & Peterson, L. (1990a) Anthropometric characteristics, passive hip flexion, and spinal mobility in relation to back pain in athletes. *Spine* **15**, 376–382.

Swärd, L., Hellstrom, M., Jacobsson, B. & Peterson, L. (1990b) Back pain and radiologic changes in the thoraco-lumbar spine of athletes. *Spine* **15**, 124–129.

Tall, R.L. & DeVault, W. (1993) Spinal injury in sport: epidemiologic considerations. *Clinics in Sports Medicine* **12**, 441–448.

Van Gheluwe, B. & Hebbelinck, M. (1986) Muscle actions and ground reaction forces in tennis. *International Journal of Sports Biomechanics* **2**, 88–99.

Verspeelt, P. (1995) A retrospective review of all tennis related injuries over the last 8 years in young Flemish high-level tennis players. In: Krahl, H., Pieper, H.-G., Kibler, W.B. & Renström, P.A., eds. *Tennis: Sports Medicine and Science*, pp. 47–51. Rau-Verlag, Düsseldorf.

Waldis, M.F. (1989) Der Eingriff nach G. Hohmann am Ellenbogen—operative Behandlung eines Symptoms? *Zeitschrift für Orthopädie und ihre Grenzgebiete* **127**, 606–610.

Wanivenhaus, A. (1986) Differentialdiagnose der Epicondylitis humeri radialis. *Zeitschrift für Orthopädie und ihre Grenzgebiete* **124**, 775–779.

Winge, S., Jorgensen, U. & Lassen-Nielsen, A. (1989) Epidemiology of injuries in Danish championship tennis. *International Journal of Sports Medicine* **10**, 368–371.

Yoshizawa, M., Itani, T. & Jonsson, B. (1987) Muscular load in shoulder and forearm muscles in tennis players with different levels of skill. In: Jonsson, B., ed. *International Series on Biomechanics*, pp. 621–628. Human Kinetics, Champaign, IL.

Young, J.L. (1996) *Back pain in tennis: is only the disk at risk?* Hand-out at the Third International Conference on Sports Medicine and Science in Tennis, Melbourne, Australia, January.

Chapter 18

Hand and wrist injuries in tennis

Epidemiology

The incidence of upper extremity injuries in tennis varies from 20% as reported in Australia (Reece *et al.* 1986) to 45% as reported prospectively by Winge *et al.* (1989). In a 6-year study of the United States Tennis Association (USTA) Boys' Championships (Hutchinson *et al.* 1995), 27% of injuries involved the upper extremity and 2% involved the wrist. Kibler *et al.* (1988) has noted that the majority of tennis injuries are of the overload variety. This applies to injuries of both the upper and lower extremities.

Anatomy and biomechanics

The wrist functions as a stable, mobile base for positioning the hand in space to allow for pinching, grasping and gripping activities. The goal of treatment for any wrist problem is to restore the wrist to a pain-free, stable unit with adequate motion.

Anatomically, the wrist is divided into two carpal rows, both geometrically and intrinsically unstable. Stability is provided by a series of intrinsic and extrinsic ligaments (Fig. 18.1). The major extrinsic ligaments are located on the volar side of the wrist and include the radioscaphocapitate, radiolunotriquetral, and radioscapholunate ligaments. The ulna lunate and ulna triquetral ligaments also serve to anchor the volar ulnar aspect of the carpus. Another ligament, the 'V' ligament, connects the proximal distal carpal rows and extends from the capitate to both the triquetrum and the scaphoid bone. Intrinsic ligaments serve to hold the carpal bones together. The most important are the scapholunate and triquetrolunate ligaments, which connect the bones of the proximal row.

The study of wrist biomechanics in tennis is in its early stages, but certain observations have been made. W.B. Kibler *et al.* (unpublished observations) have calculated that, during the service motion, approximately 10% of the force and 15% of the energy involved in the stroke is dissipated across the wrist joint. The power from these strokes emanates primarily from the trunk and lower body musculature and not from the shoulder, elbow and wrist. Maintaining normal biomechanics of the trunk and lower body in these athletes may help prevent wrist injuries.

Using a biaxial flexible goniometer, D. Tokunaga and J. Ryu *et al.* (unpublished observations) have quantified range of motion (ROM) of the wrist during various strokes by players of varying skill levels. They concluded that the service stroke involved the greatest ROM, encompassing an arc of 90° to 100° of flexion/extension. The forehand encompassed a 40° excursion and the backhand 37°. They also noted that the wrist was in extension at the time of impact on all strokes. Furthermore, the wrist was in ulnar deviation at impact in the serve. During both the forehand and forehand volley, the wrist position ranged from 15° to 30° ulnar deviation. In the backhand and backhand volley, the wrist was in neutral to 2–5° of radial deviation.

It was noted that advanced players demonstrate more extension at impact than do beginners. Maximum

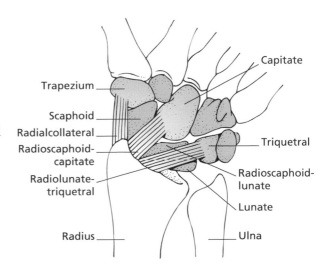

Fig. 18.1 Extrinsic radiocarpal ligaments. (Reproduced with permission from Mooney, J.F. III (1992) *Clinics in Sports Medicine* 11, 1.)

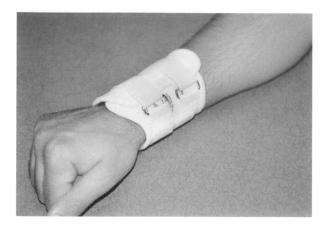

Fig. 18.2 Nirschl brace.

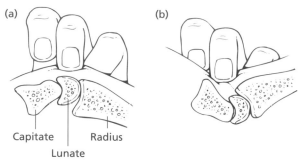

Fig. 18.3 Clinical assessment of lunate and scaphoid articular surfaces by palpation. (a) Flexion presents the articular surfaces dorsally. (b) In extension, they are inaccessible.

radial/ulnar deviation occurs more in beginners than in advanced players.

Implications of these biomechanical studies may be that ulnar deviation on impact may account for the frequency of ulnar-sided wrist injuries. Also, the limited motion required for strokes might indicate that return to play may be possible following reconstructive wrist procedures, which result in limited range of motion. Third, these studies may explain the effectiveness of a restricted motion brace such as a Nirschl brace (Fig. 18.2).

Evaluation of the tennis player with wrist pain

Wrist or hand injuries in tennis may occur from direct trauma, such as a fall, or an acute rotational force, as in a single miss-hit or maximum effort during a stroke. Most injuries to the hand and wrist, however, result from chronic overuse. It is important to establish: (i) whether the onset was sudden or insidious; (ii) how long the symptoms have existed; and (iii) whether or not they are progressive.

To determine how the athlete perceives the severity of his or her injury, the examiner must first assess the athlete's desire to return to play. Next, the examiner must determine the severity of symptoms, mechanical complaints, and the presence of clicking, catching or locking. It also should be noted what prior treatment the patient has received and what effect this treatment may have had on his or her symptoms.

Physical examination

The clinician needs to localize the point or points of maximum tenderness and at least localize the pain to the ulnar or radial aspect of the wrist. A definite diagnosis is more easily established if maximum point tenderness is identified. In dorsal wrist pain, the areas of tenderness can best be palpated by palmar flexing the wrist thus bringing the palpating finger closer to the underlying structures (Fig. 18.3).

The clinician also must note the degree of swelling, range of motion, sensation and the bilateral grip strength. Decreased values on grip may simply be due to pain or weakness secondary to muscle or neurovascular malfunction.

Imaging studies

Plain roentgenograms of the wrist always should be obtained. We recommend use of standard four-view: anteroposterior, ulnar deviation and neutral, a true lateral, and oblique. Instability series should be obtained if an instability problem is suspected.

In evaluating tennis injuries in the wrist, plain radiographs are frequently normal. In such instances, special imaging studies may be indicated to further evaluate the pathology.

A technetium bone scan may be utilized to evaluate whether or not a fracture is present and to rule out a bony ligamentous injury.

Arthrography of the wrist frequently is performed in tennis athletes primarily to look for tears of the triangular fibrocartilage, triquetrolunate or scapholunate ligaments. The three-compartment arthrogram, in which dye is selectively injected into the mid-carpal, radial carpal and distal radial ulnar joints, has been the most reliable technique in diagnosing tears.

A computed tomography (CT) scan also may be obtained to evaluate bony structures. It is particularly helpful in assessing small avulsion fractures and fractures of the hook of the hamate.

The use of magnetic resonance imaging (MRI) has become more popular recently and may be helpful if an experienced radiologist is present and a specific wrist surface coil is utilized.

Specific injuries of the wrist and hand

Tendon injuries

Tendinopathy frequently is the result of an overstretching phenomenon. The athlete will generally seek care after recent initiation of an unaccustomed motion or activity. The sudden deceleration of the musculotendinous unit as the racket strikes the ball is usually the common underlying factor in producing tendon pain.

An overuse syndrome is defined as the level of repetitive microtrauma that is sufficient to overwhelm the tissues' ability to adapt (Kiefhaber & Stern 1992). Tendons may fail in two ways: tension overload which may occur at any point in a musculotendinous unit, or shear stress which results in microtrauma at any point between a moving musculotendinous structure and a fixed structure.

De Quervain's stenosing tenosynovitis is one the most common tendon problems seen in tennis players. It is an example of shear trauma and occurs at the level of the radial styloid as the abductor pollicis longus and the extensor pollicis brevis tendons pass through the first dorsal compartment. This is thought to be caused by repetitive ulnar deviation, which occurs in the tennis stroke.

Physical examination of de Quervain's syndrome reveals point tenderness over the radial styloid and first dorsal compartment. A positive Finkelstein's test, in which the thumb is adducted into the palm and the wrist passively ulnarly deviated, is diagnostic for this condition (Fig. 18.4).

Treatment of de Quervain's syndrome involves an initial period of splinting and non-steroidal anti-

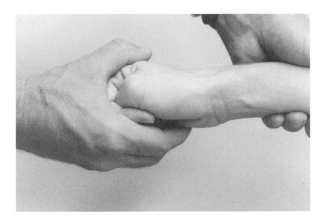

Fig. 18.4 Finkelstein's test. The thumb is adducted into the palm and the wrist passively ulnarly deviated. Reproduction of pain over the radial styloid indicates a positive test.

inflammatory medications, which generally result in an 80% reduction of symptoms. If this treatment fails, an intracompartment injection of corticosteroid is usually curative for these patients. Although rarely indicated, surgical decompression of the first dorsal compartment may be employed if the above measures are not successful. Return to racket sports may be anticipated at approximately 8 weeks following surgical decompression.

Other tendon problems occurring at the wrist in a tennis player include *extensor carpi radialis longus* and *brevis tendinopathy*. This is usually an insertional-type problem associated frequently with a carpal metacarpal boss lesion. The player may present with a tender, bony bump at the base of the second or third metacarpals, which may be treated by rest, splinting and an eccentric exercise programme. In recalcitrant cases, steroid injections near the insertion of the tendon may be performed. This should be done with care and the athlete should be aware of possible complications from such an injection.

Extensor communis tendinopathy may occur and is most common in the index and small finger due to their oblique course across the wrist. Extensor pollicis longus tendon may be involved as it abuts the Lister's tubercle, although this is rare in racket sports. Insertional tendinitis of the dorsal interossei into the base of the proximal phalanges may occur in the tennis player from repeated gripping. It presents as a vague pain in the metacarpophalangeal joint region exacerbated by grasping.

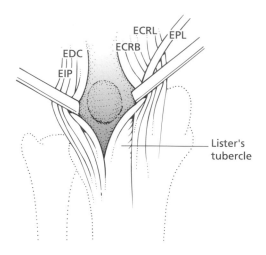

EDC
EIP
ECRL EPL
ECRB
EDC

Lister's tubercle

Fig. 18.5 Ganglion. The dorsal ganglion exposed and mobilized between the extensor pollicis longus (EPL), the extensor carpi radialis longus (ECRL), the extensor carpi radialis brevis (ECRB), the extensor digitorum communis (EDC) and the extensor indicis proprius (EIP) ulnarly. (Reproduced with permission from Angelides, A.C. (1988) *Operative Hand Surgery*, 2nd edn. Churchill Livingstone, New York.)

Compression and impingement syndromes may also occur at the wrist. The most common cause of radial wrist pain in the tennis player is most likely an occult dorsal ganglion, which should be suspected when point tenderness exists over the dorsum of the scapholunate articulation. This results from degeneration of the scapholunate ligament with the formation of a ganglion cyst (Fig. 18.5).

The patient usually has pain at the extremes of dorsiflexion and palmar flexion and has point tenderness in the scapholunate area. Usually, no mass is palpable.

Initial treatment is rest and splinting. An occasional diagnostic or even therapeutic injection also is curative in some cases. In recalcitrant cases, however, exploration and excision of the occult ganglion is curative.

Ulnar wrist pain

The most common problem encountered in tennis players is ulnar wrist pain. This can be caused by a number of clinical entities, namely extensor carpi ulnaris tendinopathy, subluxing extensor carpi ulnaris tendon, ulnar carpal impingement, which may include a tear of the triangular fibrocartilage and tear of the triquetrolunate ligament, and chondromalacia

of the lunate, triquetrum and ulnar seat. Triquetral hamate impingement is rare but also may be a cause of ulnar wrist pain as well as a stress fracture of the hook of the hamate. Both must be included in the differential diagnosis of ulnar wrist pain in tennis players. Final causes of ulnar wrist pain are abnormalities of the pisiform bone or pisotriquetral arthrosis.

Extensor carpi ulnaris problems

Extensor carpi ulnaris tendinopathy is due in most cases to simple overuse or technique flaws. Although it usually is a primary diagnosis, underlying pathological conditions such as a triangular fibrocartilage tear or ulnar carpal impingement always should be considered.

Extensor carpi ulnaris tendinopathy is seen most commonly in the non-dominant wrist of the player using the two-handed backhand. It is speculated that this is due to the extreme position of ulnar deviation utilized in the take-back portion of the stroke for the two-handed backhand.

Treatment of primary extensor carpi ulnaris tendinopathy involves rest, splinting, non-steroidal anti-inflammatory medication and attention to technique modification and, rarely, corticosteroid and lidocaine (lignocaine) injection of the sheath.

Subluxation of the extensor carpi ulnaris results from rupture of the ulnar wall of the sheath of the extensor carpi ulnaris tunnel usually due to sudden volar flexion, ulnar deviation and supination force such as in hitting a low forehand in tennis. This injury has been reported in golf, tennis, weightlifting and bronco riding (Fig. 18.6) (Rayan 1993).

The diagnosis should be suspected in patients who complain of clicking on the ulnar side of the wrist and with a history of sudden pain following the tennis stroke, particularly a low forehand.

Physical examination findings include tenderness over the extensor carpi ulnaris tendon. The hallmark of the diagnosis involves observing the tendon as the supinated wrist is actively taken from radial to ulnar deviation. In this position, one can readily observe and palpate the extensor carpi ulnaris to sublux or jump over the head of the ulna. An injection of lidocaine hydrochloride into the sheath may be diagnostic if this completely relieves the discomfort. Again, underlying wrist pathology such as ulnar carpal impingement should be suspected.

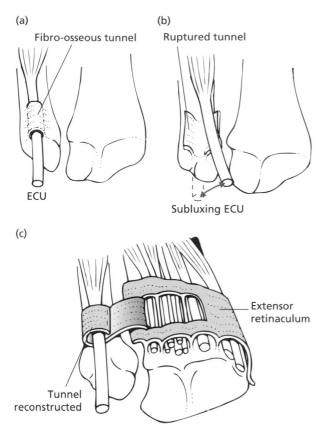

(a) Fibro-osseous tunnel

ECU

(b) Ruptured tunnel

Subluxing ECU

(c)

Extensor retinaculum

Tunnel reconstructed

Fig. 18.6 (a) Anatomic drawing of the extensor carpi ulnaris (ECU) in its fibro-osseous tunnel. (b) When ruptured, the tendon subluxes ulnarly on rotatory motion. (c) Reconstruction creates a new tunnel from a slip of extensor retinaculum.

Treatment of acute subluxation of the extensor carpi ulnaris tendon is either placement in a long arm cast in supination and radial deviation for 6 weeks or direct primary repair. In the chronic subluxing extensor carpi ulnaris case, surgical reconstruction is indicated if the symptoms prohibit play. We have found that a fibrous rim typically is present over the ulnar aspect of the tendon and reconstruction using local retinacular tissue is usually possible.

Ulnar carpal impingement

Ulnar carpal impingement refers to impingement of the ulnar aspect of the carpus against the head of the distal ulna. Individuals are predisposed to this problem due to their anatomy in that most have a positive ulnar variance. The ulnar variance is

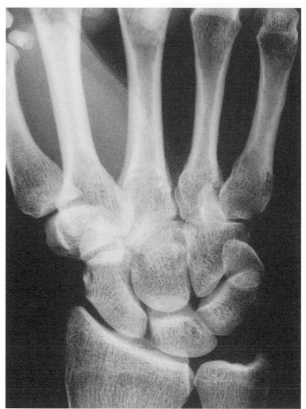

Fig. 18.7 Neutral rotation, anteroposterior wrist radiograph.

determined by a wrist radiograph. The length of the distal aspect of the ulna is compared to that of the radius. Normally, the distal ulna is shorter than the distal radius by at least 1 mm. If it is equal to or longer than the subchondral bone of the distal radius, a positive ulnar variance exists. This radiograph view is certainly the most important in evaluating wrist pain in a tennis player (Fig. 18.7).

Ulnar carpal impingement frequently is the underlying problem for a variety of other pathological conditions such as triangular fibrocartilage injuries, triquetrolunate ligament tears and degeneration of the proximal lunate and triquetrum.

A variant of ulnar carpal impingement is ulnar styloid carpal impingement in which the tip of the ulnar styloid is longer than normal and impinges on the triquetrum in ulnar deviation and supination.

A clinical test for this is pain in full supination and ulnar deviation at the styloid carpal impingement area (Topper *et al.* 1997). A diagnostic injection of lidocaine into this region may confirm the diagnosis. The symptoms may be resolved with simple excision of the tip of the ulnar styloid.

Triangular fibrocartilage injuries

Triangular fibrocartilage complex (TFCC) functions as a major stabilizer of the distal radial ulnar joint and acts as a cushion for load-bearing between the ulnar carpus and distal ulna. It is known that the axially loaded forearm bears approximately 80% of the load through the radius and 20% through the ulna (Palmer & Werner 1984). It should be noted that the thickness of the triangular fibrocartilage varies inversely with a positive ulnar variance. Triangular fibrocartilage injuries should be classified, evaluated and treated according to whether they are present in an ulnar positive or ulnar negative wrist and if they are accompanied by other pathology such as a triquetrolunate ligament tear.

A TFCC injury should be suspected when the patient complains of ulnar wrist pain and a click with active ulnar deviation. The physical examination reveals point tenderness just distal to the ulnar styloid in the area of the TFCC. Pain may be elicited by passively pronating and supinating the wrist with the examining fingers at the wrist level.

The hallmark of diagnosis of a complete tear of the TFCC resides with wrist arthroscopy, although the use of MRI has become more popular in recent years.

Palmer (1989) has classified lesions of the TFCC into traumatic and degenerative types. Traumatic injuries may result from a fall on an outstretched upper extremity or a hyper-rotation injury to the forearm such as in the tennis stroke. The degenerative type is due to repetitive loading of the TFCC due to repetitive forearm rotation, which also is frequently seen in tennis.

Traumatic types of TFCC tears may be divided into three categories: (i) the most common in which a central or radial tear is present; (ii) a peripheral or distal tear in which the TFCC is torn from the base of the ulnar styloid or associated with a styloid fracture; and (iii) those associated with an ulnar carpal ligament tear. A peripheral tear may render the distal radial ulnar joint unstable.

Palmer and Werner (1984) contend that treatment should be based on the stability of the distal radial

ulnar joint. If no instability exists, casting or splinting for 4 weeks in slight flexion and ulnar deviation may be utilized. If the distal radial ulnar joint is unstable or the ligamentous structures cannot be approximated by wrist positioning, they recommend arthroscopic evaluation.

If the stable wrist remains symptomatic after immobilization, arthroscopy may be indicated. It is known that central tears are amenable to arthroscopic debridement. Biomechanically, no effect on the load-bearing or stabilizing effect of the TFCC has been shown and Osterman *et al.* (1988) have noted excellent clinical results following centrum excision, with return to sports in 4–6 weeks.

If the distal radial ulnar joint is unstable, arthroscopy should be performed and repair of the peripheral tear is indicated in order to provide a stable distal radial ulnar joint.

In degenerative triangular fibrocartilage tears, a stellate-type central tear is usually present. This may be accompanied by chondromalacia or roughening of the cartilage on the lunate and/or head of the ulna. It also may be associated with lunotriquetral ligament injury and, in severe cases, with ulnar carpal arthrosis.

Treatment of the degenerative-type TFCC injuries involves arthroscopic debridement of the tear and of the chondromalacia of the ulna. If a positive ulnar variance exists, symptoms frequently will not resolve until some type of ulnar shortening is performed.

Triquetrolunate ligament tears

Another form of ulnar wrist pain may be due to a triquetrolunate ligament tear. This may occur with or without ulnar carpal impingement. An acute triquetral ligament tear may occur from a fall or from a rotational injury. A diagnosis is suspected by point tenderness over the triquetrolunate ligament as well as by the Reagan Shuck test (Fig. 18.8). In this test, one hand grasps the lunate and the other one grasps the triquetrum, and the two bones are shucked one against the other. If this produces the pain the player is complaining of, it supports the diagnosis. Arthrography is the imaging study of choice to confirm the diagnosis.

Treatment in the acute injury (if diagnosis is made within 3–4 weeks) may include arthroscopic

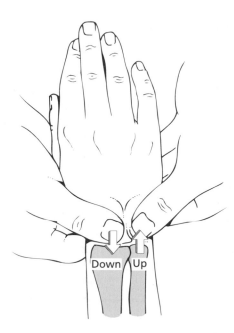

Fig. 18.8 The Reagan Shuck test. The pisiform and triquetrum are passively translated dorsally and toward the volar relative to the lunate. Positioning the wrist in slight flexion improves the examiner's grip on the lunate. (Reproduced with permission from Whipple, T.L. (1992) *Arthroscopic Surgery: The Wrist*. J.P. Lippincott, Philadelphia, PA.)

reduction and pinning, with or without repair, if obvious instability exists. In the chronic setting, an injection combined with immobilization may be tried. If this is unsuccessful, arthroscopy, debridement and arthroscopic-assisted percutaneous pinning may be indicated. The goal of this procedure is to produce an arthrofibrosis between the triquetrum and lunate in order to stabilize the joint. If this is unsuccessful, a triquetrolunate arthrodesis may be performed.

Hook of the hamate fractures

Another entity, which should be considered in the tennis player complaining of ulnar wrist pain, is a fracture of the hook of the hamate. This may occur in a tennis player due to constant abutment of the hypothenar eminence by the end of the racket handle (Fig. 18.9). Stark *et al.* (1989) described 62 patients with this entity; the majority of which occurred in baseball, golf and tennis.

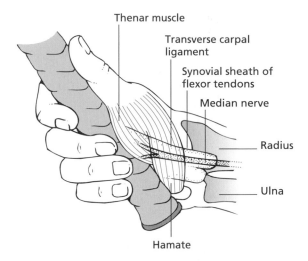

Fig. 18.9 Fractures of the hook of hamate characteristically occur in the hand that grips the butt end of the racket. (Reproduced with permission from Aulicino, P.L. (1990) *Hand Clinics* **6**, 3.)

The diagnosis should be made on the basis of a high index of suspicion. Physical findings include tenderness over the hook of the hamate, although the tenderness may also be palpated dorsally in the area of the hamate bone.

Plain radiographs usually are not helpful in the diagnosis of this condition, although carpal tunnel views or supinated oblique views may be of some help. A bone scan and CT scan are usually obtained if the diagnosis is considered and are diagnostic in most cases (Fig. 18.10).

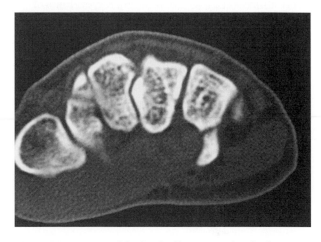

Fig. 18.10 Fracture of the hook of hamate is clearly shown on computed tomography.

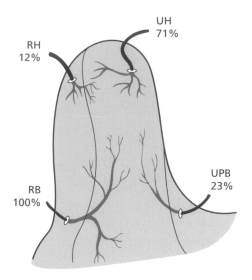

Fig. 18.11 Hook of hamate with vascular channels shown at the radial base (RB), ulnar (proximal) base (UPB), ulnar hook tip (UH), and radial hook tip (RH). (Reproduced with permission from Failla, J.M. (1993) *Journal of Hand Clinics* **18A**, 6.)

Treatment options for hook of the hamate fracture are cast immobilization, internal fixation and excision.

Most commonly, these injuries are treated by means of excision in that there is a very poor healing potential for the hook of the hamate. It has been shown in a cadaver study that 20% of hamate hooks had no vessels entering the bone distal to the base thus substantiating the poor healing potential of this fracture (Fig. 18.11). Many athletes complain of prodromal symptoms of pain prior to the actual fracture, and it is our feeling that these fractures have even less potential for healing than those caused by acute traumatic injuries.

Complications of non-operative treatment include persistent, symptomatic non-union and ulnar neuropathy due to the proximity of the ulnar nerve to the fracture. Rupture of the flexor tendon to the small finger also has been reported.

We recommend excision of the fracture fragment with immediate motion. The average return to sport is 7–10 weeks.

Triquetrohamate impingement

Triquetrohamate impingement is a rare cause of ulnar wrist pain in the tennis player and is due to impaction of the proximal pole of the hamate on the triquetrum or chondromalacia on the proximal portion of the lunate.

The diagnosis of this entity is made by point tenderness over the base of the hamate, and definitive diagnosis can be made only by arthroscopy. Treatment is arthroscopic debridement of the chondromalacia area.

Pisiform lesions

Chondromalacia of the pisiform also has been reported in racket sports (Helal 1978; Osterman *et al.* 1988). It is seen more commonly in racketball than in tennis, but may be a cause of ulnar wrist pain and should be suspected when tenderness of the pisiform and tenderness at the pisotriquetral articulation is present. Injection of lidocaine hydrochloride may be diagnostic and excision of the pisiform is usually curative with return to racket sports at 8–10 weeks.

Neurovascular injuries

Nerve injuries also may occur in tennis players. *Carpal tunnel syndrome* may occur and is frequently due to tenosynovitis of the flexor tendons. Most will resolve with rest and anti-inflammatory medications. Surgery usually is not indicated.

Guyon's canal syndrome is compression of the ulnar nerve as it passes between the pisiform and hook of the hamate. It is more common in the tennis player due to the abutment of the hypothenar area by the end of the racket handle (Rettig 1994). This condition frequently will resolve with rest. Sometimes, the use of a padded glove for playing will help prevent this condition from recurring when tennis is resumed. Surgical decompression of Guyon's canal may be indicated in certain cases.

An entity called *hypothenar hammer syndrome* may also be present in the tennis player due to repetitive abutment of the racket handle on the hypothenar region. This is an injury to the ulnar artery due to frequent repetitive trauma. The wall of the vessel may become injured resulting in stenosis. This may give a resultant circulatory symptom such as cold intolerance and recurrent ulnar wrist pain. Diagnosis by means of the Allen's test for ulnar artery patency may be utilized. Doppler studies or even arteriography may be necessary to confirm the diagnosis. If significant symptoms are present, exploration and resection of a portion of the ulnar artery with a vein graft may be indicated.

Digital nerve compression, particularly of the index finger, may occur at the radial digital nerve due to pressure between the metacarpal head and the racket handle. This is similar to compression of the ulnar digital nerve of the thumb, known as bowler's thumb. Usually, it responds to padding. However, neurolysis and nerve transfer to a less vulnerable area occasionally may be indicated.

Stress fractures

Stress fractures are rare in the upper extremity; however, stress fractures of the distal radius, ulnar shaft (Bollen *et al.* 1993) and second metacarpal have been reported in tennis players.

Ulnar shaft stress fractures are more commonly seen in the non-dominant extremity of a player with a two-handed backhand (Bollen *et al.* 1993). Recurrence of these injuries may be due to repeated impact loading at the ball strike or to repeated pronation of the effected forearm. Differential stress between the muscles originating at the ulna (the flexor digitorum profundus in the thumb outcropping muscles) may also be a cause.

Stress fractures of the ulna usually resolve with splinting and play may resume with a fracture brace in 2–3 weeks. Usually, healing is complete by 6 weeks and, to date, no cases of non-union have been reported.

Stress fractures of the metacarpals account for only 0.5% of all sports stress fractures. The aetiology is a combination of elements of stroke mechanics, racket structure and training intensity. The fractures reported were located at the base of the second metacarpal, which is the focal point about which the racket rotates.

All stress fractures reported in the literature resolved with rest and all returned to tennis in 4–6 weeks. Attention to utilization of proper technique should be emphasized when returning to the sport.

Return to play

After any of these injuries is reported, return to tennis is permitted when grip strength is within normal limits and range of motion is within normal limits, or at least within the limits required for tennis. We encourage players to use a motion-controlled brace such as designed by Nirschl when they initially return to sport (see Fig. 18.2).

We recommend stretching before and ice after practice and play. Proper technique should be emphasized and we encourage the club player to take a lesson prior to getting back to play to see if any technique flaws may be detected. The equipment, namely the racket, should be carefully selected and should be done on an individual basis.

Pre-participation stretching for prevention of recurrence of these injuries is also highly recommended (Figs 18.12 and 18.13). General conditioning throughout

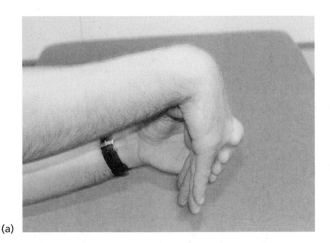

(a)

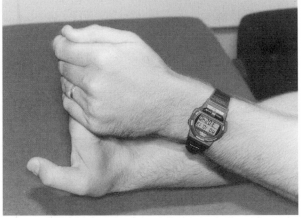

(b)

Fig. 18.12 Pre-participation stretching for prevention of recurrence of injuries. (a) Flexion; (b) extension.

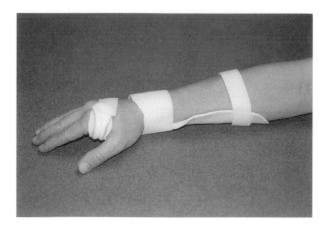

Fig. 18.13 Resting splint.

the rehabilitation period is also quite important as emphasized by Nirschl (1979) in order to maintain proper vascularity to the effected extremity.

In summary, wrist and hand injuries in tennis players are common and are responsible for a significant amount of time out of the sport. It is helpful to be familiar with the most common types of wrist problems we see in tennis players in order to know how to better evaluate and treat these athletes.

References

Bollen, S.R., Robinson, D.G., Crichton, K.J. & Cross, M.J. (1993) Stress fractures of the ulna in tennis players using a double-handed backhand stroke. *American Journal of Sports Medicine* **21** (5), 751–752.

Helal, B. (1978) Racquet players pisiform. *Hand* **10** (1), 87.

Hutchinson, M.R., Laprade, R.F., Burnett, Q.M. II, Moss, R. & Terpstra, J. (1995) Injury surveillance at the USTA boys' tennis championships: a 6-year study. *Medicine and Science in Sports and Exercise* **27** (6), 826–830.

Kibler, W.B., McQueen, C. & Uhl, T. (1988) Fitness evaluations and fitness findings in competitive junior tennis players. *Clinics in Sports Medicine* **7** (2), 403–416.

Kiefhaber, T.R. & Stern, P.J. (1992) Upper extremity tendinitis and overuse syndromes in the athlete. *Clinics in Sports Medicine* **11**, 39–55.

Nirschl, R.P. (1979) Prevention and treatment of elbow and shoulder injuries in tennis. *Clinics in Sports Medicine* **7**, 289–308.

Osterman, A.L., Moskow, L. & Low, D.W. (1988) Soft tissue injuries of the hand and wrist in racquet sports. *Clinics in Sports Medicine* **7** (2), 329–348.

Palmer, A.K. (1989) Triangular fibrocartilage complex lesions: a classification. *Journal of Hand Surgery* **14A**, 594.

Palmer, A.K. & Werner, F.W. (1984) Biomechanics of the distal radioulnar joint. *Clinical Orthopaedics and Related Research* **187**, 26–35.

Rayan, G.M. (1993) Recurrent dislocation of the extensor carpi ulnaris in athletes. *American Journal of Sports Medicine* **11**, 183.

Reece, L.A., Fricker, P.A. & Maguire, K.F. (1986) Injuries to elite young tennis players at the Australian Institute of Sport. *Australian Journal of Science and Medicine in Sports* **118**, 11–15.

Rettig, A.C. (1994) Wrist problems in the tennis player. *Medicine and Science in Sports and Exercise* **26** (10), 1207–1212.

Stark, H., Chai, E. & Zemel, N.P. (1989) Fracture of the hook of the hamate. *Journal of Bone and Joint Surgery* **71A**, 1202–1207.

Topper, S.M., Wood, M.B. & Ruby, L.K. (1997) Ulnar styloid impaction syndrome. *Journal of Hand Surgery* **22A**, 699–704.

Winge, S., Jorgenson, U. & Nielson, L. (1989) Epidemiology of injuries in Danish championship tennis. *International Journal of Sports Medicine* **10**, 368–371.

Chapter 19

Elbow injuries in tennis

Tennis is played today by millions of people around the world. Towards the end of the 1970s, more than 40 million Americans played tennis. Top-level tennis is played in more countries around the world than almost any other sport. Tennis is played by all age groups, as it is a sport which in general does not produce severe medical problems. Some of the major problems in tennis occur, however, in the elbow region exemplified by the so-called 'tennis elbow'. Pain near the lateral epicondyle of the humerus (upper arm) was described by Runge (1873), and was called 'writer's cramp'. Later it was called 'washer women's elbow'. As it also occurred in tennis, it was soon called 'tennis elbow'. It should, however, be remembered that only 5% of people suffering from tennis elbow relate the injury to tennis. This injury is more common in industry and activities of daily living and occurs in other racket sports. There are, however, many other injuries that may occur in the elbow region related to tennis. The different injuries causing elbow pain and their diagnosis, treatment and rehabilitation will be discussed below.

Functional anatomy of the elbow

The stability of the elbow is provided by the collateral ligaments, but also by the bones and their articulations and the muscles and tendons. The medial ulnar ligament is well developed and forms three distinct bands: the anterior oblique, a small transverse, non-functional ligament, and the posterior oblique ligament. The anterior oblique ligament is very strong and is taut through the entire arc of elbow flexion and is the primary constraint of valgus stress of the elbow. The posterior oblique ligament is taut in flexion and lax in extension and does not play a primary role in elbow stability. The lateral–collateral ligament is not clinically important as it has only a few non-functional weak fibres.

The anconeus muscle appears to provide lateral support, as does the forearm extensor muscles. The extensor carpi radialis brevis and longus, digitorum communis, digiti minimi and carpiradialis originate at the lateral epicondyle and are mainly wrist extensors (Fig. 19.1). The three primary flexor muscles of the elbow are the biceps brachii, the brachioradialis and the brachialis. The most important pronator muscles of the elbow are the pronator teres and the pronator quadratus. The triceps is the only effective extensor of the elbow.

The radial nerve runs anterior lateral of the elbow and divides into the posterior interosseous nerve and the lateral cutaneous nerve of the forearm, and especially the former can be entrapped. The medial nerves remain anterior of the elbow in its course and pass between the two heads of the pronator muscle and can also become entrapped. The ulnar nerve travels through the triceps fascia, as it approaches the cubital tunnel on the medial posterior aspect where it can be compressed and cause distal problems.

The elbow is a joint that can be moved about a longitudinal and transverse axis. Flexion–extension is provided by the humeral–ulnar joint. The rotational motion is provided by the unique articulation of the radius with the capitellum portion of the humerus so that forearm pronation and supination can be carried out.

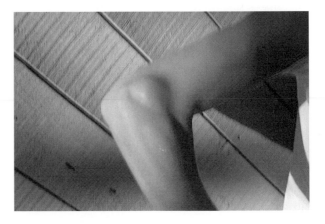

Fig. 19.1 The forearm muscles are very well developed in top level tennis players.

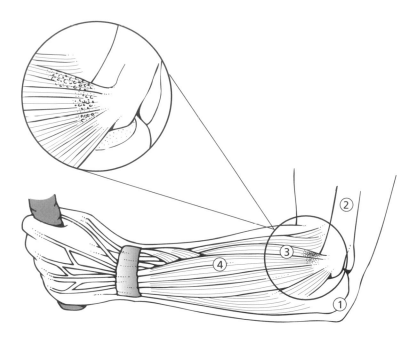

Fig. 19.2 The tennis elbow pathology is often located in the carpi radialis brevis. 1, Ulna; 2, humerus; 3, extensor carpi radialis brevis; 4, extensor digitorum communis. (From Peterson, L. & Renström, P. (2000) *Sport Injuries: Their Prevention and Treatment*, p. 163. Martin Dunitz, London.)

The normal range of motion of the elbow is flexion and extension 0–145° with a functional arc of 0–130°. Constraints to elbow extension and flexion can be seen in Fig. 19.2. Pronation and supination can be carried out with 70° of pronation to 80° of supination. The axial rotation is around the centre radial head to the centre of the distal ulna.

There is a valgus carrying angle of 10–15° in full extension and 8° varus in full flexion. The internal rotation is 5° during early flexion and external 5° during terminal flexion.

Injuries to the elbow

Injuries can occur in the elbow depending on the type of activity. In tennis they are most commonly localized to the lateral epicondyle such as lateral elbow tendinopathy ('tennis elbow'—formerly lateral epicondylitis). Tennis can also cause medial elbow tendinosis (formerly medial epicondylitis) and extensor overload can cause posterior tennis elbow.

Lateral elbow tendinopathy ('tennis elbow', formerly lateral epicondylitis)

Lateral elbow tendinopathy is most common in tennis players of 35–50 years of age. This group is often characterized by a high activity level and they often play tennis three times per week or more of at least 30 min or greater per session. Forty-five per cent of the athletes who play tennis daily, or 20% of those who play twice per week, may at certain stages suffer from lateral elbow tendinopathy. Frequency of play has a direct relationship with pain. The more frequently a person plays, the greater the incidence of pain. Players of higher ability, which means players that play longer and practice more, have more commonly a history of elbow pain.

Persons most likely to sustain lateral elbow tendinopathy are those that have demanding techniques and inadequate fitness levels. It is well established that faulty technique is one of the most common causes for lateral elbow tendinopathy, especially a faulty backhand. The serve is also associated with elbow pain. Studies have shown an association of tennis elbow with repetitive hobbies such as house decorating, gardening and knitting, and industrial activities involving wrist motions of different kinds.

In a study of average players, Priest *et al.* (1980) found that 31% of a group of 2633 players suffered elbow pain at some time during their career. Thirty-seven per cent of 84 top-level players had elbow pain, which can be compared to 22% of 41 players in another study. In top-level players, however, the clinical observation is that they more commonly have elbow pain localized to the medial side.

Pathology

The lateral elbow tendinopathy related to tennis involves primarily extensor carpi radialis brevis and secondary extensor digitorum communis. Figure 19.2 shows the anatomical relations near the lateral epicondyle. The bellies of the relevant muscles are all located in the forearm, while the long tendons bridge the elbow and wrist joints, and insert on the metacarpals (mid-hand) or phalanges (the lateral epicondyle of the humerus forms a common origin for at least parts of all the extensors of the wrist and fingers).

The *pathology* represents a degenerative process that is secondary to tensile overuse fatigue, weakness and possible avascular (poor circulation) changes. Degeneration is characterized by microtears, fragmentation and poor orientation of the collagen. Microscopic tendon tears of the extensor origin is present primarily in the extensor brevis tendon. The likely sequence of events is: 'avascular compromise, an altered nutrition state, and forced overload cause angiofibroblastic changes and ultimate rupture of these vulnerable tissues' (Nirschl 1992). There are usually no inflammatory cells present. The term tendinopathy has therefore been replacing the term tendinitis. This means that tennis elbow should be called lateral elbow tendinopathy.

Symptoms

• The onset and diagnosis of symptoms can be sudden or gradual. In most instances, there is no predisposing activity that can be found. Sometimes there is a history of repetitive activity or overuse, such as playing tennis intensively at a training camp or going back to tennis activity after a period of no activity.
• Lateral elbow tendinopathy is characterized by pain and often weakness localized to the lateral part of the elbow. Sometimes this pain can radiate distally or not-so-commonly more proximally.
• There is palpable tenderness over the lateral epicondyle. This tenderness is mostly localized over the extensor brevis tendon insertion, which is slightly on the anterior aspect of the epicondyle.

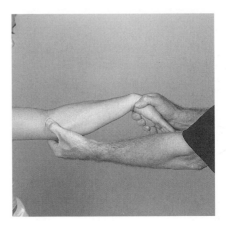

Fig. 19.3 Diagnostic test. Assisted wrist extension causes pain of the elbow.

• The coffee cup test, which means picking up a full cup of coffee, will produce localized pain at the lateral epicondylar area. This test is more or less pathognomonic for lateral epicondylitis.
• There is pain with resistance stress tests by dorsiflexion of the wrist (Fig. 19.3) or the middle finger (Fig. 19.4), localized to the elbow confirming the area of abnormality. Involvement of the extensor carpi radialis brevis is typical for tennis players. This involves pain at the elbow on resistance stress test by dorsiflexion of the wrist. When lateral elbow tendinopathy is caused by industrial work, it seems according to the author's experience, that extensor digitorum communis is mostly involved. This can also generate a positive middle finger test, i.e. pain at the elbow on

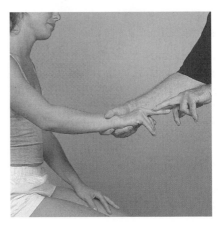

Fig. 19.4 Middle finger test—resisted finger extension causes pain at the elbow.

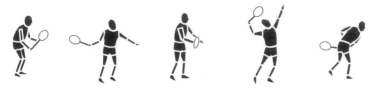

Phase I	Mild pain after exercise activity, resolves within 24 h
Phase II	Pain after exercise activity, exceeds 48 h, resolves with warm-up
Phase III	Pain after exercise activity that does not alter activity
Phase IV	Pain with exercise activity that alters activity
Phase V	Pain caused by heavy activities of daily living
Phase VI	Intermittent pain at rest that does not disturb sleep
	Pain caused by light activities of daily living
Phase VII	Constant rest pain (dull aching) and pain that disturbs sleep

Table 19.1 Tendinosis phases of pain. (From Nirschl 1992.)

resistance at dorsiflexion of the middle finger. In other words, it seems clinically that there may be two different aetiologies in lateral elbow tendinopathy with somewhat different locations of the problems.

• An accurate diagnosis of tendinosis changes includes an evaluation of the magnitude of pathological change, which is helpful as a prognostic predictor, as well as formulating the treatment protocol.

• The patient's description of time and intensity of pain is the best guideline to evaluate the amount of problems. A grading system concerning the tendinosis phase of pain is outlined in Table 19.1.

Contributing factors (aetiology)

AGE AND SEX

Epidemiological studies have identified age as a contributing factor associated with the occurrence of tennis elbow, with onset more common after age 30 (Table 19.2).

Results concerning the incidence of tennis elbow between sexes is somewhat conflicting. Some have found no statistical difference between male and female tennis players and some found that women were affected more often than men.

	10–19	20–29	30–39	40–49	50–59	60 +	Total
Men							
In last year	1	2	3	8	7	0	21
>1 year ago	0	2	10	21	32	24	89
Never	11	2	17	23	11	13	77
Women							
In last year	1	0	3	2	0	0	6
>1 year ago	0	1	9	12	8	2	32
Never	7	3	12	10	2	1	35
Total	20	10	54	76	60	40	260

Table 19.2 Incidence of tennis elbow by age group (*n* = 260). (From Kamien 1989.)

STRENGTH AND FLEXIBILITY

Inadequate strength, primarily of the forearm muscle, is considered to play a role in causing tennis elbow as well as inadequate wrist flexibility. This is because a tight wrist will affect the muscle flexibility of the forearm, which may result in lateral epicondyle tendon strain.

In tennis players, there are statistically significant increases in forearm muscle, girth and grip strength, and decreases in the range of motion of playing extremities. The increase in forearm girth is approximately twice that of the upper arm. Statistically significant increases in the humerus bone were found for nearly all the dimensions in the playing arm. The significance of this is not known.

PLAYING TIME

Increased playing time has been shown to increase the incidence of tennis elbow up to 3.5 times for people over the age of 40. The players who play more than 2 h a day are more susceptible than those who play less than 2 h a week. The incidence of elbow pain increases with playing frequency.

It has been shown that the number of people who have had tennis elbow during their careers increased with the number of years they had played. Experience can influence the prevalence of elbow pain and the presence of a history of elbow pain. Increased playing experience has been shown to be associated with a lower incidence of tennis elbow for those players under 40 years of age. Players over 40 years of age who had played tennis for many years had a higher incidence of tennis elbow. Increased incidence of tennis elbow among the better tennis players is probably due to increased playing time rather than a deficiency in their ability. Inexperienced players more often use improper stroke techniques, and are more prone to miss-hit the ball. Either of these, or the combination of the two, result in greater mechanical stress on the elbow joint.

MOTIONS INVOLVED

Tennis elbow is generally combined with an improperly executed backhand stroke technique. Out of 75% of players with tennis elbow, 40% have reported the use of a faulty backhand in combination with muscle weakness. Fifty per cent of female and 30% of male professional tennis players with tennis elbow

problems get tennis elbow by overuse of the forehand and/or backhand. The player with a faulty backhand can often compensate with the use of a forehand grip or a fist-list grip with the thumb extended behind the handle for more power. The faulty backhand stroke usually starts with a high backswing with the bodyweight on the back leg. The power is generated at the wrist and elbow. As the elbow extends, the wrist strongly hooks into ulnar deviation, which is a motion commonly used for opening doors, chopping wood, and so on. The combination of extended elbow and the ulnar hooking of the wrist causes the extensor mass, especially the deep extensor carpi radialis brevis, to rub and roll over the lateral epicondyle and the lateral head. Microtears are present, and as a result of the rubbing, rolling and the microtears, a painful elbow evolves. In an attempt to heal the damage, granulation tissue forms, which can swell, stretch and become painful.

Adhesions can also form between the annular ligament and the joint capsule. The pain worsens from the constant strain of the faulty backhand.

Twenty-five per cent of the players in one study identified the serve as the most painful tennis stroke. Overhead stroke, and especially the serve, caused pain in 29% of players with elbow pain. Epidemiological studies have linked the serving action with injuries to the elbows.

THE RACKET

Factors of importance for the racket are torsion and centre of percussion—the sweet spot. The centre of percussion can be defined as the point on the racket which, when hit, will keep vibrational impact from being transferred to the hand, and consequently will maximize the energy available to the ball. One primary goal when designing a racket would be to have as large a sweet spot as possible. Secondly, it would be desirable to have the sweet spot as powerful as possible, with the delivery power as uniform as possible from the centre of the sweet spot to its outer edge. These goals are achieved differently, and result in various designs of rackets and frames. Modern frame designs have made it possible to enlarge the sweet spot and increase its power.

There is a popular belief that tennis elbow is the result of transmitted vibration caused by hitting heavy tennis balls. This view is supported by 8 years of experience of an English Sports Medicine Clinic, which found upper limb injuries to be more frequent in tennis players than in badminton players. The role of vibration is still unclear.

Considerably worse strain has been seen occurring on the forearm muscles from hitting balls off-centre along the vertical axis of any racket. These off-centre impact vibrations have been shown to be best absorbed by oversized rackets. Kamien (1989) suggested that tennis elbow may result from using an oversized aluminium racket. In interviews, some players in his study blame oversized aluminium rackets for the cause of their elbow pain, while other players gave it credit for their cure. Occurrence of tennis elbow by composition, size, weight of racket, grip size, tension and type of strings is shown in Table 19.3.

Tennis elbow is more likely to occur in players who use a heavy racket than in players who use a light racket. Other studies indicate that the weight of the rackets does not influence the incidence of tennis elbow. The heavier the racket, the greater the momentum. The heavier and stiffer rackets increase the muscle force that is required during the swing of impact; while also increasing the stress on the elbow. It is recommended that recreational players should use evenly balanced light rackets.

Racket materials may be a factor in the incidence of tennis elbow. Metal rackets have been considered to be too stiff to absorb the shock waves transmitted at ball impact. Bernhang *et al.* (1974) found that tennis players who use aluminium rackets are afflicted with tennis elbow almost twice as much as players who use wooden rackets. Other studies have been inconclusive over this point. Frames made of fibreglass, different composite materials, and so on, are supposed to reduce the vibration with increasing stiffness; however, definite evidence for this does not exist.

Table 19.3 Occurrence of tennis elbow by composition, size and weight of racket, grip size, tension and type of strings. (From Kamien 1989.)

	Tennis elbow		
	In last year $n = 27$ (%)	Past history $n = 121$ (%)	Never $n = 112$ (%)
Racket material			
Wood	22	13	28
Aluminium	30	49.5	28
Graphite	18.5	13	24
Composite	18.5	13	15
Other	11	8	5
Racket size			
Standard	22	23	38
Mid-size	45	30	42
Oversize (Jumbo)	33	47	20
Racket weight			
Light	11	19	24
Light medium	30	28	33
Medium	33	35	18
Not sure	26	32	25
Grip size			
Correct	55	50	49
Small	4	9	11
Large	30	29	26
Not sure	11	12	14
Type of strings			
Gut	33	26	21
Synthetic	67	74	79
Tension of strings			
Tight	44	37	50
Moderately tight	52	60	44
Low tension	4	3	6

GRIP SIZE

There have been several studies correlating the incidence of tennis elbow with different grip sizes. Some have indicated that too large (10.2 cm (4 inches) and 12.7 cm (5 inches)) or too small (10.8 cm (4.25 inches)) a grip is associated with a very high incidence rate of tennis elbow (Hang & Peng 1984). Of players over 40 years of age, those who used a large grip size had an incidence rate of over six times that for those who used a smaller grip size. It is not immediately evident,

however, that the grip size relates to the pathology of tennis elbow. Bernhang *et al.* (1974) compared hand size with grip size, calculating whether a grip size was correct or incorrect for that player. No association was found between the incidence of tennis elbow and the use of a grip that is too large or too small for the player's hand. An electromyographic (EMG) study of muscle activity generated in the forearm and shoulder muscles of a player using different size grips concluded that the force change in the muscles was not significant enough to suggest the need for a change in racket grip size. Bernhang concluded that using the largest grip size that is comfortable is an effective prophylaxis against developing tennis elbow. Further verification of this point in his study is required. A player can determine his or her grip size by measuring from the proximal palmar crease to the top of the ring finger along the medial side of the ring finger.

STRINGS

Strings are either made of gut or nylon. Gut is manufactured from the smooth-muscle portion of sheep or cows. Gut provides better control, higher ball velocities, lower levels of vibration transmission to the hand and improved playing characteristics according to player evaluation. In addition, tests measuring ball velocity favoured gut string over synthetic string when strung at the same tension.

Ball velocities following impact are superior in rackets with gut string. The looser the strings are, the higher the postimpact ball velocity. This may be of some importance in tennis elbow treatment. The stringing patterns can also vary and can be trampoline, fishnet or pulley-like.

How does string tension affect control? One effect is that an increase in string tension causes the ball to flatten out during impact. A second is that a trampoline effect occurs at low string tensions, where the ball is on the racket face for a longer period of time.

At higher tensions, the ball is on the racket face for a shorter period of time. Therefore, if a ball is hit off-centre, the racket will have more time to rotate during impact, sending the ball in an errant direction. This provides less control and also higher rotational accelerations. A recommendation is that a racket should not be strung too tightly, usually between 50 and 55 pounds (25–27 kg) of tension in order to avoid tennis elbow. In general, more tightly strung rackets will give better control, whereas looser strung rackets will give more force. However, the tension in the strings will decrease within a short time. Gut string is rather resilient when freshly strung, whereas nylon string will last longer and is more economical.

BALLS

Heavy balls should be avoided, as well as dead, wet or pressureless balls. Use of these will increase the impact against the tennis racket thereby increasing the risk of tennis elbow.

COURTS

The condition of the court can also be a factor for the incidence of tennis elbow. Irregularities in the court may be possible factors in the development of tennis elbow. These irregularities cause the ball to bounce unexpectedly and, consequently, the stroke may be incorrectly timed, and result in strain due to the faulty technique. On the other hand, a slow court decreases the velocity of the ball, thereby minimizing the impact and torsional forces during impact. It is for this reason that the use of slow courts is suggested for players with tennis elbow problems.

BACKGROUND—VIBRATION AND MUSCLE ACTIVITY

Brody (1987) compared the oscillations of a hand-held racket with a clamped tennis racket. It was concluded that the hand-held racket showed vibrational modes similar to those of free rackets, while being very different from clamped rackets. He stated that 'a free racket's lowest frequency of oscillation is about 100–175 Hz, which is similar to the higher frequency of the clamped racket'. He further compared tennis racket vibration damping in hand-held rackets with freely suspended rackets. He found that the hand-held rackets clamped out racket vibration a magnitude shorter than freely suspended rackets. Two other important points were mentioned in his study, one being that the time required to clamp the amplitude of oscillations to hold its value is dependent upon how tightly the racket is gripped.

The other important point in Brody's study is that the vibrations of a tennis racket that are the most disturbing are caused by the first harmonic mode of oscillation. The frequency of this mode is from about 120–200 Hz. The highest magnitudes to occur at low frequencies are around 1 Hz. The muscle resonance is between 20 and 25 Hz and elbow resonance is between 0.5 and 1.0 Hz. In view of this and the information from the hand power tool studies, it has been theorized that low-frequency vibrations travel up the arm and this event is a contributing factor to the cause of tennis elbow. Miniature accelerometers at the wrist and elbow in 24 tennis players in a simulated backhand stroke were used to study vibration. They found more than four-fold reduction in acceleration amplitude and integral between wrist and elbow. Off-centre impacts resulted in approximately three times increased acceleration values. Increased racket head size was found to reduce arm vibration. In summary, they found that hitting close to the centre of the racket phase, a better skill level of the players, and increased resonance frequency of the racket were identified as the main factors for a reduction of acceleration of the wrist and elbow.

Due to the discussions of the effects of racket vibration, vibration dampeners have been developed. Although these dampeners work well for damping string vibration, they do not seem to aid in damping harmful frame vibration caused by off-centre shots.

In summary, it seems that the vibration from the racket stays at the level of the hand. It seems that mishits, which produce racket torsion and result in increased lower arm muscle activity, most likely are a main contributor to the tennis elbow pain syndrome. Vibration probably does not cause tennis elbow, but may aggravate the condition once a player has the injury.

Concepts for treatment

The treatment should follow the healing response and stimulate healing. The relief of pain and limitation of inflammation in the acute phase can be carried out with rest, protection, ice, compression and elevation. Rest is defined as absence from abuse, but this does not mean that pain-free activities cannot be carried out. Sometimes modalities and anti-inflammatory medication can be helpful.

In the chronic phase there is little inflammation but mostly generative changes. In this setting, exercise is a key treatment, sometimes combined with braces and modalities such as electrical stimulation, ultrasound or acupuncture. If this is not effective for at least 6–12 weeks or a couple of months, shock wave therapy can be tried. Cortisone injection can be tried if everything else fails and finally surgery may be needed.

EXERCISES
Exercises are a key treatment for tennis elbow as the main cause for the chronic problems is tendon degeneration which means micro tears of the tendon fibres, poor orientation of the collagen, weakened cross-links between the collagen fibres and biomechanical changes which altogether will weaken the tendon. The real cause why this is painful is

unknown. The main therapy for degeneration is exercise in a planned fashion often under the guidance of a well-qualified physiotherapist.

The training programme should include the following:
• Isometric strength training of the wrist extensors is carried out with the wrist in three positions: first fully flexed downwards, then in a neutral position and finally flexed upwards. The exercise should be carried out 30 times a day. The wrist may be flexed for 10 s at a time with muscle contraction. When these exercises can be carried out without major pain, a load of 0.5–1 kg (1–2 lbs) can be introduced.
• Dynamic strength training can be carried out by using an elastic band over the ends of the fingers. An attempt to spread the fingers against its resistance can then be made. Another technique is to extend (concentric contraction) and flex (eccentric action) the wrist with a load of 1–2 kg (2–4 lbs) 20 times a day.
• Flexibility exercises of the wrist should be carried out with the elbow of the injured arm held extended and the forearm pronated. The bent wrist is stretched to almost maximum and is held there for 10–20 s (Fig. 9.23b). The exercise is repeated 15 times 2–3 times a day.
• Exercises including strength and mobility of the shoulder and arm should be included. Endurance training can be carried out with many repetitions and low resistance. General body conditioning is important.
• It should be pointed out that the dynamic strength training involving flexing the wrist with weights is a so-called eccentric exercise which is very effective in managing degenerative tendinopathy. It should be the main element of the exercise treatment.

MODALITIES
Modalities include many different types of equipment generating heat in different ways.

Ultrasound has been used for many years and may be helpful. *Electrical stimulation* has become very popular and is used widely today not the least by the ATP medical service.

Shock wave treatment involves giving high-energy ultrasound pulses to the affected area. In the past, it has been tried extensively and been shown in some prospective randomized clinical trials to be an effective modality for chronic tennis elbow. It creates an area with increased circulation and thereby a stimulus to healing. The healing time is at least

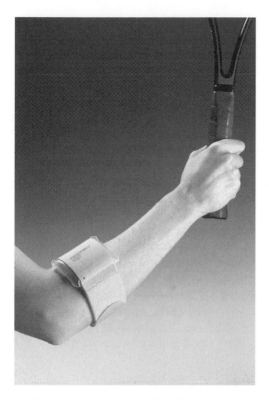

Fig. 19.5 Tennis elbow brace with localized pressure is often helpful.

1–2 months with this type of treatment. It should be pointed out that a scientific support for the current management of tennis elbow with modalities is not convincing.

BRACES

The proximal forearm band and the counterforce brace are the most commonly used types. Counter-force bracing, which constrains key muscle groups for maintaining muscle balance, decrease in the angular acceleration of the wrist and elbow during the serve and of the elbow during the backhand. An air-filled bladder (Aircast, Inc.) (Fig. 19.5) has been developed as a counter-pressure element. Snyder-Mackler and Epler (1989) found that this constrictive band caused a significant reduction in integrated EMG of the extensor carpi radialis brevis and the extensor digitor communis when compared with controlled values and a standard band. The decrease in integrated EMG effected by the bands was more marked in the extensor digitorum than in the extensor carpi radialis brevis. This could be a result of the location, relative depth, or cross-sectional area of the muscles under the band. More research is needed to confirm the effect of braces for the treatment of tennis elbow. Clinical experience, including the author's, indicates, however, that the use of tennis elbow braces is a valuable complementary tool in the treatment of tennis elbow. The elbow bands can be combined with heat-retaining neoprene sleeves to add the positive effects of heat in stimulating healing.

CORTISONE INJECTION

This can occasionally be given in very chronic cases when other methods fail. Small doses of 1 ml can be injected at the insertion. The athlete should rest for a couple of days and then continue with the exercises. The effect of cortisone injection is short—often only 6 weeks.

ACUPUNCTURE

The acupuncture technique applied to acupuncture points related to the elbow can be a valuable method in the treatment of tennis elbow. Low-energy laser and pulsed ultrasound are not effective.

FAILED HEALING

This is considered to occur if there are chronic symptoms of phase VI tendinosis pain (see Table 19.1) or greater, exceeding a duration of 1 year. If there is poor response to a quality rehabilitation programme, if there is a history of persistent pain of phase IV or greater, or if the patient has not been able to return to an acceptable quality of life, failed healing is suspected and surgery may be indicated.

SURGERY

This is sometimes indicated. During surgery it has been found that the tissue involved in tennis elbow is extensor carpi radialis brevis in 100% of cases. Extensor digitorum communis and especially the anterior edge is involved in 35% and there is an osteophyte formation of the lateral epicondyle in 20% (Nirschl 1992). The surgery consists of identification of the pathological tissue, which is resected. The attachment of normal tissues should be maintained and the normal tissues protected. There should then be quality postoperative rehabilitation. The elbow is protected at 90° for 1-week in a counter-force elbow immobilizer. Strength and endurance resistance exercises usually start at 3 weeks after surgery. Modified sports technique patterns are often initiated starting at 6 weeks after surgery. Eighty-five per cent of people experience complete pain relief and return to full strength after surgery.

There is a recurrence rate of 18–66%. The degree of pain prior to treatment is the most important predictor of complete recovery. The greater the pain, the more likely the complete success of the treatments. This means that there is no need for treating cases early to elicit the most favourable outcomes of the treatment regimen.

Summary of tennis elbow management

It should be pointed out that the management of tennis elbow is very difficult and may be time consuming. The key treatment technique is using eccentric exercises to manage the effects of degeneration. The exercise programme should be carried out in cooperation with a well educated physiotherapist. Modalities can be used and are probably helpful. Shock wave treatment seems to be a breakthrough in the management of these chronic tendinopathies.

The normal time for rehabilitation of a chronic tennis elbow is 3–5 months give or take a month. It is therefore important to inform the player that management of chronic tennis elbow takes time, is difficult, requires patience and teamwork.

Differential diagnosis

Cervical nerve root compression of C6 and C7, as well as cervical osteoarthritis may cause lateral elbow pain and mimic lateral tennis elbow. This is, however, something that is rare and is seen in the elderly.

The radial nerve and posterior interosseous or superficial radial nerve branches are vulnerable to compression from distal to the level of the lateral head of the triceps through the arcade of Frohse. A point of tenderness with this nerve entrapment is usually localized directly over the area of nerve entrapment. EMG and nerve conduction studies may be helpful in differentiation of which motor segment is involved. Pain on resistive extension and testing of the long finger are sometimes associated with findings of posterior interosseous nerve compression. This injury is present in not more than 1–2% of the cases with lateral elbow pain.

Medial elbow tendinosis ('thrower's elbow' and 'golfer's elbow', formerly medial epicondylitis)

The primary pathological changes involved in medial tennis elbow are present in the origin of the pronator teres, palmaris longus and flexor carpi radialis close to the attachment to the medial epicondyle. Occasionally pathological changes also occur in the flexor carpi ulnaris.

The aetiology of medial tennis elbow is the same as in lateral tennis elbow. The most common cause is technical errors. The player can hit the ball hard with too much topspin on the forehand stroke, or a hard first flat serve or overhead stroke. The basic principles for treating medial tennis elbow are the same as treating the lateral tennis elbow.

The prognosis for healing for medial tennis elbow is, however, worse and the healing time is longer than for the lateral side. It can sometimes take 6–12 months before return to tennis. The patients should be told this so that their expectations are realistic.

Valgus stress overload syndrome

During an extensive serve or, even more so, during a pitching motion, there is a tremendous valgus (lower arm is directed outwards in relation to the upper arm) stress upon the elbow causing distraction and tension of the medial aspect of elbow and compression of the lateral aspect (Fig. 19.6). Compression of the lateral compartment, which often occurs in the so-called cocking phase, can result in fracture of the capitellum or deformation of the radial head. An associated problem can be chondromalacia, synovitis, osteophytic (bony) spurs and loose fragments. In the medial compartment there can be additional strain and rupture and valgus instability of the elbow can occur.

Elbow instability

The valgus stress overload syndrome can cause medial tension which means tension of the medial–collateral ligaments (MCLs) (Fig. 19.7).

The MCL, especially the anterior band, is of great importance for elbow stability and is composed of two parts. The origin of the anterior band is posterior to the axis of elbow rotation. The origin of the posterior band is just posterior to the above. The increased

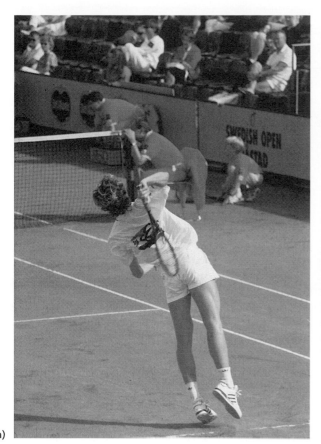

(a)

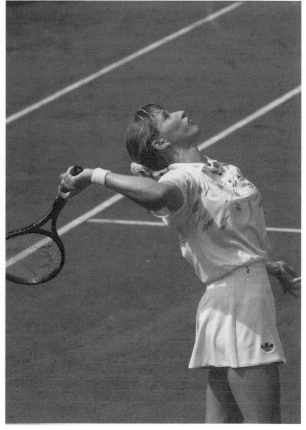

(b)

(c)

Ulnar nerve

Fig. 19.6 (a,b) A serving motion showing valgus overload of the elbow. (c) Valgus overload results in medial tension and lateral compression. (From Hunter, S.C. (1985) Little leaguer's elbow. In: Zarin, B., Andrews, J.F. & Carson, W.G., eds. *Injuries to the Throwing Arm*, p. 229. WB Saunders, Philadelphia, PA.)

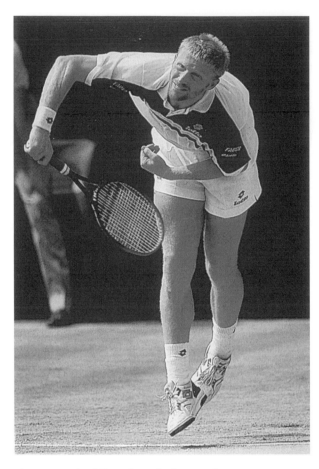

Fig. 19.7 In the follow-through phase in the serve, hyperextension of the elbow is common.

distance from origin to insertion of this ligament with flexion is from 0° to 120°. The posterior portion of the MCL contributes little to valgus stability. The radial head contributes on the other hand significantly to stability at 0°, 45° and 90° of flexion, but the MCL is the most important stabilizer except at full extension. The anterior band is the major stabilizer from 20 to 120 degrees of flexion.

Symptoms and treatment

When the patients have MCL instability, there is pain on the medial side of the arm during throwing or serving. There is a sensation of elbow opening or giving way.

There is a valgus instabilty with the arm flexed 30°, which can be confirmed on stress radiographs or arthroscopy.

The injury involves oedema and inflammation or scar formation within the ligament. There can also be calcific densities within the scar or ossifications (bone formation) within the ligament. Ruptures can also occur. These changes can be verified on an MRI.

The treatment includes rest and ice and generally rehabilitation with strengthening exercises as the main focus. Surgery is indicated if failure with conservative therapy is present after 6 months and occasionally in acute ruptures.

Ulnar neuritis

The majority of nerve lesions in athletes can be described as neuropraxia, which is the mildest form of nerve injury. It is characterized by a conduction block along a nerve where all nerve elements (axon) and connective tissue remain in continuity. Prognosis for complete recovery is good if organ damage has not occurred owing to long-standing compression. Severe injuries can be axonal injury and distal axon degeneration without disruption of the supporting sleeve of connective tissue, or complete nerve disruption, which is rare in athletes.

The peripheral nerves in athletes can be injured by compression, tension (traction) or a combination of both. Acute compression nerve damage occurs when any heavy force compresses a nerve against an unyielding structure, e.g. ulnar compression at the wrist of bicyclists. Chronic nerve compression, which can cause irreversible damage, and nerve fibrosis can occur in the wrist in the form of carpal tunnel syndrome.

Peripheral nerves are also susceptible to stretch injury. Nerves may stretch up to 20% before damage occurs. Valgus extension overload during serving, as well as pitching, creates significant tensile overload on the medial elbow ligament structures, and compressive loads laterally. The ulnar nerve can elongate 4.7 mm during extension to full flexion. It can be moved 7 mm medially by the triceps. These tensile loads also affect the ulnar nerve as it crosses through the cubital tunnel, causing nerve irritation and compression. The nerve may become unstable as the elbow is flexed.

Ulnar nerve entrapment can be found in 60% of surgical cases of medial tennis elbow. These entrapments are found distal to the medial epicondyle at the medial and muscular septum, as a nerve enters the flexor carpi ulnaris. The nerve entrapment may be secondary to elbow instability, spurs, synovitis and more proximal compression.

Symptoms

The symptoms are often pain or numbness down into the little finger region, i.e. ulnar nerve innervated regions. The diagnosis is set by history and palpation tenderness over the medial epicondyle, or just posterior of the medial epicondyle, as well as pain on palmar flexion of the wrist against resistance.

Treatment

The treatment consists of rest, ice and immobilization in the acute phase. Anti-inflammatory medication can be of value. Strengthening and stretching programmes should start as early as possible. In a chronic phase, the nerve can be treated surgically with transposition (moving) of the nerve beneath the flexors and decompression for at least 5 cm distal to the epicondyle.

Ulnar nerve problems are in the author's opinion probably more common in tennis than earlier observed. Damage to this nerve should be suspected in tennis players with long-lasting elbow problems on the medial side.

Osteochondritis dissecans (loose pieces of bone–cartilage)

Osteochondritis dissecans (OCD) is an injury to the articular cartilage and the bone. It usually occurs on the anterolateral surface of the capitellum (lateral elbow) because of the compression secondary to the valgus stress. An osteochondritis dissecans occurs most commonly in men in their second decade.

This injury causes pain and limitation of extension, swelling and locking. A reattaching or excision of the fragmented portion of the capitellum and drilling of the base of the lesion to help the bleeding bone give satisfactory results and can be performed through the arthroscope.

Loose fragments can also occur, often secondary to osteochondritis dissecans. They can also be composed of cartilaginous or fibrous tissue. These loose bodies can be removed through arthroscopy.

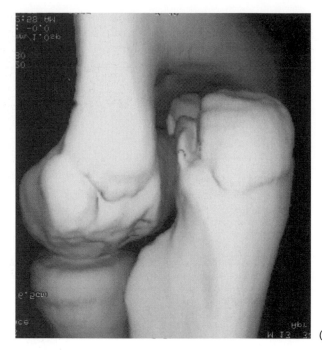

(a)

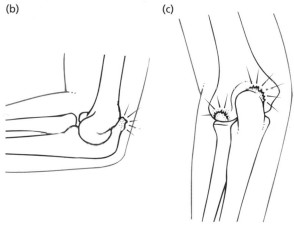

(b)   (c)

Fig. 19.8 The hyperextension during the serve can cause compression of the olecranon against the humerus and form bone spurs and loose bodies. (a) CT scan of posterior elbow; (b,c) formation of osteophytes, posterior or medial to the olecranon tip. (From Peterson, L. & Renström, P. (2000) *Sport Injuries: Their Prevention and Treatment*, p. 174. Martin Dunitz, London.)

Posterior tennis elbow

During the serve motion there may be an aggressive elbow extension during the follow-through phase (Fig. 19.8). The olecranon can impinge with the

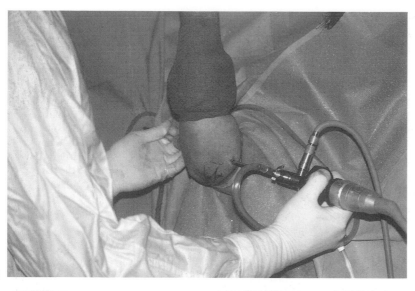

(a)

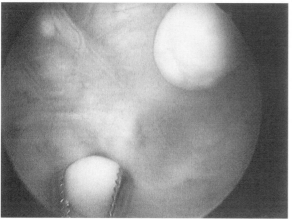

(b)

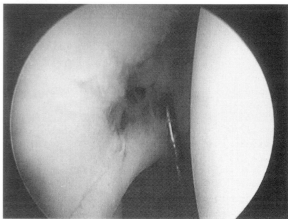

(c)

Fig. 19.9 (a) Arthroscopy of the elbow with (b) removal of loose bodies. (c) Articular cartilage damage at the lateral aspect of the elbow.

posterior aspect of the humerus and cause problems with posterior elbow pain on extension. Triceps tendinosis can occur. Osteophytes can form on the olecranon by forced hyperextension of the olecranon into the olecranon fossa, or by shear forces between the olecranon and the olecranon fossa secondary to the valgus movement placed on the elbow during the serve (Fig. 19.8).

The pathology of the posterior compartment can be evaluated through arthroscopy with a posterior lateral portal (Fig. 19.9). The osteophytes or loose bodies are usually located on the posterior medial aspect of the olecranon. The treatment is usually conservative, but occasionally surgery is needed.

Conclusions

Elbow injuries in tennis players are common. When they occur they are often of overuse character and can often be chronic and give long-lasting problems.

The most common injury is the so-called tennis elbow, which remains an enigma and a great clinical problem as still little is known about its pathophysiology and aetiology. It seems that a tennis player's chance of eventually getting a tennis elbow is more than one in two, and this means that more focus should be directed towards prevention. It appears that the type of racket grip, and so on, are not important in producing tennis elbow, but these factors are probably important in the rehabilitation after tennis elbow and to avoid reinjury. Factors such as using gut string, low string tension, light balls and pain-free strokes may allow return to competitive tennis earlier. The natural history for tennis elbow is good and most patients will get better regardless of treatment used. Exercises that promote healing, and a forearm brace are key factors in the treatments and return to tennis. The healing time of overuse syndromes in the elbow is long. Tennis elbow may cause pain for between 1 week and 18 months with a mean of about 36 weeks. Because of the long treatment time and limited treatment alternatives, these problems continue to be frustrating for both the patient and the doctor. The key to successful treatment is also a correct diagnosis and therefore the treating doctor must be aware of the available differential diagnosis.

References

Bernhang, A.M., Dehner, W. & Fogarty, C. (1974) Tennis elbow: a biomechanical approach. *American Journal of Sports Medicine* **2**, 235–260.

Brody, H. (1987) *Tennis Science for Tennis Players*. University of Pennsylvania Press, Philadelphia, PA.

Hang, Y.S. & Peng, S.M. (1984) An epidemiologic study of upper extremity injury in tennis players with a particular reference to tennis elbow. *Journal of the Formosan Medical Association* **83**, 307–315.

Kamien, M. (1989) The incidence of tennis elbow and other injuries in tennis players at the Royal Kings Park Tennis Club of Western Australia from October 1983 to September 1984. *Australian Journal of Science and Medicine in Sports* **21**, 18–22.

Nirschl, R.P. (1992) Elbow tendinosis/tennis elbow. *Clinics in Sports Medicine* **11**, 851–870.

Priest, J.D., Braden, V. & Gerberich, S.G. (1980) The elbow and tennis, part 2: a study of players with pain. *The Physician and Sportsmedicine* **8**, 77–84.

Runge, F. (1873) Zur genese und behandlung des schreibekrampfes. *Berliner Klinische Wochenschrift* **10**, 245–248.

Snyder-Mackler, L. & Epler, M. (1989) Effect of standard and Aircast tennis elbow bands on integrated electromyography of forearm extensor musculature proximal to the bands. *American Journal of Sports Medicine* **17**, 278–281.

Recommended reading

Boddeker, I. & Haake, M. (2000) Extracorporeal shockwave therapy in treatment of epicondylitis humeri radialis. A current overview. *Orthopäde* **29**, 463–469.

Boyer, M.I. & Hastings, H. II (1999) Lateral tennis elbow: 'is there any science out there?'. *Journal of Shoulder and Elbow Surgery* **8**, 481–491.

Groppel, J. & Nirschl, R.P. (1986) A mechanical and electromyographical analysis of the effects of various joint counterforce braces on the tennis player. *American Journal of Sports Medicine* **14**, 195–200.

Haker, E. & Lundeberg, T. (1990) Acupuncture treatment in epicondylalgia: a comparative study of two acupuncture techniques. *Clinical Journal of Pain* **6**, 221–226.

Khan, K.M., Cook, J.L., Bonar, F., Harcourt, P. & Astrom, M. (1999) Histopathology of common tendinopathies. Update and implications for clinical management. *Sports Medicine* **27**, 393–408.

Kraushaar, B.S. & Nirschl, R.P. (1999) Tendinosis of the elbow (tennis elbow). Clinical features and findings of histological, immunohistochemical, and electron microscopy studies. *Journal of Bone and Joint Surgery of America* **81**, 259–278.

Sevier, T.L. & Wilson, J.K. (1999) Treating lateral epicondylitis. *Sports Medicine* **28**, 375–380.

Chapter 20

Shoulder injuries in tennis

Shoulder injuries in tennis players are not uncommon. Fortunately, the majority are easily reversible and resolve with simple treatments such as diminution of playing time and gentle exercise. However, even benign injuries can become complex if neglected. In these situations muscle atrophy occurs, tendon or ligament injury progression occurs, and the athlete begins a process of maladaptation to the injury. Maladaptation refers to the change in stroke production that occurs in the tennis athlete who tries to 'play through' a shoulder injury. We have found that this type of reaction to shoulder injury is more common in tennis than other overhead sports, such as baseball and volleyball. There appear to be two reasons for this. First, tennis is an individual sport making time away for treatment of injury costly in the case of the professional. Secondly, and perhaps more significantly, is the nature of the game, which, with its large number of stroke types and multiple strategic options, allows room for changes in the way an individual plays the game. These changes, or adaptations, permit the player with an injured shoulder to continue to participate. Over time, however, these changes often become maladaptive as they diminish the player's performance level and eventually worsen the original injury.

The common denominator of all tennis shoulder injuries is repetitive microtrauma with gradual tissue failure. The three areas of frequent injury are tendon, ligament and labrum. Two other possible sites of injury are bone and articular cartilage. Probably the most important determinant of injury is the player's age. Tennis, alongside golf, is a sport that spans an enormous age range. For the sake of this discussion we will divide the players into three age groups: adolescent, adult and senior. In addition there are, to some degree, injury differences that occur between players of different skill levels. These differences will be discussed within each age group.

The goals of this chapter are to familiarize the reader with the spectrum of shoulder injuries seen in tennis players, to improve the reader's understanding of the causes of these injuries, to help the reader learn methods of injury prevention, and finally, how to treat these injuries.

Pathophysiology

Shoulder injuries are not uncommon in overhead athletes. When compared to other overhead sports there are several features that are unique to tennis. First and perhaps most importantly, is the length of time needed to establish an appropriate skill level and the length of time needed to complete a match. Of the five tennis strokes (forehand, backhand, volley, overhead and serve), clearly the groundstrokes are the most frequently struck. These are generally considered to be less likely to cause shoulder injury than the serve and overhead. Due to the frequency and violence with which they are struck, they contribute to fatigue of the shoulder girdle musculature.

Stability of the glenohumeral joint relies on two systems: the static and dynamic stabilizers. The static stabilizers consist of the bony architecture, the articular cartilage, and the glenoid labrum and glenohumeral ligaments. The dynamic stabilizers are the deltoid, rotator cuff, biceps, latissimus and scapular musculature. These systems interact in a complex fashion to centre the humeral head on the glenoid during shoulder motion. Fatigue of, or injury to, a portion of this system places excessive load on the other uninjured segments increasing their risk of injury over time. In cases of microtraumatic injury to the shoulder it is not uncommon then to find multiple sites of injury or deficiency.

As stated previously, most shoulder injuries in tennis players begin insidiously as simple tissue fatigue, most often of the muscular type. A classic example is an injury to the rotator cuff. When the muscular function of the rotator cuff weakens, the deltoid relatively overpowers the rotator cuff and the humeral head migrates superiorly on the glenoid during active overhead elevation of the arm. If left untreated, eventually the tendon of the rotator cuff will begin to rub on the undersurface of the coracoacromial arch

(Deutsch *et al.* 1997). In turn, this 'impingement' of the rotator cuff tendon further weakens the rotator cuff, whose function then further deteriorates. As the impingement worsens, structural changes can take place in both the tendon and coracoacromial arch that may ultimately require surgical correction. This example points out that what begins as a simple case of muscular overload, if neglected, can result in serious injury.

A similar mechanism is responsible for the development of glenohumeral instability in the tennis athlete. The tennis player over time often develops stretching of the anterior capsular ligaments. This can allow a pathological increase in glenohumeral translation, which in turn increases the stress on both the glenoid labrum and rotator cuff. Over time this can result in tearing of the labrum and degeneration or tearing of the undersurface of the rotator cuff.

Shoulder injury in the adolescent tennis player

Adolescent refers to ages 11–16, 16 being a typical age by which skeletal maturity is reached. Although muscular and tendon injuries are rare in the adolescent they do occasionally occur. These injuries are typically self-limited and reversible with simple rest.

Epiphyseal injury

If the player complains of disabling shoulder pain refractory to rest, the physician should consider the possibility of injury to the proximal humeral epiphysis (growth plate). The player typically complains of chronic anterolateral shoulder pain of insidious onset. Physical examination demonstrates a full range of motion without bursal crepitation. Pain is reproduced by rotator cuff resistance. Typical impingement signs do not reproduce pain. The key to the diagnosis is the anteroposterior radiograph, which demonstrates widening of the humeral physis. To avoid confusion a comparison radiograph should be made of the contralateral shoulder.

Treatment

This injury is treated by rest from all pain-producing activities. The period of time typically required is 6 weeks. During this interval the player should work

on exercises that promote aerobic conditioning, trunk strength and leg strength. Healing is confirmed by complete absence of symptoms; radiographic evidence of healing typically lags behind and therefore is not a reliable sign.

Instability

The second disabling problem encountered in the shoulder of adolescents is instability. It has been shown that shoulder laxity peaks in adolescence (Emery & Mullaji 1991). In some sporting adolescents who participate in overhead sports, symptomatic shoulder instability can develop on the basis of capsular laxity, without any discrete trauma. This occurrence is more common in girls than boys (Emery & Mullaji 1991). The player will usually complain that the shoulder slips in and out on occasion while serving or while hitting an overhead. Rarely do individuals with this type of instability have frank dislocations requiring manipulative reductions.

Physical examination of adolescent tennis players complaining of shoulder subluxation usually reveals evidence of generalized ligamentous laxity. This laxity can be demonstrated by hyperextension of the hand metacarpophalangeal (MCP) joints, hyperextension of the elbow and an ability to touch the thumb to the forearm. The shoulder examination demonstrates multidirectional laxity, while apprehension signs, which are typically present in patients with traumatic instability, are notably absent.

Treatment

The cornerstone of treatment for this type of shoulder instability in adolescent tennis players is strengthening of the dynamic stabilizers. Over time this gradual increase in shoulder girdle, rotator cuff strength and endurance should allow the player to compensate for the excessive laxity present. The ultimate prognosis for this condition is good. Shoulder laxity decreases with age, usually resulting in resolution of instability symptoms (Emery & Mullaji 1991).

Shoulder injury in adult tennis players

Adulthood is defined by skeletal maturity, reached from 15–17 years of age in most individuals. The shoulder injuries in this age category involve the rotator cuff, capsular ligaments and labrum. Only rarely in this group are the bony elements or articular cartilage involved.

Rotator cuff injuries

The term 'rotator cuff injury' encompasses a broad range of injuries ranging from minor strains to complete tears of the rotator cuff tendon. The diagnosis of rotator cuff injury can usually be made by history and physical examination, but imaging studies may be necessary to stage the degree of injury.

The rotator cuff refers to a group of muscle tendon units divided into four segments. The largest is the subscapularis, which travels from the anterior portion of the scapula to insert on the lesser tuberosity of the humerus. The subscapularis functions generally to stabilize the humeral head in the glenoid fossa. Specifically the subscapularis helps to accelerate the arm in internal rotation and to add anterior stability during the cocking phase of serving. The subscapularis is innervated by the subscapular nerves in which injuries have not been reported in tennis players. Unlike the other tendons of the rotator cuff, the subscapularis is rarely injured from repetitive microtrauma. The usual causes of injury are violent trauma in a position of humeral external rotation or, more commonly, degeneration due to ageing. In fact, subscapularis injuries are rare in the adult player and will be discussed in the section on senior tennis players.

The supraspinatus, infraspinatus and teres minor originate from the posterior portion of the scapula and insert via a common tendon onto the greater tuberosity of the humerus. These tendons function to stabilize the humeral head into the glenoid fossa, to assist in arm elevation, and to externally rotate the humerus. The supraspinatus and infraspinatus are innervated by the suprascapular nerve while the teres minor is innervated by a branch of the axillary nerve.

Symptoms

The most common complaint of players with rotator cuff injury is pain. The location of the pain may be anterolateral, lateral or posterior. In general the location of the symptoms corresponds to the location

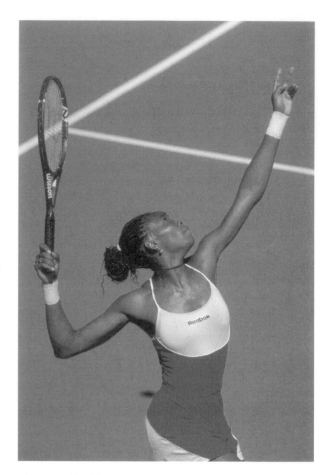

Fig. 20.1 Shoulder injuries commonly occur during the service action. Photo © Allsport/C. Brunskill.

of the tendon injury. Anterior pain stems from the subscapularis or anterior supraspinatus; lateral pain stems from the supraspinatus or anterior infraspinatus; posterior pain stems from the infraspinatus or teres minor. The pain typically is intermittent but is most often present during the serve (Fig. 20.1), when lifting objects overhead, and at night when attempting to sleep. Surprisingly, groundstrokes, particularly when struck with the proper mechanics, are often not painful unless severe injury is present. Tennis players will frequently note that moderate use makes the shoulder feel better. However, vigorous use causes pain and the pain is often present after use.

In addition to pain, tennis players with rotator cuff injuries will complain of weakness and clicking. The weakness is often pronounced on certain activities such as the backhand and backhand volley. Players with one-handed backhands often complain of a loss of power on that stroke. The clicking sensation is often non-specific and is due to either a thickened bursa or torn tendon end.

Physical examination of players with suspected rotator cuff injury should begin with inspection. In particular the examiner should focus on the infra-spinatus fossa. Atrophy in this zone in the young adult suggests suprascapular neuropathy (nerve injury), which is surprisingly common in elite players.

After a thorough inspection of the affected shoulder, the examiner palpates for tenderness. Particular attention is paid to the acromioclavicular (A-C) joint, acromion and the tuberosity insertion of the rotator cuff. If A-C joint tenderness is present, the examiner should adduct the arm to see if this manual com-pression of the A-C joint reproduces the pain at the joint. Adding downward pressure on the arm in the horizontally adducted position will maximize the pressure on the A-C joint and increase any potential symptoms (O'Brien *et al.* 1998).

Acromial tenderness is not common, and its presence should suggest a possible os acromiale (unfused acromial epiphysis—growth plate), and radiographic corroboration is needed.

With the examiner standing behind the player, active range of motion is assessed in both shoulders. The examiner should evaluate the scapular rhythm. Possible abnormalities include shrugging (excessive scapular elevation), which is usually due to weakness of the scapular stabilizers. Passive motion is assessed in all planes: forward flexion, abduction, external and internal humeral rotation both with the arm at the side and abducted to 90°. The non-dominant arm in most instances is used as the control.

Differences between both active and passive motion in the affected shoulder as well as between the affected and non-dominant shoulder should be noted. Numerous studies have documented that the dominant shoulder in tennis players will exhibit a loss of internal rotation and increase in external rotation when compared with the non-dominant side. Symptomatic shoulders with rotator cuff injuries, in our experience, often demonstrate further limita-tion of internal rotation. This is known to be an adaptive change that occurs, but it is not known whether this is a pathological or healthy adaptation

(Chandler *et al.* 1990). It is recognized that tightness of the posterior capsule and posterior cuff muscles will have profound effects on glenohumeral translation. Individuals with such contractures will demonstrate increased anterosuperior humeral head translation during arm elevation. In theory this would increase the strain on the anterior labrum and anterior capsule, possibly predisposing the individual to anterior instability. Rotation, both internal and external should be checked both with the arm adducted and abducted to 90°.

The rotator cuff is directly assessed by testing for impingement in the overhead position and by testing rotator cuff strength. If these manoeuvres reproduce the player's symptoms then rotator cuff injury is likely to be present.

In players less than 30 years of age, rotator cuff injury is often associated with injury to the capsular ligaments and the glenoid labrum. The physical examination findings of these problems will be dis-cussed below.

Radiographs of the shoulder should be obtained. In players less than 30 years of age, bony abnormal-ities associated with rotator cuff disease are rare. In older players, abnormalities of the acromion can occur, with spur formation at the anterior margin. Magnetic resonance imaging (MRI) is useful to stage the degree of tendon injury. Injury ranges from intrasubstance tearing or degeneration, partial tear on the articular or bursal side, to full-thickness tears of the tendon.

Treatment

Treatment of rotator cuff injury, of course, depends on the exact injury. Although in non-active indi-viduals such injuries may be tolerated with minimal treatment, the high demands on the shoulder often require the tennis player to undergo extensive treatment.

Two principles lie at the core of all treatment plans. The first is to reduce pain. This is accomplished with non-steroidal anti-inflammatory agents, ice and a reduc-tion in overhead activity. The second is muscular rehabilitation. There are several components to this. The first is to strengthen the scapular stabilizers. Weakness of these muscles may precede the rotator cuff injury rendering the shoulder more vulnerable

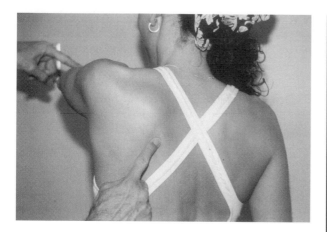

Fig. 20.2 Photo demonstrating scapular muscles essential for scapular stabilization.

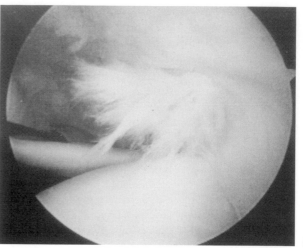

(a)

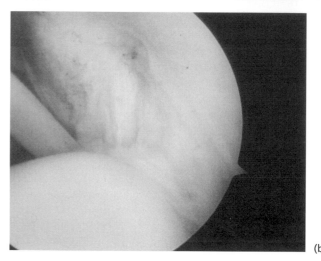

(b)

Fig. 20.3 (a) Intraoperative photo of a partial undersurface rotator cuff tear. (b) Partial rotator cuff tear after operative debridement.

(Fig. 20.2). Scapular weakness may also occur as the result of the rotator cuff injury due to involuntary or voluntary splinting. Scapular strengthening is easily performed with the player using elastic tubing.

The second component of the programme involves direct strengthening of the rotator cuff in external rotation and abduction. This should be performed using only light resistance, being careful to avoid pain. If possible these exercises are progressed gradually until the player can resume practising. A time frame for a successful conservative programme is approximately 3 months. Return to competitive play can take up to 6 months with a proper rehabilitation programme.

Surgical treatment

If the rehabilitation programme fails and the player wishes to return to tennis, a surgical approach may be taken. The surgery is performed under scalene block anaesthesia. The shoulder is examined for evidence of instability. A complete diagnostic arthroscopy of the intra-articular and subacromial spaces is performed. For younger players with intrasubstance tears or partial tears, a debridement of visibly torn rotator tissue is performed (Fig. 20.3). The remaining tendon is then carefully examined. If the depth of the tear is judged to be less than 50%, debridement alone is performed. If the tear depth exceeds 50% in young

players, a repair is performed (repair technique will be discussed below). Any concurrent labral lesions if frayed are debrided, or repaired if detached. The capsular ligaments are examined for tearing or stretching. If instability exists on examination under anaesthesia and ligamentous attentuation is determined arthroscopically, an instability repair is performed (see instability section below).

The subacromial space is evaluated for the presence or absence of bursal hypertrophy. All abnormally

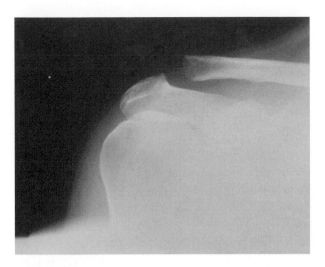

Fig. 20.4 Postoperative radiograph of a distal clavicle resection.

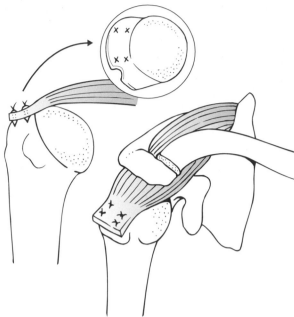

Fig. 20.5 The mini-open rotator cuff repair technique.

thickened bursal tissue is debrided. The superior rotator cuff surface is then examined for tears. As stated previously, minor (<50%) tears are debrided while major (>50%) tears are repaired.

Finally, the coracoacromial arch is evaluated. If narrowing of the anterior outlet of the subacromial space has occurred by soft-tissue hypertrophy usually involving the coracoacromial ligament, the ligament is debrided. If the acromial bone has hypertrophied and is contributing to the outlet impingement, an acromioplasty is arthroscopically performed.

The A-C joint is entered only in cases where large spurs are present on the undersurface of the distal clavicle, adding to the outlet impingement or when the player has distinct pain at the A-C joint. If spurs are present but no A-C joint pain or tenderness can be elicited preoperatively, only the inferior spurs are removed. In cases of a painful A-C joint reproduced by adduction manoeuvres, the distal clavicle is excised arthroscopically. Distal clavicular bone removal is performed so that the A-C joint space is at least 12 mm wide (Fig. 20.4).

Rotator cuff repair is performed using a 'mini-open' technique (Blevins *et al*. 1996). This allows an ideal combination of minimal trauma and maximal stabilization of the torn tendon (Fig. 20.5).

Postoperative rehabilitation follows similar guidelines to the conservative programme. The initial goals are to minimize pain and swelling and to prevent the formation of adhesions. The second phase of rehabilitation works to restore active motion, the third phase to restore balanced shoulder girdle strength while the fourth phase emphasizes return to play activities such as plyometrics. Throughout the entire duration of the rehabilitation protocol an effort is made to maintain cardiovascular fitness as well as lower body and trunk strength.

Suprascapular neuropathy (nerve injury)

This unusual injury is known to be caused by two mechanisms. The most common is traction neuropathy. The second cause is a ganglionic cyst (sac with viscous fluid), which occurs in or around the suprascapular notch. The cause of these cysts is not precisely known but may on occasion be associated with tears of the superior labrum (Fig. 20.6).

All players with suprascapular neuropathy present with posterior pain in the region of the scapula. The pain subsides over a period of 1–2 weeks and the player notices shoulder weakness and the onset of infraspinatus atrophy (decreased muscle volume).

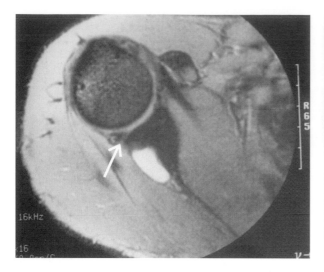

Fig. 20.6 Magnetic resonance image demonstrating a labral tear (arrow) with a glenoid cyst (white tissue).

Treatment

Controversy exists over the management of chronic cases of suprascapular neuropathy. Most experienced authors agree that when the lesion has been present for greater than 6 months, operative measures are unlikely to succeed (Martin *et al.* 1993).

When acute, our experience suggests that significant improvement in rotator cuff strength can be made if operative treatment is instituted. If a ganglionic cyst is present, the shoulder should be arthroscoped to evaluate the superior labrum. If a labral detachment is present, this is repaired arthroscopically using a device to repair the labrum to the surgically abraded humeral neck.

Once evaluation and/or labral surgery is completed, the surgeon must decide whether the ganglion projects close enough to the capsule so that it is accessible arthroscopically. In these cases the capsule (usually posterosuperior) is incised under arthroscopic vision and the cyst is entered and decompressed into the joint. The surgeon must confirm that the typical 'yellowish mucoid' cyst fluid is visualized. With the arthroscope, the surgeon can generally enter the cyst to break up any locculations.

If the cyst cannot be entered arthroscopically or if no cyst is present and the surgeon wishes to decompress the nerve at the suprascapular notch, an open procedure is employed.

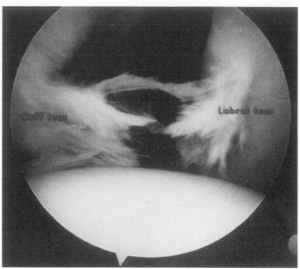

Fig. 20.7 An intraoperative photo of the lesion of internal impingement showing a partial tear of the rotator cuff (left) and tear of the posterior labrum (right).

Shoulder instability including labral tears

Shoulder instability is defined as shoulder dysfunction due to a pathological increase in glenohumeral translation due to injury. The dysfunction may manifest itself as pain, weakness, dead arm syndrome or, if severe, frank instability. The injury is often microtraumatic but may be the result of a single traumatic event.

The diagnosis of shoulder instability is made through a combination of history, physical examination and imaging studies. The examiner should enquire as to which motion and arm positions in particular reproduce the player's symptoms. The acceleration phase of serving is typically symptomatic in players with anterior instability, while the follow-through phase is typically symptomatic in players with posterior labral tears or posterior instability. Internal impingement, which is due to a collision of the posterior rotator cuff and posterosuperior labrum, typically produces posterior pain at the joint line during the maximal cocking phase of serving (Fig. 20.7).

The player should be specifically asked if he or she senses the shoulder coming apart, a 'dead arm', or frank instability. However, the examiner should be aware that the most common complaint among this group of patients is simply shoulder pain.

Physical examination

Physical examination should include, as aforementioned, inspection for atrophy, observation of active and passive motion, and tests for rotator cuff integrity. Again, it is not uncommon for the rotator cuff to suffer injury along with the capsular ligaments and labrum. Instability and labral specific tests are performed as described.

First an assessment is made of the overall laxity of the patient by checking for thumb hyperextension, elbow hyperextension and thumb to forearm distance. Shoulder laxity is determined in three planes: inferior, anterior and posterior, and in two positions: that of adduction and 90° of abduction. Inferior testing is performed first in adduction by pulling the humerus downward. The amount of inferior displacement is reflected by the size of 'sulcus' that appears below the lateral margin of the acromion (Fig. 20.8). A large sulcus is considered to be greater than 2 cm. Anteroposterior testing in adduction is performed by shifting the humeral head in both directions. This test is often unrevealing.

Anterior and posterior testing is performed more precisely in the functional position of 90° of abduction. With the player supine, the examiner kneels behind and grasps the humerus with both hands, at the elbow and proximally. The humerus is maintained in neutral rotation and in the scapular plane while the proximal hand shifts the humerus anteriorly and posteriorly. The examiner must judge what displacement occurs relative to the glenoid: 1+ onto the glenoid rim, 2+ over the glenoid rim, 3+ completely dislocated (able to be locked) over the glenoid rim. The examiner should also be aware of whether this specifically reproduces the player's symptoms, causes grinding or pain.

While in this position two other tests are performed. The apprehension test is performed anteriorly by maximally abducting and externally rotating the humerus. In addition, the examiner adds an 'anterior' load by pushing the humeral head anteriorly. Players with moderate to severe anterior instability will complain of apprehension to instability in this position. The relocation test evaluates for internal impingement and mild anterior instability (Jobe *et al.* 1989). To perform the relocation test, the examiner simply 'relocates' the humeral head from the apprehension position by placing a posteriorly directed force with

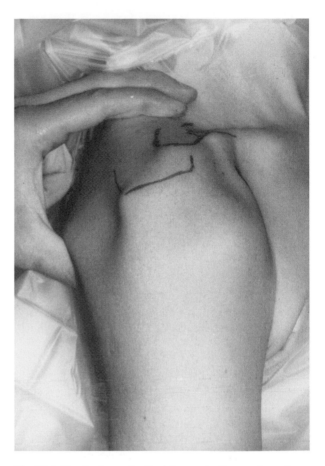

Fig. 20.8 Physical examination demonstrating a sulcus sign.

his or her hand on the anterior aspect of the proximal humerus. If this relieves the symptoms of posterior joint line pain, then it is likely that the player has internal impingement. If apprehension is relieved, it is likely the player has anterior instability.

Plain radiographs are often normal in this group of athletes with shoulder instability. Rarely will there be a glenoid erosion, bony Bankart lesion or humeral defect (Hill–Sachs lesion).

MRI scanning is useful for large labral tears, labral avulsion and associated partial thickness rotator cuff tears (Fig. 20.9).

Conservative treatment

The cornerstone of treatment of shoulder instability is rehabilitation. The essence of the rehabilitation programme is to develop the proprioceptive and

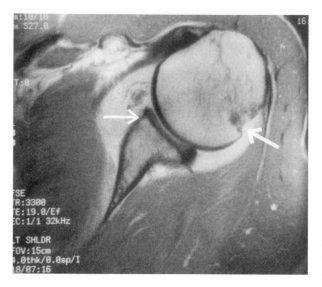

Fig. 20.9 Axial magnetic resonance image status post anterior instability demonstrating posterior Hill–Sachs lesion (thick arrow) and anterior Bankart lesion (thin arrow).

muscular symptoms to compensate for the injuries present. This approach is based on the concept that injury to the stabilizing structures (the rotator cuff, the labrum and the capsular ligaments) will result in a pathological increase in glenohumeral translation, i.e. shoulder instability. The goal of the rehabilitation is to develop the athlete's shoulder girdle musculature to allow him or her to compensate. The parameters are that this process will take time and will require a skilled and knowledgeable therapist.

Surgical treatment

Surgical treatment is reserved for athletes who have failed conservative treatment. The surgeon must identify the following factors in choosing the proper candidates for surgery:
• the athlete's symptoms have not been reduced by conservative treatment to the degree that he or she can compete at the necessary level;
• the surgeon can identify by perioperative testing that a lesion or lesions are present which the surgeon feels are repairable;
• the surgeon is confident that the athlete can attempt a painful, lengthy and intermittently discouraging recovery process;

• the surgeon is confident that the surgical trauma required to 'fix' the problem can be minimized to the degree such that the chances of recovery are maximized.

Surgical procedure

Anaesthesia is generally intrascalene block. The first step in the surgical procedure is a thorough examination under anaesthesia. This is performed in the same position as the preoperative stability examination. The data from this is a crucial step in deciding what the surgical procedure will be.

The goal of surgery in the tennis player is to affect repair of the labrum, capsule and rotator cuff such that, with extensive strengthening, the athlete can return to sports at the preinjury level. This represents a true challenge for the surgeon and the athlete.

In the case of the tennis player the final surgical plan is made after the examination under anaesthesia and the diagnostic arthroscopy. This information is combined with the data from the history and awake physical examination. Factors, that are weighted particularly, are: (i) does the athlete complain of a distinct sense of subluxation? If this is present the surgical procedure will usually require labral repair, capsular tightening or both; (ii) does the athlete have distinct, persistent rotator cuff weakness on examination with MRI evidence of a significant (50% thickness) rotator cuff tear? This situation will usually require direct repair of the rotator cuff.

The surgical procedure is begun after a complete examination under anaesthesia. The glenohumeral stability is assessed in inferior, anterior and posterior directions replicating the awake stability examination. 'Normal' stability for a tennis player athlete will demonstrate a 2+ posterior laxity and 1+ anterior laxity with a 1–2+ sulcus. Laxity of 3+ in the posterior direction or 2+ or greater in the anterior direction should raise suspicion that capsulolabral repair will be required.

Diagnostic arthroscopy is then performed in the beach-chair position (Skyhar *et al.* 1988). Beginning with the arthroscope in the posterior portal the surgeon visualizes the biceps and biceps anchor. This area of the labrum is often meniscoid in shape and can have a recessed attachment at the supraglenoid tubercle.

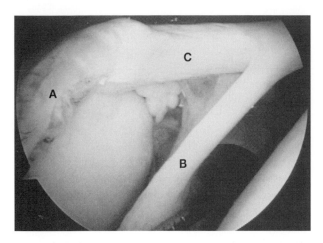

Fig. 20.10 Intraoperative photo of a SLAP tear of the superior labrum which extends into the biceps tendon: A, superior labrum; B, split fragment of the biceps and labrum; C, biceps tendon.

Next the anterosuperior labrum is visualized (Fig. 20.10). This area is important from a stability point of view because it represents the attachment site of the superior and middle glenohumeral ligaments. Confusion can arise due to the variations of ligament attachment and labral morphology in this region. Two important variations exist. The first is a 'band-like' middle glenohumeral ligament, which is usually accompanied by a complete absence of anterosuperior labral tissue. The second is a 'sublabral hole'—a defect in the anterosuperior labrum occurring below the attachment site of the middle glenohumeral ligament. In both of these cases it is important to recognize the difference between these normal variants and injury. As in the prior case, labral detachment usually has accompanying distinct evidence of injury such as fraying or tearing of the labrum. If 'repair' is performed without actual injury, i.e. in the case of normal variants, this will result in overtightening of the middle glenohumeral ligament and the athlete will lose glenohumeral external rotation.

Upon completing the evaluation of the anterosuperior labrum, the arthroscopic view is shifted inferiorly. The anteroinferior labrum has minimal variability. This portion of the labrum is normally attached securely to the glenoid margin. Any detachments in this region are pathological.

Evaluation of the integrity of the anterior portion of the inferior glenohumeral ligament is complex and somewhat subjective. Ideally the anterior band of this ligament as described by O'Brien *et al.* (1990) is a distinct, robust structure, which takes up tension quickly as the arm is externally rotated. As stretch injury occurs the anterior band loses a robust appearance and the ligament fails to tighten with external rotation. Warren has described the 'drive through' sign as a tool to evaluate the degree of ligament stretch (Warner & Warren 1991; Pagnani & Warren 1993). The inferior glenohumeral ligament must also be evaluated for the presence of tears, which are rare but do occur.

After completion of evaluation of the anterior labrum and capsule, attention is directed to the rotator cuff. While evaluating the anterior capsule, the superior tendon of the subscapularis is clearly evident. Injury to the subscapularis has rarely been reported in a young throwing athlete. Most injuries to the subscapularis that we have seen have been muscular 'sprains' rather than tendon tears.

The supraspinatus attachment to the tuberosity is visualized by placing the humerus in the plane of the scapula with distal traction. Undersurface tears are commonly seen and all frayed tissue must be thoroughly debrided to allow visualization of the remaining tendon. Conflicting data has been reported about the results of debridement (Andrews 1997; Payne *et al.* 1997). Tears greater than 50% of the thickness of the tendon should undergo repair to maximize the potential for symptom relief and return to function.

Once the supraspinatus has been evaluated, the arthroscope is switched to an anterior portal and the infraspinatus tendon and posterior labrum are evaluated. A not infrequent injury encountered in this region is that of internal impingement. This is evidenced by partial tearing of the infraspinatus and fraying without detachment of the posterosuperior labrum (see Fig. 20.7). Again, debridement is performed to remove all frayed tissue to evaluate the integrity of the remaining tendon and labrum. In cases of internal impingement where posterior joint line pain is reproduced with the position of humeral abduction and external rotation, simple debridement is often adequate treatment unless coexistent anterior instability is present.

Posterior labral detachment is less common but can occur in conjunction with posterior instability. These lesions are present in the inferior half of the posterior labrum and are evident after probing.

The final step of the diagnostic arthroscopy is to evaluate the subacromial space. The bursa is pre-distended with adrenaline (epinephrine) solution from a lateral position ensuring that the needle is anterior enough to penetrate the subacromial bursa. The arthroscopic trocar is then placed from the posterior portal and should be felt to 'pop' through the posterior bursal wall. The status of the bursa is evaluated first. A normal bursa will be a large open space and the coracoacromial ligament will be clearly visible. If the bursa is abnormal, criss-crossing adhesions will be present, the tissue will be thickened and the coracoacromial ligament will usually not be visible. All abnormal bursal tissue is debrided with a full radius resector until the coracoacromial ligament and superior surface of the rotator cuff are clearly evident, which will demonstrate fraying and degeneration if impingement is present. In the young athlete, bony spurs on the acromion are rare. If the bursa is abnormal indicating the presence of subacromial impingement, the coracoacromial ligament should be carefully evaluated. In some athletes the ligament will hypertrophy and may contribute to impingement. In these cases partial, if not complete, debridement of the ligament is indicated (Bigliani *et al.* 1995).

Surgical procedure for instability in the tennis player

The following algorithm should guide the choice of surgical procedures.

Type I

Athlete complains of pain with no discernible symptoms of true instability.

I-A

Minor rotator cuff injury, subacromial bursitis with or without a thickened coracoacromial ligament. In this case minor 'dynamic' instability is occurring because of chronic rotator cuff dysfunction.

SURGICAL TREATMENT. Debridement of undersurface cuff tear and arthroscopic subacromial decompression.

I-B

Rotator cuff injury is severe (>50% of the tendon thickness); the anterior capsule and labrum are intact.

A mini-open repair is performed on the torn portion of the rotator cuff.

I-C: INTERNAL IMPINGEMENT

Athletes with posterior pain that is reproduced by the position of abduction and external rotation. Arthroscopy reveals the typical lesion of internal impingement.

I-D: SLAP LESION

Athletes with joint line pain (at the coracoid or posterior joint line) in association with an MRI confirms a SLAP lesion.

SURGICAL TREATMENT OF SLAP LESIONS. Surgical treatment involves debridement or repair of the labrum, depending upon whether the labrum is torn or detached. Labral repair is performed with an absorbable Suretac (Acufex Microsurgical Inc., Norwood, MA).

Type II

This group of athletes is felt to have anterior instability. Symptomatically they complain primarily of pain but may, if questioned, admit that the shoulder feels excessively loose, that the shoulder 'comes apart' during the acceleration phase of serving. Examination under anaesthesia reveals 2–3+ anterior laxity and arthroscopy reveals a loose anterior capsule with a large 'drive-through'.

II-A: CAPSULAR LAXITY WITHOUT ROTATOR CUFF TEAR

The surgeon's goal in this type of patient is to tighten the anterior capsule such that the humeral head remains centred on the glenoid during the act of serving (Figs 20.11 and 20.12). The difficulty facing the surgeon is that errors in capsular tensioning, even slight, lead to restriction of motion and can cause significant disability in the throwing athlete. This procedure has been used in a large series of competitive pitchers with results of 69% returning to prior level of play (Montgomery & Jobe 1994).

II-B: CAPSULAR LAXITY WITH ROTATOR CUFF TEAR

If the athlete demonstrates anterior instability on the basis of capsular laxity and a rotator cuff tear,

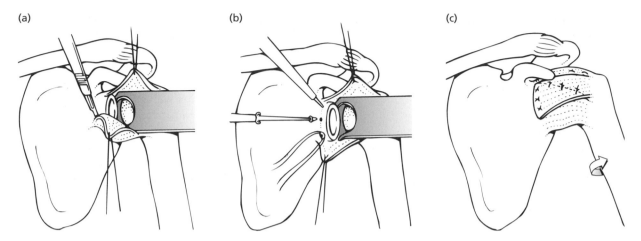

Fig. 20.11 Technique for capsulolabral reconstruction, particularly when marked anterior capsular laxity is present. (a) The capsule is incised horizontally and then (b) T'd along the vertical margin of the glenoid. (c) Labral repair can be performed where necessary and a large capsular shift can be performed along the glenoid neck.

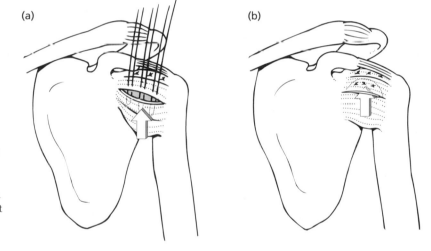

Fig. 20.12 A modification of the capsulolabral reconstruction, which utilizes only a horizontal incision. The labrum may be repaired at the medial aspect of the incision when necessary. The capsule is shifted in a north–south fashion, but the degree of capsular shift is more limited than in the previous procedure.

both issues must be addressed surgically. The rotator cuff is assessed as described previously in this chapter. If the tear is felt to extend greater than 50% of the tendon thickness, repair is performed as previously outlined using a mini-open approach. Concomitant subacromial decompression (removal of part of the acromion) is performed only if distinct arthroscopic evidence of subacromial impingement is present as previously described in this chapter. We have found that subacromial decompression is rarely

necessary in the group of patients who have distinct instability.

II-C: CAPSULAR TEAR WITH OR WITHOUT ROTATOR CUFF TEAR

Capsular tears can occur in tennis athletes but are not common. Such injuries usually involve the anterior portion of the inferior glenohumeral ligament. Conservative treatment does not ameliorate the symptoms and surgical repair is indicated for definitive treatment of this injury. Operative repair can be difficult particularly if the injury is chronic. Arthroscopy is used to confirm the injury.

Postoperative management

The first principle of postoperative management of the tennis player is restoration of motion. Although a sling may be used for protection, motion exercises must begin on postoperative day 1 and are progressed in a steady fashion. The exact details of each pro-gramme depend on the procedure performed. In general, basic motion, that is full forward flexion with 90° of external rotation, should be restored no later than 8 weeks postoperatively.

Strengthening begins with the scapular musculature and progresses to the rotator cuff muscles. Simul-taneously trunk, buttock and leg muscles groups are trained.

Hitting is begun when motion is full and muscle strength around the shoulder is at approximately 80% of normal. The hitting is progressed gradually over a period of months until the athlete is prepared to return to competitive tennis. The time frame for postoperative rehabilitation of a tennis player to full return is lengthy. We have found that 6 months of rehabilitation are needed for minor shoulder procedures and 12 months or more for major surgery, such as stabilization or rotator cuff repair.

Shoulder injuries in the senior tennis player

As is true of the older population in general, elderly tennis players more commonly develop symptoms related to rotator cuff injury. Underlying degenerat-ive disease of the glenohumeral or A-C joints can also cause symptoms primarily or can predispose to impingement symptoms. Management of impinge-ment symptoms involves pursuing standard rehabil-itative protocols. However, the increased functional demands of many of these patients often dictate a more aggressive approach to management. For middle-aged to elderly tennis players with impingement-related symptoms, a 6-week to 3-month period of rehabilita-tion is recommended, with the addition of a shoulder MRI for those patients who do not respond to this exercise regimen or in whom a rotator cuff tear is suspected. Also, for those players who do report a specific injury to the shoulder and in whom an MRI shows a rotator cuff tear, consideration should be given to early repair.

Elderly tennis players, although only rarely symptomatic from problems attributable to shoulder instability, are far more likely to experience symp-toms related to degenerative arthritis in the shoulder or A-C joint than are young adults. Treatment of symptoms due to these degenerative changes, such as stiffness and pain, is primarily accomplished through range of motion and strengthening exercises. Non-steroidal anti-inflammatory medications are generally reserved for patients with more significant disease or for patients who fail to respond to exercises alone. Arthroscopic debridement may help some patients with refractory pain. For cases of severe arthritis, total shoulder replacement is performed. Older patients with total shoulder arthroplasty can return to tennis.

Summary

Shoulder injury in the tennis player is unfortunately common. The most frequent cause is overuse. We believe that the best treatment is prevention in the form of proper preparation for play and moderation of playing time. Preparation for play should include a whole-body conditioning programme as well as thorough shoulder strengthening. Also players should be encouraged to seek professional advice on improv-ing stroke mechanics. It is clear that better mechanics may decrease the abnormal loads on the shoulder and help to prevent injury. If injury does occur, players should be encouraged to seek treatment and prevent the development of a chronic problem.

References

Andrews, J.R. (1997) Rotator cuff repairs in the throwing athlete. In: *AAOS Shoulder and Knee Course: The Athletic Perspective to Treatment, Controversies and Problem Solving*. Steamboat Springs, CO.

Bigliani, L.U., Rodsky, M.W., Newton, P.D. *et al.* (1995) Arthroscopic coracoacromial ligament resection for impingement in the overhead athlete. *Journal of Shoulder and Elbow Surgery* **4** (1), S54.

Blevins, F.T., Warren, R.F., Cavo, C. *et al.* (1996) Arthroscopic assisted rotator cuff repair. Results using a mini-open deltoid splitting approach. *Arthroscopy* **12** (1), 50–59.

Chandler, T.J., Kibler, W.B., Uhl, T.L. *et al.* (1990) Flexibility comparisions of junior elite tennis players to other athletes. *American Journal of Sports Medicine* **18**, 134.

Deutsch, A., Altchek, D.W., Veltri, D.M., Potter, H.G. & Warren, R.F. (1997) Traumatic tears of the subscapularis tendon. Clinical diagnosis, magnetic resonance imaging findings, and operative treatment. *American Journal of Sports Medicine* **25** (1), 13–22.

Emery, R.J.H. & Mullaji, A.B. (1991) Glenohumeral joint instability in normal adolescents. Incidence and significance. *Journal of Bone and Joint Surgery* **73B** (3), 406–408.

Jobe, F.W., Kvitne, R.S. & Giangarra, C.E. (1989) Shoulder pain in the overhand or throwing athlete. The relationship of anterior instability and rotator cuff impingement. *Orthopaedic Review* **18**, 963–975.

Martin, S.D., Warren, R.F., Guion, T.L. *et al.* (1993) Suprascapular neuropathy. A protocol of conservative treatment with selected late surgical decompression. *Journal of Shoulder and Elbow Surgery* **2** (1), S27.

Montgomery, W.H. III & Jobe, F.W. (1994) Functional outcomes in athletes after modified anterior capsulolabral reconstruction. *American Journal of Sports Medicine* **22**, 352–358.

O'Brien, S.J., Neves, M.C., Arnoczky, S.P. *et al.* (1990) The anatomy and histology of the inferior glenohumeral ligament complex of the shoulder. *American Journal of Sports Medicine* **18**, 449–456.

O'Brien, S.J., Pagnani, M.J., McGlynn, S.R., Fealy, S. & Wilson, J.B. (1998) The active compression test. A new and effective test for diagnosing labral tears and acromioclavicular joint pathology. *American Journal of Sports Medicine* **26** (5), 610–613.

Pagnani, M. & Warren, R. (1993) Arthroscopic shoulder stabilization. *Operative Techniques in Sports Medicine* **1**, 276–284.

Payne, L.Z., Altchek, D.W., Craig, E.V. & Warren, R.F. (1997) Arthroscopic treatment of partial rotator cuff tears in young athletes. A preliminary report. *American Journal of Sports Medicine* **25**, 299–305.

Skyhar, M.J., Altchek, D.W., Warren, R.F. *et al.* (1988) Shoulder arthroscopy with the patient in the beach-chair position. *Arthroscopy* **4**, 256–259.

Warner, J.J.P. & Warren, R.F. (1991) Arthroscopic Bankart repair using a cannulated absorbable fixation device. *Operative Techniques in Orthopaedic Surgery* **1**, 192–198.

Chapter 21

Rehabilitation principles

of injuries in tennis

Introduction

Adequate rehabilitation is the key to restoration of athletic function after tennis injury. Most of the common tennis injuries can be successfully treated by non-surgical means. In some athletes' and coaches' minds, this implies that little rehabilitation must be done. To the contrary, these injuries require precise rehabilitation due to the complexity of tennis demands and the many alterations that frequently exist due to the pathophysiology of microtrauma injuries, the most common type of injury in tennis.

This chapter will outline guidelines for efficacious rehabilitation of tennis-related injuries. It will emphasize the principles underlying the diagnosis and the practices implementing the principle, rather than detailed protocols for each injury. Several references are available for detailed protocols (Wilk 1994; Pink *et al.* 1996; Kibler *et al.* 1998). However, at the end of the chapter, protocols for shoulder and knee rehabilitation are presented as illustrative examples of the guidelines.

Guideline 1: Set up goals for rehabilitation

Principle

The goal of rehabilitation is to restore function to as near normal as possible. In tennis, due to the relatively mild nature of the injuries, normal function can often be achieved.

Practice

Rehabilitation must be carried out beyond the resolution of symptoms to the restoration of function. Optimum function occurs when normal anatomy is present, and normal physiological patterns and organization allows normal biomechanics. Rehabilitation is mostly knowing what normal physiology and biomechanics is required for each sport or activity, and then rehabilitating the entire body towards normal function.

Guideline 2: Make the complete and accurate diagnosis

Principle

Injuries create alterations in the normal functions of the shoulder, either due to the process of injury, or as a consequence of treatment. Most tennis injuries result from chronic repetitive microtrauma, in which a wide variety of tissue alterations can be seen. These include rotational inflexibilities, muscle tears, ligamentous damage, muscle strength imbalances and changes in biomechanical function. These can occur locally or at any point in the kinetic link activation sequence. Macrotrauma injuries, a one-time event, create alterations due to the injury and to treatment. These include fractures, ligament or muscle tears, and immobilization or surgical-related stiffness and muscle weakness.

From a rehabilitation standpoint, it is often more important to know the extent of the alterations in the tissues or in the biomechanics than to know a specific anatomy-based diagnosis. For example, the anatomical 'diagnosis' of shoulder impingement does not convey enough information to allow a successful rehabilitation programme. Because impingement is a clinical sign or symptom associated with many tissue alterations that may create the impingement syndrome, some of these alterations, such as glenohumeral instability, scapular dyskinesis or lumbar hyperlordosis, have little relationship to subacromial pathology.

In summary, the rehabilitation programme can only be as good as the diagnosis. Too often, diagnosis of shoulder injuries is incomplete due to the complexity of the factors that determine shoulder function.

Practice

The diagnosis must not only include the local anatomical deficit, such as rotator cuff tear, ankle sprain, ligament injury or fracture, but also the local

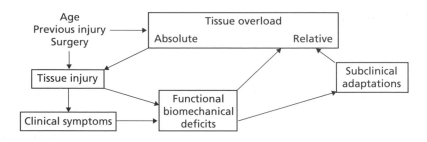

Fig. 21.1 The negative feedback vicious cycle.

biomechanical deficits that exist either as a result of the injury or as the result of treatment. These would include: inflexibility of shoulder internal or external rotation or adduction; force couple imbalance of the quadriceps/hamstrings or ankle dorsiflexors/plantar flexors; or acquired alterations in joint position such as dropping the arm in the throwing position because of impingement or not extending the knee in patellar tendinitis. In addition, the regional deficits that may occur around the joint must be evaluated. The acromioclavicular (A-C) joint can have sprains or instability in shoulder problems. Hip muscle strength may be weak in anterior knee pain patients, or shoulder rotation strength may be weak in elbow tendinitis patients. The scapula is a very important link in the shoulder joint function. The position, motion and strength of the scapula and its muscles should be evaluated. Whether or not there is any dyskinesis, winging, abnormal motion or decreased strength in the muscles should be considered in the diagnosis.

Finally, distant deficits should be evaluated as well. Back and hip inflexibility, injuries or strength imbalances should be evaluated. It is very common to see inflexibilities of hip rotation, hamstring flexibility or of back flexibility as contributors to shoulder pathology. In addition, alterations in mechanics, whether it be hyperlordosis of the back, lack of rotation of the hip or trunk, or alteration of the plant leg in throwing, need to be evaluated as well.

By making a complete and accurate diagnosis, we are utilizing the negative feedback vicious cycle (Fig. 21.1) to understand the clinical symptoms that are present and the tissues that are injured, the tissues that are overloaded, the functional biomechanical deficits that exist, and the subclinical adaptations that the athlete uses to try to maintain performance. Rehabilitation will require normalization of all of these components of the complete and accurate diagnosis.

Guideline 3: Completing all of the phases of rehabilitation

Principle

The phases of rehabilitation must match the biological stages of healing and the tissue's ability to accept loads to progress at optimal efficiency. Our functional rehabilitation programme is divided into three phases, each based on the resolution of certain aspects of the tissue injuries or alterations that exist in the tennis injury. These are specific goals, activity progressions and criteria for movement to the next phase. Because this is a function-based programme, all of the protocols tend to progress to some common end points in the later phases, regardless of the starting point.

Practice

The phases are the acute, recovery and functional phases.

Acute phase

The acute phase begins with the onset of clinical symptoms of injury or when the patient is seen for rehabilitation. This corresponds to the inflammatory phase of wound healing. Patient injuries will vary widely, from acute fracture or dislocation, to a postoperative repair, to an overload tendinitis. In each instance, attention will focus on resolving the clinical symptom and the tissue-injury complexes of the vicious cycle evaluation. This phase will be the most diverse because of the wide spectrum of clinical symptoms and tissue injuries, and the variety of treatments that are necessary. The objective of this phase is to create stable, healing tissues and improve joint health to allow more advanced rehabilitation. Early motion is allowed, but should be kept within pain-free limits. Modalities and medications are appropriate in this phase. Very little tensile load is applied to the healing tissues. However, maintenance of fitness in other parts of the athlete's body is continued.

Recovery phase

The recovery phase will continue rehabilitation of the tissue injury complex but will address the tissue overloads and functional biomechanical deficits. This phase corresponds to the proliferative phase of wound healing. Entry into this phase assumes that the injured tissues may be loaded in tension and compression so that normal strength and flexibility may be reached. Tensile loading, first in one plane, then in multiple planes, promotes collagen organization so that higher ultimate strength may be achieved. This phase is frequently the longest and most complex because of the large amount of work required to restore all of the alterations, both locally and distantly. Force couple restoration, full range of motion, joint stability and kinetic chain restoration are addressed in this phase. Normal physiological motor organization is achieved by this integration. By the end of this phase, most of the protocols will be merging towards the common goals of gaining full motion and muscular balance.

Functional phase

The functional phase will address any of the remaining functional biomechanical deficits, correct any subclinical adaptations that may have developed, and use functional progressions to return to play. This phase corresponds to the remodelling phase of wound repair. This is the final common pathway of all of the protocols. Plyometric exercises for power development are a key component. The athlete may start some modified physical activity, such as jogging or throwing a limited number of pitches, but functional progressions of running, throwing, hitting or serving need to be completed before full competition is allowed. These progressions test all of the mechanical parts of the motions required in the sport or activity. Very few deviations from normal mechanics should be allowed since these deviations

will create extra stress when the athlete has to meet the normal demands inherent in the sport.

The functional phase should also be used to instruct the athlete in preventative activities, or 'prehabilitation'. The athlete who is injured as a result of participating in a sport will usually return to that sport and its demands after the injury is rehabilitated. A maintenance programme of stretching, muscle balance exercises, power exercises and kinetic chain exercise, all designed to improve the athlete's ability to withstand sports demands, is the best method of conditioning to prevent the overload injuries that are common in tennis.

Guideline 4: Integration of the kinetic chain into rehabilitation

Principle

The kinetic chain needs to be restored early in the rehabilitation process as a basis for joint activity and joint strength. All of the activities of a joint in tennis work off a kinetic chain linkage from the ground through the trunk to the hand and racket. While the local area is recovering from the injury or surgery, exercises can be instituted for the distant components, the legs, trunk, shoulder or arm, so that when the local injury is ready for rehabilitation the kinetic chain base is also ready for link activity. After the local injury is ready for rehabilitation, activation of the kinetic chain patterns from the legs through the back to the shoulder and arm restores the normal physiological motor activation patterns and restores normal biomechanical positions. This then allows for normal sequencing of links for generation of velocity and force.

Practice

Inflexibilities of the hamstrings, hip, trunk and shoulder, and strength weakness or imbalances of the rotators of the trunk, flexors and extensors of the trunk, hip and shoulder rotators, and any subclinical adaptations of stance patterns, gait pattern or throwing mechanics should be corrected before starting formal strength rehabilitation. These adaptations will have been evaluated in the evaluation stage prior to initiation of rehabilitation.

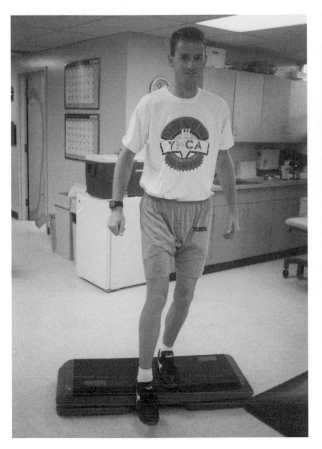

Fig. 21.2 Step-down exercises to emphasize load absorption. They may be started without weights, and then weights may be added.

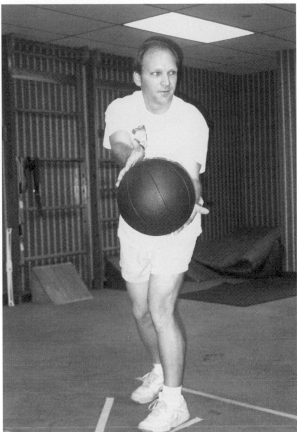

Fig. 21.3 Rotational exercises using the medicine ball.

Rehabilitation of the legs and hips should be concerned with generating appropriate sport-specific force and velocity from the lower extremity, and should be performed in a closed-chain fashion. This pattern, which is done with the foot on the ground, simulates the patterns that exist in the throwing or hitting activities. Eccentric patterns should also be emphasized to absorb the load from jumping forward movement or stopping of the plant leg in the baseball throw (Fig. 21.2). Combined patterns of hip and trunk rotation in both directions, hip and shoulder diagonal patterns from the left hip to the right shoulder and from the right hip to the left shoulder, and rotation from one hip to the other, should also be emphasized as most physical activities involve rotation and diagonal patterns (Fig. 21.3). An excellent exercise involves jumping on a mini-trampoline and simul-

taneously extending the hips and scapula upon landing (Fig. 21.4). This extensor pattern allows for hip extension, trunk extension and scapular retraction in the same pattern that exists in the cocking phase of throwing activities. Integration of the scapular retraction muscles to the hips is very important because these actions tend to be coupled in the cocking phases of throwing. Reversal of the thoracic kyphosis and neck lordosis also should be accomplished in this preliminary phase to allow normal positioning of the scapula.

Endurance activities in the legs should also be emphasized at this time. Both aerobic endurance for recovery from exercise bouts and anaerobic endurance for agility and power work should be emphasized. These can be achieved through the use of mini-trampoline exercises, agility drills with running and jumping, jumping jacks and slider or fitter boards.

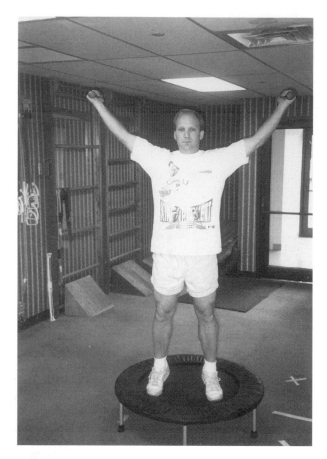

Fig. 21.4 Extensor exercise for hip, scapula and shoulders.

Guideline 5: Rehabilitation of the scapula in arm injuries and hip in leg injuries

Principle

The scapula is the base upon which all shoulder activities rest. Four main roles of the scapula include: (i) retraction and protraction in the different phases of throwing motion; (ii) elevation of the acromion in abduction of the arm; (iii) acting as a socket for the glenohumeral joint; and (iv) acting as a base of origin for all of the intrinsic muscles of the rotator cuff and the extrinsic muscles of the deltoid, biceps and triceps. In addition, the scapula acts as a platform upon which shoulder rotation and arm activities are based. In biomechanics, the glenohumeral joint has been described as a golf ball on a tee due to the size relationships. A more accurate biomechanical description would be of the ball on a seal's nose. As the ball or humeral socket moves, the seal's nose or the scapula needs to move to maintain the position of the ball on the glenoid.

Acromial elevation and scapular stabilization is often jeopardized early in the injury process due to pain-based inhibition of the serratus anterior and lower trapezius and due to subclinical adaptations altering the position of the scapula to accommodate injury patterns in subluxation or impingement.

Practice

Evaluation of the scapula should take a high priority before rehabilitation. The motion and position of the scapula should be evaluated in various phases of the throwing motion, and muscular strength and scapular stabilization should be evaluated (Kibler 1998). Exercises that can be performed early in the rehabilitation process for scapular control include scapular pinch, an isometric activity in which the scapulae are retracted toward the midline. Integration of scapular retraction with hip rotation, back extension and rotator cuff co-contractions allows a more normal physiological pattern to redevelop.

Principle

The hip acts as the stable base for the pelvis in one-legged stance, such as in throwing or kicking. Lack of stance leg hip flexor or abductor strength, creating a Trendelenburg posture, or tightness of the hip flexors, decreases or alters pelvic stability, creating abnormal biomechanics. Also, a stable hip is important to create normal knee kinematics and load absorption. Hip stability decreases anterior knee force and creates stiffness of the entire leg in the face of normal sports demands of running, jumping and kicking.

Practice

Evaluation of hip posture should include one-legged stance (Fig. 21.5), stair stepping and one-legged squat. If the Trendelenburg position occurs with these tests, hip abduction and extension should be emphasized as part of the rehabilitation. A large number of patients with ankle and knee microtrauma overload injuries will demonstrate these alterations.

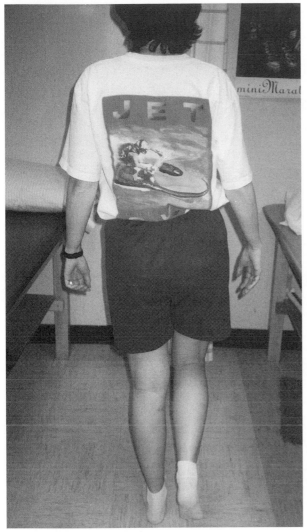 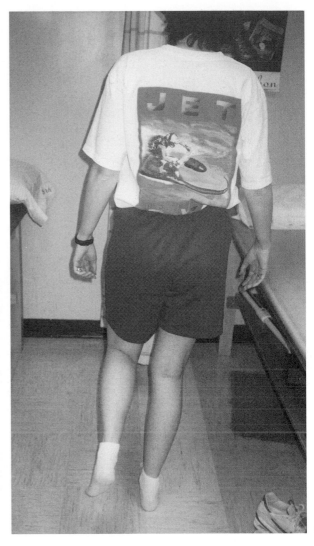

(a)   (b)

Fig. 21.5 One-legged stance testing: (a) standing on left leg, normal pelvic tilt; (b) standing on right leg, Trendelenburg posture.

Guideline 6: Closed-chain rehabilitation

Principle

Closed-chain exercises are very effective in lower extremity injury rehabilitation. They decrease strain and shear on anterior cruciate ligament reconstructions by hamstring/quadriceps coactivation; they simulate concurrent shift, the agonist/antagonist muscle activation pattern seen in walking or running; they provide normal proprioceptive feedback; and they activate all of the links in the kinetic chain of the leg. They also allow specificity of training in that most athletic activities are performed with the foot on the ground.

Practice

Emphasis should be placed on starting most exercises with the foot on the ground or on a solid, stable object (Fig. 21.6). Squats, leg presses, lunges and agility exercises can be based on this stance as tissue healing allows.

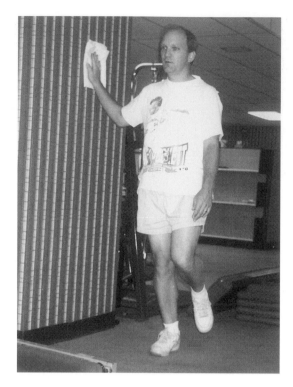

Fig. 21.6 Early closed-chain exercise for the leg.

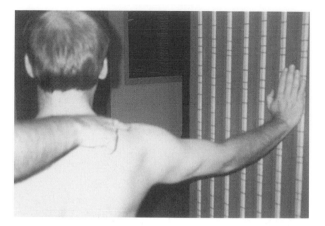

Fig. 21.7 Early closed-chain exercise for the shoulder. The hand is against the wall and the scapula moves from protraction to retraction.

Principle

The predominant method of muscle activation organization around the shoulder articulation is a closed-chain activity emphasizing co-contraction force couples at the scapulothoracic and glenohumeral joints. This results in proper scapular position and stability, and allows the rotator cuff to work as a 'compressor cuff', conferring concavity–compression and a stable instant centre of rotation. Closed-chain activity also simulates the normal proprioceptive pathways that exist in the throwing motion, and allows feedback from the muscle spindles and Golgi tendon organs in their proper anatomical positions. Closed-chain activity replicates the normal ball and socket kinematics, minimizing translation in the mid ranges of motion. Finally, by decreasing deltoid activation, these activities decrease the tendency for superior humeral migration if the rotator cuff is weak.

Practice

The exercises are started at levels below 90° of abduction in the early phases of rehabilitation to allow for healing of the tissues. They may be started at 45° of abduction and 60° of flexion and then proceed to 90° of abduction as tolerated. The hand is placed against some object, such as a table, a ball or the wall, and resistance is generated through the activities of the scapula and shoulder. When the arm can be safely positioned at 90° of abduction, it is placed in either abduction or flexion, and a specific progression is started. The closed-chain activities are first started with scapular stabilization. Patterns of retraction and protraction of the scapula are started in single planes and then progress to elevation and depression of the entire scapula and then selective elevation of the acromion (Fig. 21.7). The next progression is one of rotator cuff activity. Joint compression with contraction into the shoulder joint is followed by 'clock' exercises in which the hand is moved to the various positions on the clock face, ranging from 8 o'clock on around to 4 o'clock. This allows for rotation of the humerus with the arm at 90° of abduction, which replicates rotator cuff activity throughout all components of the rotator cuff. These activities are first performed against fixed resistance such as a wall and then can be moved to moveable resistance such as a ball or some other moveable

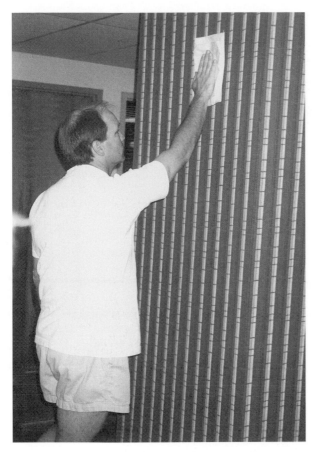

Fig. 21.8 Closed chain with moveable resistance for humeral elevation.

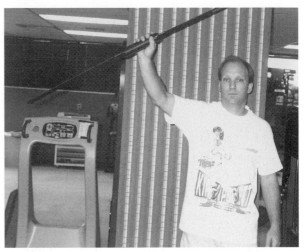

Fig. 21.10 Advanced closed chain—'body blade' vibrates, providing resistance and proprioceptive feedback.

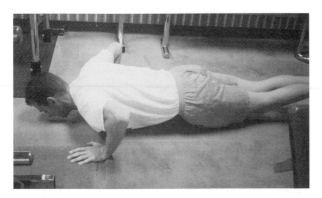

Fig. 21.9 Advanced closed chain—push-ups with wide hand placement.

implement (Fig. 21.8). These exercises may be done early in the rehabilitation as they do not put shear on the joint and allow rotator cuff muscles to be activated without being inhibited by pain or deltoid overactivity.

Closed-chain progressions may be used in later phases of rehabilitation. They include: various types of push-ups, i.e. wall leans, knee push-ups, and regular push-ups (Fig. 21.9); and blade exercises (Fig. 21.10).

Guideline 7: Plyometric exercises

Principle

Most sporting activities involve development of power. Power is the rate of doing work and, therefore, has a time component. For most sports, this time component is relatively rapid. Plyometric activities develop the athlete's ability to generate power. Plyometrics are open-chain exercises that involve a stretch–shortening cycle in which the muscle is eccentrically stretched and slowly loaded. This pre-tensioning phase is followed by a rapid concentric contraction to develop a large amount of momentum and force. Because these exercises develop a large amount of strain in the eccentric phase of the activity, and force in the

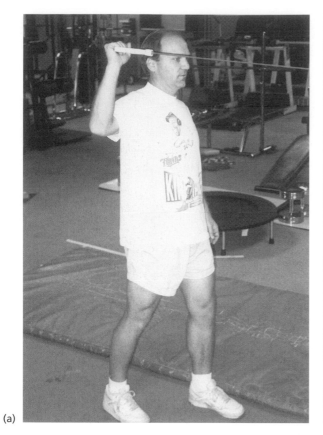
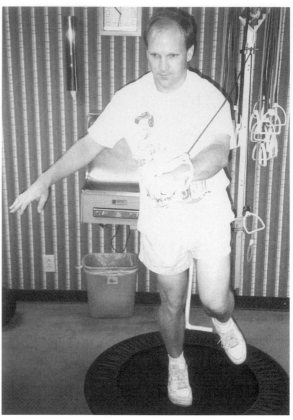

(a)

(b)

Fig. 21.11 Tubing plyometric exercises: (a) stretch–shortening cycle for external rotation with feet on ground; (b) stretch–shortening cycle for internal rotation. This may be combined with one-legged stance to emphasize diagonal kinetic chain activation.

concentric phase of the activity, these exercises should be performed when complete anatomical healing has occurred. Similarly, because large ranges of motion are required, full range of motion should be obtained before the plyometrics are started. These stretch–shortening activation sequences are part of the normal physiological patterns that are present in skilled athletes.

Practice

Plyometrics should be performed for all body segments involved in the activity. Hip rotation, knee flexion/extension, trunk rotation and shoulder rotation are all power activities that require plyometric activation. Plyometric activities for the non-injured areas can be

performed in the early phases of rehabilitation, but plyometric exercises for the injured areas should be instituted in the later phases of rehabilitation. Many different activities and devices can be utilized in plyometric exercises. Rubber tubing is a very effective plyometric device (Fig. 21.11). The arm or leg can be positioned exactly in the position of the physical activity, and then the motion can be replicated by use of the rubber tubing. Medicine balls are also excellent plyometric devices. The weight of the ball creates a prestretch as the ball is caught, and creates resistance for contraction forces (Fig. 21.12). Light weights can also be used for plyometric activities, but caution must be used in using heavier weights in a plyometric fashion due to the forces applied on the joint. Plyometric activities with larger weights

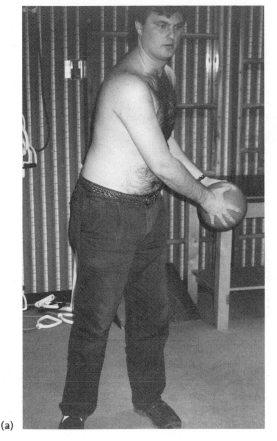
(a)

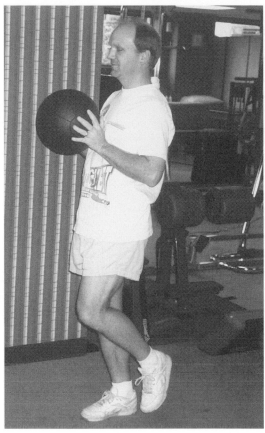
(b)

Fig. 21.12 Medicine ball plyometrics: (a) Rotational plyometrics, catching the ball, then returning it. This simulates a backhand stroke pattern. (b) Medicine ball push. This is combined with one-legged stance to emphasize kinetic chain activation.

can be performed more easily in the lower extremity than the upper extremity. By reproducing these stretch–shortening cycles at positions of physiological function, these plyometric activities also stimulate proprioceptive feedback to fine-tune the muscle activity patterns. Machines are another type of open-chain plyometric activity (Fig. 21.13). Plyometric exercises are the most appropriate open-chain exercises for functional rehabilitation.

Conclusions

These guidelines have been shown to be very effective in our clinical practice. They emphasize the entire sequence of rehabilitation and all of the functional deficits that may occur in association with shoulder

pathology. Many types of therapeutic exercises can be used to fulfil each of the guidelines. The exact protocol may be based on the patient's presentation, the clinical examination, the therapist's skill and the therapist's imagination. Adherence to this programme does require patient education and guidance from the physician and physical therapist on the techniques of rehabilitation. However, most of the physical therapy can be done by home programmes once the exercises have been taught appropriately. We use physical therapy office visits for assessment of achievement of the individual goals for the rehabilitation sequence, instruction in the exercises to be performed in the next phase, and specific guidance as to goals to achieve for the next rehabilitation phase. We find that modalities, such as ice, electrogalvanic stimulation, ultrasound or heat,

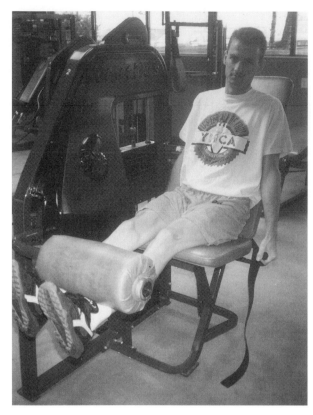

Fig. 21.13 Stretch–shortening for quad extension using knee extension machine.

are very rarely needed after the initial stages of pain reduction.

Putting it all together: specific rehabilitation protocols

Shoulder rehabilitation protocol

This general protocol will illustrate principles for rehabilitation of any non-operative or post-operative shoulder problem. This protocol assumes stable repair of the labrum, capsule or rotator cuff, and ability to achieve 90° abduction without impingement or excessive capsular stretch. Our postoperative goal is to progress our postoperative labral repairs, shoulder reconstructions and acromioplasties to 90° of passive or active assisted abduction by 3 weeks, and our rotator cuff repairs

to 90° passive or active assisted abduction by 4–6 weeks.

Acute phase

GOALS
1 Tissue healing.
2 Reduce pain and inflammation.
3 Re-establish non-painful range of motion below 90° abduction.
4 Retard muscle atrophy.
5 Scapular control.
6 Maintain fitness of other components of kinetic chain.

TISSUE HEALING
Combination of:
1 rest;
2 short-term immobilization;
3 modalities;
4 surgery.

PAIN AND INFLAMMATION
Aggressive treatment to control pain to decrease inhibition-based muscle atrophy and decrease scapular instability due to serratus and/or trapezius inhibition.
1 Medications, either non-steroidal or judicious use of steroids orally or by injection.
2 Modalities, usually ultrasound, two per week, for 2 weeks.
3 Cold compression devices.
4 Joint protection, usually by sling or swathe, with gradual progression out of sling.

RANGE OF MOTION
Should be started in pain-free arcs, kept below 90° abduction, and may be passive or active assisted. The degree of movement will be guided by the stability of the operative repair.
1 Codman's or other pendulum exercises.
2 Manual capsular stretching and cross-fibre massage.
3 T-bar or ropes and pulleys.

MUSCLE ATROPHY
1 Isometric exercises, with arm below 90° abduction and 90° flexion. These should be performed by labral or capsular repair patients, but not in rotator cuff patients.

SCAPULAR CONTROL

1 Isometric scapular pinches and scapular elevation.
2 Closed-chain weight shifts, with hands on table, shoulder flexed <60°, abducted <45°.
3 Tilt board or circular board weight shifts with same limitations.

FITNESS OF REST OF KINETIC CHAIN

1 Aerobic exercises such as running, bicycling or stepping.
2 Anaerobic agility drills.
3 Lower extremity strengthening, by machines, squat exercises or open-chain leg lifts.
4 Elbow and wrist strengthening by isometrics or rubber tubing.
5 Flexibility exercises, especially areas that are shown to be tight on the evaluation.
6 Integration of the kinetic chain by leg and trunk stabilization on a ball, employing rotational and oblique patterns of contraction.

CRITERIA FOR MOVEMENT OUT OF ACUTE PHASE

1 Progression of tissue healing (healed or sufficiently stabilized for active motion and tissue loading).
2 Passive range of motion 66–75% of opposite side.
3 Minimal pain.
4 Manual muscle strength in non-pathological areas 4+/5.
5 Scapular control, with dominant side/non-dominant side scapular asymmetry <1.5 cm.
6 Kinetic chain function and integration.

Recovery phase

GOALS

1 Normal active and passive shoulder and glenohumeral motion.
2 Improve scapular control.
3 Normal upper extremity strength and strength balance.
4 Normal shoulder arthrokinematics in single, then multiple planes of motion.
5 Normal kinetic chain and force generation patterns.

RANGE OF MOTION

1 Active assisted motion above 90° abduction with wand.

2 Active assisted, then active motion in internal and external with scapula stabilized. In this manner, glenohumeral rotation is normalized without substitution movements from the scapula.

SCAPULAR CONTROL

1 Scapular proprioceptive neuromuscular facilitation (PNF) patterns, in diagonals.
2 Closed-chain exercises at 90° flexion/90° abduction—scapular retraction/protraction and scapular elevation/depression (see Fig. 21.7).
3 Modified push-ups.
4 Regular push-ups (see Fig. 21.9).
5 Medicine ball catch and push (see Fig. 21.12).
6 Dips.

UPPER EXTREMITY STRENGTH AND STRENGTH BALANCE

1 Glenohumeral PNF patterns.
2 Closed-chain exercises at 90° flexion then 90° abduction—glenohumeral depressors and glenohumeral internal/external rotators (see Fig. 21.8).
3 Forearm curls.
4 Isolated rotator cuff exercises.
5 Machines or weights for light bench press, military press and pull-downs. The resistance should initially be light, then progress as strength improves. Emphasis is placed on proper mechanics, proper technique and joint stabilization.

NORMAL SHOULDER ARTHROKINEMATICS

1 Range of motion with arm at 90° abduction. This is the position where most throwing and serving activities occur. The periarticular soft tissues must be completely loose and balanced at this position.
2 Muscle activity at 90° abduction. Normal muscle firing patterns must be re-established at this position, both in organization of force generation and force regulation patterns and in proprioceptive sensory feedback. Closed-chain patterns are an excellent method to re-establish the normal neurological patterns for joint stabilization.
3 Open-chain exercises, including mild plyometric exercises, may be built upon the base of the closed-chain stabilization to allow normal control of joint mobility.

NORMAL KINETIC CHAIN AND FORCE GENERATION
1 Normalization of all inflexibilities throughout chain.
2 Normal agonist/antagonist force couples in legs by squats, plyometric depth jumps, lunges and hip extensions.
3 Trunk rotation exercises, with medicine ball or tubing (see Fig. 21.3).
4 Integrated exercises with leg and trunk stabilization—rotations, diagonal patterns from hip to shoulder (Fig. 21.12) and medicine ball throws.
5 Rotator cuff strength 4+/5 or higher.
6 Normal kinetic chain function.

Functional phase

GOALS
1 Increase power and endurance in the upper extremity.
2 Increase normal multiple-plane neuromuscular control; locally, regionally and in entire kinetic chain.
3 Instruction in prehabilitation activities.
4 Sport-specific activity.

POWER AND ENDURANCE IN UPPER EXTREMITY
Power is the rate of doing work. Work may be done to move the joint and the extremity, or it may be done to absorb a load and stabilize the joint or extremity. Power has a time component, and for shoulder activity, quick movements and quick reactions are the dominant ways of doing work. These exercises should, therefore, be performed with relatively rapid movements in planes that approximate normal shoulder function (i.e. 90° abduction in shoulder, trunk rotation and diagonal arm motions, rapid external/internal rotation).
1 Diagonal and multiplanar motions with tubing (Fig. 21.11), light weights, small medicine balls and isokinetic machines.
2 Plyometrics—wall push-ups, corner push-ups, weighted ball throws and tubing. Tubing exercises may be used to mimic any of the needed motions in throwing or serving. Medicine balls are very effective plyometric devices (Fig. 21.12). The weight of the ball creates a prestretch and an eccentric load when it is caught, creates a resistance, and

demands a powerful agonist contraction to propel it forward again.

INCREASE MULTIPLE-PLANE NEUROMUSCULAR CONTROL
The force-dependent motor firing patterns should be re-established. No subclinical adaptations, such as 'opening up' (trunk rotation too far in front of shoulder rotation), three-quarter arm positioning on throwing or excessive wrist snap should be allowed. Help in this area can be obtained by watching pre-injury videos or by using a knowledgeable coach in the particular sport. Special care must be taken to integrate completely all of the components of the kinetic chain to generate and funnel the proper forces to and through the shoulder.

PREHABILITATION
The athlete who is injured while playing a sport will most often return to the same sport with the same sports demands. The body should be healed from the symptomatic standpoint, and should be prepared for resuming the stresses inherent in playing the sport. A maintenance programme is the best way to condition to prevent overload injuries and further problems in sport.
1 Flexibility—general body flexibility, with emphasis on sport-specific problems (shoulder internal rotation and elbow extension in the arm, lower back, hip rotation and hamstrings in the legs).
2 Strengthening—appropriate amount and locations of strength for sport-specific activities (quadriceps/hamstring strength for force generation, trunk rotation strength, strength balance for the shoulder).
3 Power—rapid movements in appropriate planes with light weights.
4 Endurance—mainly anaerobic exercises due to short-duration, explosive and ballistic activities seen in throwing and serving.
   These exercises should be based on the periodization principle of conditioning.

SPORT-SPECIFIC ACTIVITY
Functional progressions of throwing or serving must be completed before full competition is allowed. These progressions will gradually test all of the mechanical parts of the throwing or serving motion. Very few

deviations from normal parameters of arm motion, arm position, force generation and smoothness of all of the kinetic chain, and from preinjury form should be allowed because most of these adaptations will be biomechanically inefficient. The athlete may move through the progressions as rapidly as possible.

CRITERIA FOR RETURN TO PLAY
1 Normal clinical examination.
2 Normal shoulder arthrokinematics.
3 Normal kinetic chain integration.
4 Completed progressions.

Knee rehabilitation protocol

Acute phase

All of the local effects resulting from treatment and subsequent immobilization have to be reversed to allow functional restoration. Medications and modalities may be helpful during this phase to relieve pain and inflammation. The patella should be released from any retinacular tightness. Early restoration of normal neurological control of muscle firing is important to retard atrophy and rebuild strength. A lightweight brace can aid in controlling swelling and giving support. The upper body and opposite leg should continue to be conditioned for strength and endurance. The two most important criteria for advancement to the next phase are the elimination of swelling and the ability to straight leg raise 3.6 kg (8 lb). This indicates very little intra-articular abnormality and good neural control of motor neuron firing.

GOALS
1 Reduce effects of immobilization.
2 Retard muscle atrophy of entire lower extremity.
3 Neuromuscular control of the patella.
4 Maintain components of fitness.

EFFECTS OF IMMOBILIZATION
1 Non-steroidal, anti-inflammatory drug (NSAID) 48–96 h if needed.
2 Modalities 2–3 weeks.
3 Patellar mobilization.
4 Joint protection (brace/non-weightbearing).
5 Range of motion.

MUSCLE ATROPHY/NEUROMUSCULAR CONTROL
1 Local:
  (a) Isometrics;
  (b) Straight leg raises (avoid adduction and abduction);
  (c) Biofeedback—patellar control.
2 Distant:
  (a) Open chain—non-pathological areas (ankle, hip): (i) concentrics; (ii) eccentrics.

MAINTAIN COMPONENTS OF FITNESS
1 Aerobic endurance for upper body:
  (a) ergometer.
2 Strength for upper body and opposite leg:
  (a) weights;
  (b) machines.

CRITERIA FOR ADVANCEMENT
1 Elimination of most swelling.
2 Level II pain.
3 Healing of injured tissue to allow mild tensile stress, range of motion (ROM), weightbearing.
4 Straight leg raise 3.6 kg (8 lb).

Recovery phase

ROM should become normal in this phase. Vigorous, active ROM activities should be stressed. Likewise, vigorous strengthening can be pursued. PNF techniques are excellent ways to challenge the muscles, but require individual attention by a skilled therapist. Single-plane strengthening is a prelude to multiple-plane patterns. Open-chain activities, in which the foot moves with a weight, can be used to isolate specific muscles. Closed-chain activities are thought to be more physiological because the foot is fixed and muscle co-contractions are more common. This makes the muscles work as force couples to control the forces generated by the attached resistance. After muscle strength is obtained, tennis-specific arthrokinematic drills are instituted. Kinetic chain movement patterns that involve knee flexion and extension, hip and leg rotation around both legs, and gentle acceleration and deceleration movements such as lunges are started. These patterns start the integration of isolated muscles into purposeful tennis-specific activities. Other purposeful activities that may be started involve integrating the knee back into the kinetic chain. Easy groundstrokes may be hit, and the service motion may be practised. Both should be done with emphasis on smoothness of mechanics. Playing of points or matches should be delayed. Criteria for advancement include 75% normal strength, good quadriceps–hamstrings balance and smooth arthrokinematic motion.

GOALS

1 Re-establish non-painful active and passive ROM.
2 Regain and improve lower extremity muscle strength.
3 Improve lower extremity neuromuscular control.
4 Normal arthrokinematics in single plane of motion.

RANGE OF MOTION

1 Dependent:
   (a) patellar mobilization;
   (b) manual capsular stretch and cross-friction massage.
2 Independent:
   (a) knee flexion and extension, active and passive;
   (b) heel wall slides;
   (c) bike and rowing machine;
   (d) stretching—quadriceps, hamstring, iliotibial band, hip flexor, gastrocsoleus.

STRENGTHENING

1 Dependent:
   (a) PNF.
2 Independent single planes (avoid aggressive hamstring work after horn tear):
   (a) open chain: (i) concentric and eccentric isotonics; (ii) isokinetics; (iii) tubing and free weights.
   (b) closed chain: (i) Nautilus/Stairmaster; (ii) lifeline/tubing; (iii) free weights.

NEUROMUSCULAR CONTROL

1 Balance board.
2 Biomechanical ankle platform system.
3 Fitter and slide board.
4 Mini-trampoline.
5 Lifeline.

ARTHROKINEMATICS

1 Joint mobilization.
2 Kinetic chain movement patterns (tennis specific):
   (a) flexion and extension;
   (b) hip and leg rotation;
   (c) acceleration and deceleration.

OTHER ACTIVITIES

1 Practise service motion.
2 Hit groundstrokes.
3 No intense play.

CRITERIA FOR ADVANCEMENT

1 Nearly full active and passive non-painful ROM equal to other side.
2 Quadriceps/hamstring ratio 66% and strength 75% of non-involved side.
3 Static balance on one leg, 1 min.
4 Normal and smooth arthrokinematics with single-plane motion.

Functional phase

Tennis-specific muscle coordination patterns and tennis-specific functional progressions are the main goals of this phase. Multiple-plane motions, such as start and stop, slide lunges and directional changes simulate tennis movements. Plyometric drills, which employ relatively slow muscle lengthening followed by rapid muscle shortening, provide power and explosiveness for short bursts of activity. Examples of plyometric drills are 'depth jumps', jumping off or over a platform at varying heights; 'lunges', striding one leg forwards, backwards or sideways, with rapid recovery to the starting point; repeated vertical jumps, with knee bends between jumps; and knee–chest or foot–buttock drills, movement of the leg and hip so that the knee approaches the chest and the foot touches the buttock during running. Rope jumping and shuttle run agility drills also contain plyometric activity. Agility and footwork drills with tennis racket in hand simulates tennis-playing situations and improves neuromuscular control. Plyometric activities can achieve rapid and significant gains in power for performance, but are quite stressful to the muscle–tendon units. The potential for overload injury in these activities is quite high, especially if done when the musculoskeletal base is inadequate. Plyometric activity should be performed only twice per week, should be performed in the functional phase of rehabilitation, and is not recommended for athletes under 15 years of age. After muscle strength and coordination are optimized, functional progressions determine return-to-play suitability. The first two phases can usually be mastered quickly. The second two require normal knee anatomy and physiology. Direction changes, repeated anaerobic sprints with cutting, and jumping and landing on the rehabilitated leg should be performed. Sport-specific training should emphasize the full spectrum of tennis strokes, and play conditions should be simulated.

GOALS
1 Increase power and endurance in lower extremity.
2 Increase normal multiple-plane neuromuscular control.
3 Tennis-specific activities.

POWER AND ENDURANCE
(Avoid compressive and shear loads for 6–8 weeks)
1 Multiple-plane motions:
   (a) start and stop;
   (b) side lunges;
   (c) change of directions.
2 Plyometrics.
3 Anaerobic conditioning based on periodization.

NEUROMUSCULAR CONTROL, MULTIPLE PLANES
1 Agility drills.
2 Footwork drills.

SPORT-SPECIFIC TRAINING FUNCTIONAL PROGRESSION—TENNIS
Stage I:
1 standing on one foot;
2 jumping on two legs (forwards, backwards, sideways);
3 jumping on a mini-trampoline;
4 jumping from stool, 40 cm (one foot);
5 rope skipping on both feet;
6 balance board with both feet (forwards, side to side, 45° angle);
7 balance board with both feet (catch tennis ball).
Stage II:
1 rope skipping on one foot;
2 jumping from stool, 40 cm, land one foot;
3 jumping from stool, 80 cm, land two feet;

4 hopping one foot (forwards, backwards, sideways);
5 jogging in place;
6 jogging around court;
7 jog figure 8 (large and small);
8 jog figure 8 backward;
9 balance board with one foot (forwards, side to side).
Stage III:
1 running with direction changes;
2 Carioca running;
3 running 1–1.5 miles (1.6–2.4 km);
4 jumping: two-footed take-off, land on one foot.
Stage IV:
1 anaerobic sprints with cutting on demand.
2 split step.
3 Sport-specific training:
   (a) motions: (i) five-dot drill; (ii) hexagon drills; (iii) spider drills.
   (b) skills: (i) normal service; (ii) volleys; (iii) overheads.
   (c) match conditions.

Criteria for return to play

• Negative clinical examination.
• Normal ROM and flexibility equal to opposite side.
• Isokinetic strength 90% of normal side.
• Normal arthrokinematics in multiple plane.
• Pass functional examination—hop test, spider agility drill.

References

Kibler, W.B. (1998) The role of the scapula in athletic shoulder function. *American Journal of Sports Medicine* **26**, 325–337.

Kibler, W.B., Herring, S.A. & Press, J., eds (1998) *Functional Rehabilitation of Sports and Musculoskeletal Injuries.* Aspen, Rockville, MD.

Pink, M.M., Screnar, P.M. & Tollefson, K.D. (1996) Injury prevention and rehabilitation in the upper extremity. In: Jobe, F.W., ed. *Operative Techniques in Upper Extremity Sports Injuries*, pp. 3–15. Mosby, St Louis.

Wilk, K.E. (1994) Rehabilitation of isolated and combined ligament injuries. *Clinics in Sports Medicine* **13**, 649–675.

Chapter 22

The psychology of tennis: gaining the mental advantage

Introduction

Have you ever walked off the tennis court in disgust because you lost a match you felt you should have won? Have you ever choked at a critical point in the match? Have you ever been upset over a bad line call and lost your concentration? Does your mind ever wander and think about other things during the course of a match? Have you ever become tentative and started to push the ball during critical points in a match? Have you ever become angry and frustrated with your game and thrown your racket or called yourself names?

If you answered yes to one of more of these questions, do not despair because you have lots of company. In fact, in my experience working with tennis players and coaches, it has been extremely rare to find a tennis player who does not fall victim, at least at times, to the ravages of the mind. Nobody who has ever played or coached tennis with any degree of seriousness or passion would dispute the statement that beyond the purely physical and technical aspects to the game is a mental or emotional component that overshadows or transcends the physical aspects. All of us who play tennis can recall times when we were 'in the zone' and everything we were doing was going right as winners seem to fly effortlessly off our rackets. Unfortunately, we can also remember those times when nothing went right and every shot was an adventure. Most players and coaches believe that these good and bad days are just part of the game and some days we have it and other days we do not.

Importance of mental skills

The basic premise of this chapter is that we gain control over these mental and emotional states and thus maximize the probability that we are at our best every time we step out on the court. Of course this is easier said than done. The problem is that most tennis players and coaches focus on and practise the physical side of the game to the exclusion of the mental side (although I am pleased to say that in my work with tennis players and coaches I have observed somewhat more emphasis being recently placed on the mental aspects of tennis). This occurs despite the fact that most serious tennis players and coaches realize that the mental aspects of tennis are critical for success. For example, Jimmy Connors, one of the most successful and mentally tough players of all time, has said that 95% of the game at the professional level is mental. He reasons that at the professional level, all the players are talented in terms of physical skill although a few of the truly great players also have exceptional ability or are known for a particular shot (e.g. Andre Agassi—return of serve, Steffi Graf—forehand, Patrick Rafter—serve and volley, Pete Sampras—serve, Venus Williams—movement, Monica Seles—two-handed groundstrokes). Thus, the difference in winning and losing often is determined by a player's mental skills. This does not only apply to elite players, as we all seek out players of reasonably equal ability (e.g. 4.5 players usually play against other 4.5 players) and thus matches are often decided more by mental skills than physical skills.

The notion of the importance of mental skills in determining success is reinforced by the scoring system in tennis. That is, many matches are decided by a few key points (such as break points or tie breakers) and in fact, in a number of close matches the player who wins the most total points does not actually win the match. Being able to play the big points well has always been one of the attributes of the top players. In fact, some of the top players in the world, past and present, such as Michael Chang, Thomas Muster, Chris Evert and Arantxa Sanchez-Vicario, have reached that pinnacle due to their mental toughness and their willingness to stay out on the court as long as it takes to win. In addition to the scoring, the stop-and-go nature of tennis makes it extremely difficult from a mental perspective. For example, in a typical tennis match, only one-third of the time is actually spent playing tennis.

If we agree that the mental skills are essential for tennis success, then why do not more coaches and players practise mental skills. One simple answer to this is that most coaches do not have proper training and do not clearly understand how to teach mental skills. I have observed tennis coaches telling their players such things as 'don't choke', 'concentrate out there', 'be confident', 'stay loose' and 'be mentally tough'. However, these carry little meaning to players because there is no specific instruction concerning how to achieve these mental/emotional states. A key premise of this chapter (and of sport psychology) is that these mental or psychological skills can be learned but they need to be practised systematically like physical skills (Fig. 22.1). The ability to control your thoughts and feelings is one of the characteristics of top players who maintain consistently high levels of performance every time they go out on the court. In essence, the ability to concentrate, stay relaxed, maintain motivation, keep confident and make proper decisions are all psychological skills that can be learned by practice and repetition. The remainder of this chapter will attempt to describe the psychological state that elicits our best performance and then briefly review some of the core psychological skills essential for tennis success.

Peak performance states

> I just started feeling so confident in my game. I felt that no matter how hard I hit the ball it was going in the court. I was no longer occupied with winning and losing, but rather I was just totally focused on the match.
> (Ivan Lendl after his victory over John McEnroe in the 1985 US Open, *Dallas Morning News*, September, 1985.)

The above quote represents a great player describing his thoughts and feelings during one of the top moments in his career. Research (Jackson 1992; Jackson & Csikszentmihalyi 1999) has indicated that when tennis players (as well as athletes in all sports) are asked to describe their top performances, they consistently use the same terminology and feeling states. The relationship between these special emotional states and exceptional performances is called flow or peak experiences. In tennis terminology, this is commonly called 'playing in the zone'. A composite of the thoughts and feelings that tennis players report during outstanding or peak performances is presented below:

> I felt very relaxed but yet I was energized and feeling strong. I enjoyed the tennis competition and was not afraid to lose. In fact, I felt a sense of calmness and quiet inside and my strokes just seemed to flow automatically. I really wasn't thinking about my shots, and what I needed to do; it just seemed to happen naturally. My shots did not feel rushed, in fact the ball seemed to slow down and I felt as if I could do anything. I was totally into the match and yet I was not consciously trying to concentrate. I was aware of everything but distracted by nothing. I knew my shots were going in and I felt totally in control.

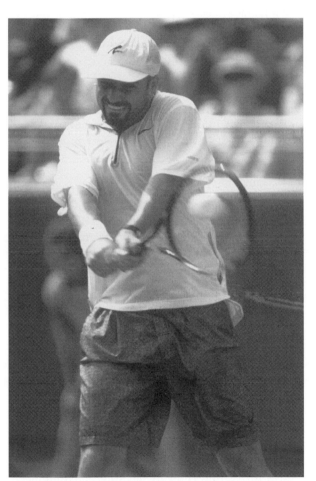

Fig. 22.1 Psychological skills can be learned and must be practised as with physical skills. Photo © Allsport/G.M. Prior.

Of course it is unusual for a tennis player to feel all these things at one point in time. The key is that what is generally called mental toughness is the ability to create and maintain the type of internal climate described above. In essence, the main components of this special internal mental state include the following:

- highly confident;
- focused concentration;
- physically relaxed;
- in control;
- motivation/enjoyment;
- effortless;
- automatic;
- lack of fear.

Being a mentally tough tennis player translates into the ability to create and maintain the proper psychological state regardless of the circumstances or situation. It is not too difficult to maintain positive thoughts and feelings when you are winning and playing well. The real challenge comes when things get tough, you are behind, the pressure is high, and everything is going wrong. If you can stay relaxed, concentrated, confident, in control and motivated under these adverse conditions, then you are well on your way to winning the mental game. The remainder of the chapter will briefly discuss some of these important mental skills including tips to help achieve these positive states, but a more detailed analysis and description can be found in Weinberg (1988).

Confidence

Of all the psychological states relating to peak performance, the most consistent mental state found in the research literature is confidence. Tennis players often describe their wins and losses by saying things such as, 'I just didn't feel confident in my backhand', 'I really felt confident in my serve', 'I felt confident I could come from behind', or 'I just felt everything I hit today would go in'. However, one of the things that distinguishes top tennis players from their less successful counterparts is that they have a strong belief in their abilities even when they are playing poorly. Although they may temporarily lose confidence in a particular stroke, they find other things to do well until they regain their confidence.

Definition of confidence

So what is this thing called confidence that seems to be critical for a tennis player's success? Simply put, confidence refers to the belief that you can successfully perform a desired behaviour (e.g. hitting a passing shot, serving an ace, beating a tough opponent). Confident players expect to be successful and believe in their capacity to perform the actions necessary to be successful. In fact, confidence can help your game in a variety of ways:

- confidence facilitates concentration;
- confidence arouses positive emotions;
- confidence increases persistence and effort;
- confidence positively affects goal setting;
- confidence affects shot selection.

For example, how many times have you seen a player (or yourself) lose confidence in a particular shot and start to push the ball on critical points in the match? But watching top players like Martina Hingis, Lleyton Hewitt, Pete Sampras and Lindsay Davenport, you notice that they continue to hit their shots on critical points, playing the percentages but not being afraid to go for the line if given the right opportunity.

Enhancing self-confidence

Many tennis players make the mistake of thinking that there is nothing they can do to build their confidence. But as noted earlier, you can build confidence through practice, planning and good old hard work. A few strategies for enhancing your confidence are provided below.

Performance accomplishments

Research (Bandura 1986) has shown that the strongest builder of self-confidence is performance accomplishments. Basically what this means is that having performed a behaviour successfully in the past will increase your confidence that you will execute it successfully in the future. The behaviour might be beating a particular opponent, coming from behind to win, hitting a down-the-line backhand passing shot under pressure or hitting a topspin lob. Building confidence through previous success is not as easy as it sounds, because how can you be confident in the first place without previous success? This dilemma is captured in a quote by former top 10 player Brian Gottfried who was in the midst of a hot streak. 'I'm winning now because I'm confident, but the reason I'm confident is because I'm winning' (Tarshis 1977, p. 21).

Think confidently

One of the most important aspects of keeping your confidence throughout a tennis match is to think confidently. If you think confidently, your body is more likely to act in a confident manner. As one tennis player who I worked with said, 'If I think I can win, I'm awfully tough to beat'. Thinking confidently, in essence, means keeping a positive attitude and eliminating all the negative things we often say to ourselves. This means stopping such negative statements as 'I'm so stupid', 'I can't beat this person', 'I can't believe I'm playing so bad', 'I hope I don't double fault', and changing them to more positive statements such as 'I can hang in there', 'one point doesn't make a match', 'keep your eye on the ball' and 'I can beat this person'. These positive statements should be instructive rather than judgemental because the body can translate these instructions into positive actions and better stokes.

Image success

Imagery will be explained in more detail later in the chapter, but in essence it refers to visualizing a particular action, event or strategy. One of the great things about imagery is that you can see yourself beating an opponent whom you have never defeated before or executing a particular shot that has been troubling you recently. For example, if you are having trouble with your passing shots you might visualize yourself hitting cross court and down the line crisp passing shots under pressure. Or you might see yourself carrying out your game plan to perfection. It can help provide you with a feeling of success and confidence that might ordinarily not be available to you.

Act confidently

One of the easiest ways to build confidence is to act confidently. Because your thoughts, feelings and behaviours all affect one another, the more you act confidently, the more likely you are to feel and think confidently. Acting confidently not only makes you feel better, but it can be very disconcerting to your opponent. Players like Chris Evert and Bjorn Borg never let their opponent know when they were not feeling confident (which probably was not often) as their expressions, movements and mannerisms were the same regardless of whether they were winning 5–1 or losing 5–1. So keep your head up, shoulders back, racket head up and facial muscles loose, indicating that you are confident and still fighting for the match. This will help your attitude as well as keep your opponent guessing as to how you are feeling.

Regulating anxiety

> Sometimes when I go out on the court to play an important match, I get so nervous that I actually have trouble breathing. My strokes feel rigid and forced instead of natural, and I feel tension in my forearm and neck. To make matters worse, when I try to run my legs feel stiff and tight and I feel really slow on the court. I start pushing my shots with little or no follow-through. It seems that I lose all my tennis instincts and I am being controlled by the fear of losing.

The above quote represents what most competitive tennis players have felt on the court at one time or another due to feelings of nervousness and anxiety. Even the top players in the world admit to being anxious from time to time when the pressure is great, but they usually have a way of coping with this fear and nervousness. This fear of failure can be really debilitating, but here is how Rod Laver, two-time Grand Slam winner, dealt with his fears.

> The thing that always worked best for me whenever I felt I was getting too tense to play good tennis was to simply remind myself that the worst thing—the very worst thing—that could happen to me was that I'd lose a bloody tennis match. That's all (Tarshis 1977, p. 87).

Surveys and interviews with athletes from a variety of sports have indicated that a wide variety of situations and circumstances can cause anxiety, although fear of failure is typically given as the number one reason for this heightened anxiety (Gould *et al.* 1992). The unfortunate aspect for most tennis players is that this increased anxiety can have negative effects on us

both physically and psychologically. From a physical perspective, these include:
- increased muscle tension;
- shallow breathing;
- reduced flexibility;
- increased fatigue;
- reduced muscle coordination.

From a mental perspective, some problems associated with excess anxiety include:
- reduced concentration;
- impaired decision making and tactical judgment;
- reduced confidence;
- giving up mentally.

Any tennis player can easily see how any of the above physical or mental manifestations of excess anxiety can be quite debilitating and certainly make the difference between winning and losing close matches. The key point then is not necessarily to eliminate these feelings of anxiety since some anxiety could be positive. Rather, it is critical that you be able to control and manage these feelings more effectively. In fact, feeling a little anxious before a big match would certainly be expected and the comments of all-time tennis great Vic Sexias underscores this point.

> Early in my career I read an article that quoted Ted Williams as saying, 'I never over-come nervousness.' That statement stuck with me throughout my career. I got to the point where I wanted my mouth to feel a little dry. I wanted to be aware of my heart pounding. It gave me the edge I needed to play my best (Tarshis 1977, p. 170).

The above comments emphasize the importance of having the ability to reduce your anxiety prior to and throughout a tennis match. Particularly imperative is trying to relax your muscles, because muscle tension not only impairs coordination and timing, it also drains your energy because your muscles are working overtime. This problem is highlighted by the comments of Wimbledon champion Arthur Ashe.

> The one thing I've learned about tension on the court that's helped me is something I got from Pancho Gonzalez. He told me once that if you can somehow learn to relax in between points, the tension won't build up in a match the way it does if you try to concentrate every second. Physical fatigue can make you mentally tired and whatever you do to minimize the tension will make choking much less likely (Tarshis 1977, p. 87).

There have been a number of relaxation techniques that have been developed to help us cope more effectively with excess anxiety and pressure. These include strategies such as progressive relaxation (Jacobson 1938) which focuses on the physical side of reducing anxiety. Specifically, it involves progressively relaxing the different major muscle groups throughout the body so that you understand the difference between muscle tension and relaxation. A technique that focuses more on the mental aspect of reducing anxiety is termed the relaxation response (Benson 1975). The idea here is that if we can relax the mind, then the body will also relax. These strategies need to be systematically practised and integrated into practices and competitions. A detailed description of how to utilize these techniques to help reduce anxiety while playing tennis is provided by Weinberg (1988).

On-court relaxation tips

In addition to a more formal relaxation programme, I would like to present a few on-court relaxation tips to help us more effectively cope with pressure.

Slow down—take time between points

One of the things that excess anxiety often does to tennis players is to cause them to play too quickly. When the pressure starts to build, and we begin to feel frustrated and angry at our erratic play, one of the easiest (but least effective) ways of coping with this pressure is to hurry up and get off the court. Because anxiety can be uncomfortable, one way to get rid of it is to remove yourself quickly from the anxiety-producing situation. Therefore, I recommend when you are feeling anxious, tense and upset, and start rushing your serves, you should walk to the ball farthest away from you, and use it for the next point. An even more effective way to slow down is to develop consistent pre-serve and pre-service returns routines. This enables you to keep composed and slow down even under great pressure.

Breath control

One of the quickest and easiest (although often overlooked) ways to cope with pressure is through proper breathing. Research across different sports has indicated that in pressure situations, athletes often hold their breath while performing (thus increasing muscle tension) instead of breathing out (thus decreasing muscle tension) in rhythm with their movements. Along these lines, tennis players under pressure often fail to coordinate their breathing patterns with their stroke production. However, some players try to accentuate breathing out when striking the ball (e.g. Monica Seles, Jimmy Connors) and these players have been termed 'grunters'. Although some players complain that this can be distracting, what these players are really doing is making sure that they breathe out at all times (especially under pressure) when they strike the ball. Furthermore, deep breathing from the diaphragm between points will also serve an important function of reducing accumulated pressure (as noted earlier by Arthur Ashe's quote) and keeping you focused and relaxed throughout a match.

Set up stressful situations in practice

A very effective way to prepare for stressful situations is to occasionally practise under pressure. As you become more accustomed to playing under these conditions, you will not be as negatively affected by pressure during actual competitions. For example, instead of simply practising groundstrokes, try to get a certain number of strokes (e.g. 10) in a row to fall past the service line as you practise keeping the ball deep. If you hit a short ball before you reach 10 you have to start all over. As you get closer to 10 the pressure starts to build, which is similar to a competitive match.

Have fun—enjoy the situation

Common to virtually all tennis players playing at the top of their games is a sense of enjoyment and fun. Most top players look forward to pressure situations instead of fearing them. Keeping the enjoyment of tennis foremost in one's mind can help to prevent burnout, especially in younger players. This involves keeping winning in perspective and focusing on the experience without undue concern for the outcome. Remember the old adage, 'it's only a game', and games are meant to be fun.

Goal setting

> Motivation depends in large part upon goal setting. The coach must have goals. The team must have goals. Each individual tennis player must have goals—real, vivid, living goals. . . . Goals keep everyone on target. Goals commit me to the work, time, pain, and whatever else is part of the price of achieving success.

The above quote by a top collegiate tennis player captures the important role that goal setting can have on a tennis player's motivation. In addition, research from both the industrial/organizational and sport psychology literatures investigating the effects of goals on enhancing performance has clearly demonstrated the impressive effects that goals can have on performance (Locke & Latham 1990; Kyllo & Landers 1995; Weinberg 1996; Burton et al. 2001). On average, research has indicated that goals have improved performance from 10–15%. Although the mental skills discussed so far are critical to achieving your potential in tennis, they probably will not do a lot of good if you are motivated to work hard and improve. Motivation is a powerful source of energy and without it your progress, will come to a halt. But as long as you see yourself moving towards meaningful goals, the chances are high that you will maintain a high level of motivation. In essence, goals provide you with a sense of purpose and direction as well as stimulating you to meet challenges. As Keith Bell (1983) aptly noted in his book *Championship Thinking*, 'Floundering in the world of sports without setting goals is like shooting without aiming. You might enjoy the blast and kick of the gun, but you probably won't bag the bird'.

Why goals work

Although we know that goals can have an extremely positive effect on increasing performance, researchers have also identified the reasons underlying why goals work. Understanding the ways in which goals work can help coaches and athletes be better goal-settters.
• Goals help determine what is important to you. In essence, goals help provide perspective on guiding you along your journey to success.
• Goals help maintain and sustain motivation over both the short and long haul.

• Goals increase effort and push you a little harder to be the best you can be.

• Goals increase the use of relevant learning strategies. To reach your goals, specific strategies (such as hitting with more topspin to keep the ball in play and reduce unforced errors) are implemented.

• Goals direct your attention and action. If your goal is to increase the consistency of your first serve, then you would focus on this aspect of your game during practices.

Goal-setting guidelines

Many tennis players (and other athletes as well) are under the mistaken impression that simply setting some goals will help enhance performance. But research has indicated that there are certain guidelines and principles that can help make your goals more effective in improving performance (see Weinberg 1988 and Gould 2001 for a more detailed description of effective goal-setting principles).

Set challenging goals

One of the strongest findings in the goal-setting literature is that goals should be difficult and challenging. Research with Olympic and collegiate athletes has indicated that high-level athletes prefer moderately difficult to very difficult goals as opposed to easy goals (Weinberg *et al.* 1993). Similarly, research has also demonstrated that the higher the goal the better the performance, as long as the goal does not exceed your ability (Locke & Latham 1990). By setting goals high, you continue to strive to reach your potential as a tennis player and hopefully always looking to improve your game.

Set short- and long-term goals

Research has indicated that both short- and long-term goals are necessary to improve performance over time (Kyllo & Landers 1995). Long-term goals provide you with direction; they give you something to shoot for in the future. But short-term goals are also important because they provide you with feedback concerning how you are progressing towards your long-term goal. In addition, short-term goals can be a source of motivation because you can see immediate improvements in performance.

Set specific measurable goals and target dates

Research (Locke & Latham 1990; Weinberg 1996) has indicated that specific, measurable goals are more effective in enhancing performance than 'do your best' goals, easy goals or no goals. The more clearly your goals are specified, the better they guide you to your long-term objective. Unfortunately, many tennis players tend to set goals that are more general in nature such as becoming mentally tougher, playing more aggressively, reducing unforced errors or improving service. While these may all be worthwhile goals, in their present form they do not provide much useful information. More specific goals such as improving your first serve percentage from 50% to 60% or reducing your unforced errors to fewer than 10 per set would be more helpful and provide a clear-cut way to compare your actual performance to your goal.

Set performance goals instead of outcome goals

In tennis (as with other sports) success is highly valued and as a result players tend to focus solely on the goal of winning. However, research in sport psychology (Duda 1993) has indicated that outcome goals (i.e. winning) are less effective than performance goals (goals relative to your own past performance). One main problem with setting only outcome goals is that reaching your goal is often not in your control. That is, you might play the best match of your life but lose a closely contested match to a player who is also playing extremely well and who happens to be a little more talented than you. If your goal was simply to win, then you might feel disappointed and frustrated. But if your goal was to play well and improve on your past performances, then you would feel satisfied and positive about the match. This does not mean that winning is unimportant or that you should not set any outcome goals. Rather, the problem occurs when tennis players focus solely on winning, then success can only be tied to winning. However, success should be seen in terms of exceeding your own goals rather than merely beating an opponent.

Identify strategies to reach your goals

In my work with tennis players, one of the major mistakes that both players and coaches often make is the failure to identify specific strategies to help players achieve their goals. Although goals can provide direction, you still have to map out a strategy on how to reach them. For example, let us take the example of setting a goal to decrease your unforced groundstroke errors from 15 per set to 10 per set in 2 months. This is a specific, measurable goal but how do you realize this goal? In essence, what are you going to do differently in practice to improve the consistency of your groundstrokes? Some potential strategies might be:

- spend an extra 15 min in practice working on your groundstrokes for depth and consistency;
- hitting with more topspin to provide a greater margin for error; or
- shortening your backswing to avoid overhitting.

In any case, strategies need to accompany goals so a specific plan is in place to help players reach their goals.

Concentration through proper attentional focus

> Very often in a tennis match, you can point to just one game where for a couple of points you lost concentration and didn't do the right thing, and the difference in the match will be right there (Tarshis 1977, p. 21).

The above quote by Bjorn Borg highlights the importance that concentration and proper attentional focus can have on the outcome of a tennis match. Figure 22.2 illustrates focused attention of a tennis player on the ball. The scoring in tennis is such that a brief lapse in concentration can cost you a match. For example, you might have won the first set and are holding serve easily in the second while your opponent is holding with difficulty. Then, serving at 4–4, 30–30, you have an easy high put-away forehand volley but out of the corner of your eye you see that your opponent is running to where you intend to hit it so at the last second you change your mind to hit behind your opponent and miss by a few centimetres. You get momentarily angry and upset with yourself and proceed to double fault. Your opponent is boosted by the break in serve and holds to win the set while you still are thinking about that high volley you missed.

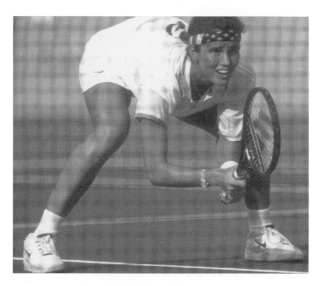

Fig. 22.2 Focused concentration is essential for optimal performance. Photo © Allsport/S. Dunn.

Definition of concentration

Concentration can be defined as the ability to focus on the relevant cues in your environment and to maintain that focus for the duration of the athletic contest. The first part of the definition refers to focusing on important cues in the tennis player's environment. The most obvious, but often overlooked, cue is watching the ball. Although players focus in the general vicinity of the ball, they often do not watch the ball intently. Other relevant cues might include the movements and racket work of your opponent, cues players give themselves before hitting the ball (e.g. racket back, follow-through, forward) or focusing between points on strategy and shot selection. But it is not enough to merely focus on these cues from time to time. Rather, it is the ability to maintain this focus over the course of a match that is especially difficult. One of the keys to Chris Evert's incredible success was her consistency and unusually low amount of unforced errors. This consistency can be traced back to her uncanny concentration ability to stay focused on the match and her shots regardless of the circumstances.

Attentional problems due to inappropriate focus

Many players have problems concentrating throughout a match and this is typically caused by inappropriate attentional focus. Some of the typical problems experienced by tennis players are provided below.

Attending to past events

A concentration problem we all have probably experienced is our inability to forget about the pervious point or game. Focusing on what happened in the past is simply inappropriate and simply undermines our ability to focus on the current point. After missing an easy shot it is often difficult to forget about the mistake and move on to the next point. This is especially difficult when that error led to a break of serve or a missed opportunity to break serve or finish off a set. In a memorable US Open match between Jimmy Connors and Paul Haarhuis, a long spectacular point was won by Connors where Haarhuis repeatedly failed to put away some overheads. That one point appeared to be the turning point in the match as it gave Connors an emotional lift (he drew energy from the partisan crowd) and Haarhuis never seemed to recover.

Attending to future events

Besides worrying about what just happened, many tennis players have attentional problems concerning attending to future events and the consequences of certain actions. Many of these thoughts start with the words 'what if'. For example, 'What if I double-fault?', 'What if I lose (win) the first set?', 'What if I lose my big lead?', 'What if I lose (win) the next point?', or 'What if I have my serve broken?'. The one commonality to all these thoughts is that they are irrelevant to the particular point on which a player should be concentrating. Worrying about what might happen acts purely as a distraction and can cause excess muscle tension and tentative play.

Paralysis by analysis

A final type of attentional problem is focusing on body mechanics during the stroke. When you are learning a new stroke or trying to refine your technique on a particular stroke, it is important to focus on body mechanics and the feel of the movement. Until you integrate this new movement pattern and stroke to the point that they become automatic, your performance is likely to suffer. In fact, this is what practice is all about; focusing on improving your strokes by getting

a better feel of the movement. The problem occurs when this type of focus occurs during a match. For example, after missing a few backhand passing shots you might start to think more about your backhand and wonder if you are following through properly, bending your knees, lifting up too soon or dropping your wrist. If you start to attend to any (or all) of these while hitting your backhand, the likelihood is that you will start thinking too much, causing a 'paralysis by analysis'.

Improving concentration

Now you are aware of some of the typical problems with proper attentional focus that can wreak havoc with your game and your ability to concentrate. To help cope effectively with these problems, several tips for improving on-court concentration are presented below.

Use cue words

One of the best ways to keep your mind focused on the match is through the use of cue words. These simply are words that can help trigger a particular response. These words can have an instructional component (e.g. racket back, firm wrist, follow-through) or they can be more motivational or emotional (relax, strong, easy, move). The key is to keep the cue words simple and let them trigger the desired response. For example, before serving, you might use the cue word, reach, to make sure you get a good extension and aggressively reach and go after the ball.

Routines

Another way to minimize distractions and keep focused is through the use of routines. Because tennis is a sport where there is a small break between each point and a little longer break between games (change-overs), opportunities exist to develop routines during these times. In particular, service and service routines can be very helpful in preparing for the next point and keeping your concentration. The beauty of routines is that no matter what the situation might be (e.g. playing in front of a hostile crowd) or how much pressure is on a particular point (e.g. set point, match point), they allow you to prepare the same exact way for every single point. With consistent practice, a routine will eventually become a habitual, automatic and natural part of your game that you can rely on regardless of the circumstances.

Focus on the seams of the ball

This idea comes from the work of Tim Gallwey (1974), in his book *Inner Game of Tennis*. You often hear players at all levels yell, 'watch the ball'. As noted earlier, many tennis players simply focus in the general vicinity of the ball without really focusing on the ball itself. Watching the seams of the ball forces us to start watching the ball intently from the moment it leaves our opponent's racket to the time it hits ours. In addition, when watching the seams of the ball, our mind becomes absorbed in watching the pattern that it forgets to think about all the other distractions and is less likely to wander. This usually results in more fluid, natural, rhythmic stroke production.

Practice with distractions present

One of the major reasons that our concentration can become erratic during matches is that we become distracted by noise, movement or other disruptions. It always amazes me how a small noise made by someone in the crowd or a little movement can destroy a tennis player's concentration, whereas athletes in other sports such as basketball and football routinely deal with all sorts of distractions and disruptive fan behaviours. One of the ways to cope better with potential distractions in a tennis match is to systematically practise with distractions present. For example, crowd noise can be generated, movement by players in adjoining courts could be created and bad line calls can be incorporated into practice. In fact, research with Olympic athletes (Gould *et al.* 1992) has found that the most successful athletes are those who mentally and physically prepare for distractions and unusual events. Thus, do not always practise under ideal conditions; rather, periodically incorporate typical distractions into practice and learn how to cope effectively with them in preparation for matches.

Play one point at a time—disregard future and past

Since attending to past and future events is one of the main problems with keeping a focused attention,

it stands to reason that playing one point at a time is essential for proper concentration. Of course, this phrase is often used but its importance still cannot be over-emphasized. When Bjorn Borg was asked 'what was the most important reason for his incredibly successful tennis career?' he replied 'it was my ability to play one point at a time and not worry and think about what just happened or what might happen. The only thing that was important was the point to be played.' Remember that playing one point at a time is one of the characteristics that tennis players note when describing their peak performances. Staying in the present requires a focused concentration; this is when our minds start to drift to future and past events. The next section on self-talk will present some suggestions for staying in the present.

Self-talk

In my work with tennis players, I probably work more on improving self-talk than on any other psychological skill. Simply put, any time you think about something, you are engaging in self-talk. Self-talk becomes an asset when it enhances self-esteem, attentional focus and performance, and is thus termed positive self-talk. Conversely, self-talk that gets in the way because it is inappropriate, increases anxiety and undermines concentration and confidence is called negative self-talk. Because we cannot usually eliminate thinking altogether, the key question is not whether to think, but how, what and when to think.

How self-talk works

It is a common misperception that events determine our physical and emotional responses. However, it has been demonstrated that our reactions to events are mediated by our interpretation of the events, not the events themselves. For example, after blowing a big lead and holding five match points before losing an important match, you might react by feeling upset, angry and frustrated. This may cause a lack of motivation and undermine your desire to work hard because despite all your practice, you still 'choke' in big matches. However, instead of putting yourself down and getting discouraged, you might say to yourself, 'I realize that I lost my concentration and I need to work on maintaining focus if I expect to be successful in the future'. In essence, you believe that you have the ability to win but just need to work a little harder in practice. This, in turn, could result in enhanced motivation and resolve to work on improving your concentration in practice.

Ways to use self-talk

There are a variety of areas in which self-talk can help tennis players. A few examples are provided below.

Self-talk to initiate action

Self-talk has been utilized to help players get started and motivated. For example, if you were not moving your feet well and getting into position, you might use words such as *move*, *quick* or *fast* to help speed up your movement on the court.

Self-talk to sustain effort

Although getting started is sometimes difficult, once you get into a match you need to work hard to maintain a high degree of effort. Of course, good conditioning is essential to enable continued high effort, but effort can also be sustained through self-talk with phrases such as '*hang in there*', '*keep it up*' and '*stay with it*'.

Self-talk for skill acquisition

Self-talk can be important when learning new skills and strokes and should be self-instructional in nature. Simple cue words such as *wrist firm*, *elbow straight* or *bend* can help in learning the appropriate sequence of action. This self-talk should be kept to a minimum, because over verbalization can cause problems and we eventually want our strokes to be automatic.

Self-talk for breaking bad habits

Unfortunately, many of us develop bad habits when learning the game of tennis and we have to try to change these at some point in order to push our game forward to higher levels. Self-talk can again help us in this process. For example, if you continue to drop your racket head on your backhand drive, you will typically hit with slice. A cue word such as *wrist firm* would reinforce the habit you are trying to make automatic.

Techniques to improve self-talk

The first step to help gain some control over your self-talk is to become more aware of what you say to yourself and when you say it. Although tennis players tend to know that they say inappropriate things at inappropriate times, they often do not know the specific details and circumstances that bring out different types of self-talk. One way to get a better understanding of the relationship between your self-talk and performance is through self-monitoring.

Self-monitoring

The best way to self-monitor your self-talk is to transcribe it as soon after you get off the court as possible, whether it is a practice or a match. You should be particularly sensitive to the types of situations that trigger destructive negative self-talk such as double-faulting, making unforced errors, losing a critical point or blowing a big lead. Once you get a handle on what situations and circumstances produce negative, destructive self-talk, you are ready to take positive steps to improve your self-talk.

Thought stopping

One way to cope with your negative thoughts is to try to stop them before they hurt your performance. One such technique is known as thought stopping. This involves concentrating on the undesired thought briefly, then using a cue or trigger to stop the thought and clear your mind. The trigger can be a simple word like *stop*, or a trigger like snapping your fingers or hitting your hand against your thigh. Each player needs to determine what works best for them. When first attempting thought stopping, it is best to restrict it to practice. Whenever you start thinking a negative thought just say *stop* out loud and then refocus on a task-related cue such as watching the ball. After you master this you could say *stop* to yourself and practise this until you are ready to use it in matches. Finally, thought stopping could also be practised by using imagery described earlier. Visualizing a situation in which you typically say negative things and then seeing yourself stopping this thought and focusing on a relevant cue will help learn the thought-stopping technique.

Table 22.1 Negative and positive self-talk.
(From Weinberg, R.S. (1988) *The Mental
ADvantage: Developing Your Psychological
Skills in Tennis*, p. 96. Human Kinetics,
Champaign, IL.)

Negative self-talk	(*change to*)	Positive self-talk
You idiot—how could you miss such an easy shot?		Everyone makes mistakes—just concentrate on the next point.
What will everyone think if I lose?		Just give it your best. Winning and losing will take care of itself.
I hope I don't choke again.		Relax and just watch the ball.
He robbed me on the line call—the ball was definitely in.		There's nothing I can do about it. If I play well I'll win anyhow.
I'll take it easy today and work out hard tomorrow.		If I work hard today then the next workout will be easier.
That was a terrible serve.		Just slow down and keep your rhythm and timing.
I'll never win this match.		Just take one point at a time.
I never play well in the wind.		It's windy on both sides of the court. This just requires extra concentration.

Changing negative self-talk to positive self-talk

Although it would be nice to eliminate all negative thoughts, this is very difficult to achieve. One way to cope effectively with these negative thoughts is to change them to positive self-talk, which should help redirect attentional focus and provide encouragement and motivation. Probably the best way to change negative to positive self-talk is to make a list of all the types of self-talk that hurt your performance. The goal is to recognize which situations produce negative self-talk and why. Then try to substitute a positive statement for a negative one. Some examples of changing negative to positive self-talk are provided in Table 22.1. Similar to thought stopping, when changing negative to positive self-talk, first try to do this in practice and also employ imagery to help in the transition. Finally, if you become aware of a negative thought, take a deep breath (because negative thoughts typically occur under stress) and as you exhale, try to relax and repeat the appropriate positive statement.

Countering irrational beliefs

Changing your negative self-talk to positive self-talk will probably not be totally effective if you still believe in the negative statements. For example, if you really believe that your opponent's bad line calls cost you the match, then telling yourself it does not matter probably will not help your performance much. Usually at the core of negative self-talk are what Albert Ellis (1962) calls *irrational beliefs*. In my work with tennis players, there are several beliefs that I have seen consistently when players describe their play. I will briefly list a few of these irrational beliefs.

• *I can play perfect tennis.* This belief leads only to frustration and disappointment. Nobody (not even Pete Sampras or Martina Hingis) plays perfect tennis and feeling that you should not make any mistakes is unrealistic and produces increased muscle tension. Accepting that everyone makes mistakes and attempting to learn from these mistakes is a much more constructive and productive approach.

• *External circumstances are responsible for my losing.* Some players like to blame the wind, court conditions, injuries, bad luck, line calls, etc. for their losses. However, when you lose (or win) you are responsible and you should focus only on things that you can control.

• *My performance on the tennis court reflects my worth as a person.* This is a particularly devastating belief that unfortunately is held too often by junior tennis players (and some adults). Some players develop their self-esteem around their tennis ability and thus they feel more worthy when they win and are depressed and down when they lose. But players should heed the comments of Boris Becker after he was upset in a first round loss at Wimbledon. When asked how he felt, Becker replied, 'Nobody died on centre court today. I only lost a tennis match, nothing more'. Thus, players need to feel good about themselves as people outside tennis and not rely on tennis results to determine their self-worth.

• *Because I played poorly early in a match, I will continue to play poorly.* Although many players believe this statement, research has indicated that early match performance is not a good predictor of later match performance. We have all seen players down a set or two and facing match point fight back to win seemingly impossible matches. And the scoring in tennis is unique in that time never runs out on you so your opponent always has to finish off the match (which is often difficult to do). In fact, if you are playing below the level of your ability, it is more likely that you will improve across a match than keep on playing poorly. So keep your head up and keep battling.

Summary

This chapter has attempted to provide a brief overview of the importance of developing psychological skills to enhance tennis performance as well as the tennis experience itself. If we want to reach our peak performance more consistently, then integrating mental training with your physical training and conditioning is essential. A number of psychological skills have been discussed and specific suggestions put forth on how to develop these skills and integrate them into your daily training regimen. It is hoped that the skills you learn will help you win the mental game. Although you may not always walk off the court a winner, you should be able to effectively control your thoughts and emotions on the court. If you can achieve this end, then you will have come a long way in reaching your physical potential as well as getting more enjoyment and fun out of the game. It is not necessarily an easy trip, but it is a worthwhile pursuit. Have a nice trip.

References

Bandura, A. (1986) *Social Foundations of Thought and Action: A Social Cognitive Theory*. Prentice Hall, Englewood Cliffs, NJ.

Bell, K. (1983) *Championship Thinking*. Prentice Hall, Englewood Cliffs, NJ.

Benson, H. (1975) *The Relaxation Response*. Morrow, New York.

Burton, D., Naylor, S. & Holliday, B. (2001) Goal setting in sport: investigating the goal effectiveness paradox. In: Singer, R., Hausenblaus, H. & Janelle, C., eds. *Handbook of Sport Psychology*, 2nd edn, pp. 497–528. John Wiley, NY.

Duda, J.L. (1993) Goals: a social cognitive approach to the study of achievement motivation in sport. In: Singer, R., Murphey, M. & Tennant, K., eds. *Handbook on Research in Sport Psychology*, pp. 421–436. Macmillian Publishing, New York.

Ellis, A. (1962) *Reason and Emotion in Psychotherapy*. Lyle Stuart, New York.

Gallwey, T. (1974) *Inner Game of Tennis*. Random House, New York.

Gould, D. (2001) Goal setting for peak performance. In: Williams, J., ed. *Applied Sport Psychology: Personal Growth to Peak Performance*, pp. 190–205. Mayfield, Mountain View, CA.

Gould, D., Eklund, R. & Jackson, S. (1992) US Olympic wrestling. I: Mental preparation, precompetitive cognition, and affect. *The Sport Psychologist* **6**, 358–382.

Jackson, S. (1992) Athletes in flow: a qualitative investigation of flow states in elite figure skaters. *Journal of Applied Sport Psychology* **4**, 161–180.

Jackson, S.A. & Csikszentmihalyi, M. (1999) *Flow in Sports*. Human Kinetics, Champaign, IL.

Jacobson, E. (1938) *Progressive Relaxation*. University of Chicago Press, Chicago.

Kyllo, L.B. & Landers, D.M. (1995) Goal setting in sport and exercise: a research synthesis to resolve the controversy. *Journal of Sport and Exercise Psychology* **17**, 117–137.

Locke, E.A. & Latham, G.P. (1990) *A Theory of Goal Setting and Task Performance*. Prentice Hall, Englewood Cliffs, NJ.

Tarshis, B. (1977) Tennis and the mind. *Tennis Magazine*, New York.

Weinberg, R.S. (1998) *The Mental ADvantage: Developing Your Psychological Skills in Tennis*. Human Kinetics, Champaign, IL.

Weinberg, R.S. (1996) Goal setting in sport and exercise: research to practice. In: Van Raalte, J.L. & Brewer, B.W., eds. *Exploring Sport and Exercise Psychology*. American Psychological Association, Washington DC.

Weinberg, R.S., Burton, D., Yukelson, D. & Weigand, D. (1993) Goal setting in competitive sport: an exploratory investigation of practices of collegiate athletes. *The Sport Psychologist* **7**, 275–289.

Chapter 23

ITF involvement in tennis medicine and science

Introduction

The purpose of this chapter is to review the International Tennis Federation's (ITF's) involvement and role in tennis medicine and science as well as to examine the different areas of work within this field.

Tennis is a game for everybody. In approximately 203 countries worldwide, 60 million regular tennis players, both male and female, from the age of 5 to 95, enjoy our great sport.

The ITF is the governing body of tennis worldwide and has several broad areas of responsibility: administering and regulating the game, organizing international competitions and structuring, developing and promoting the game.

The ITF owns the Davis Cup and the Federation Cup, manages the Olympic Tennis Event and sanctions the Hopman Cup. The ITF is also involved with the four Grand Slams—the Australian Open, Roland Garros, Wimbledon and the US Open—through its representation on the Grand Slam Committee and its relationship with the four countries' National Associations.

Within the administration and regulation of the game, the ITF has programmes and initiatives that involve technological and medical issues.

The ITF places great emphasis on medical aspects and the following areas are those in which the ITF is involved.

The ITF Sports Medical Commission

An example of the ITF's attention to medical matters has been the development of the ITF Sports Medical Commission. This Commission reviews the medical and sports science issues related to tennis. Members of the Commission include prominent medical doctors, physiotherapists and sport science experts as well as tennis coaches. It deals with the anti-doping procedures and regulations and the medical implications of the rules of tennis and tournament regulations. Among other issues over which the Commission regularly convenes is the allocation of research grants for researchers interested in studying sports science and medicine matters related to tennis.

The ITF Anti-Doping Programme

The ITF operates a Tennis Anti-Doping Programme in association with both the ATP Tour and the WTA Tour, and the National Associations. Tennis may be regarded as having both horizontal integration with the professional tours and vertical integration down to the grass roots of tennis through the inclusion of the National Associations. The fundamental principles of the Programme are to ensure the health of the players, to uphold both medical and sport ethics and to ensure equality for all competitors.

The Programme is based upon the Olympic Movement Anti-Doping Code and is operated in accordance with internationally accepted practices. The Programme is not merely concerned with deterrence through testing but it also involves education projects and the access to information through the provision of a 24-h telephone helpline. The ITF is rightfully proud of the Tennis Anti-Doping Programme and continues to develop and refine the Programme to retain a position as a world leader and example to other sports.

Olympics

Tennis returned to the Olympic Games as a full medal sport at Seoul in 1988 after an absence of 64 years.

It was one of the original sports at the first modern Olympiad in Athens in 1896 and tennis featured in all of the Olympic Games until Paris in 1924. Tennis was also a demonstration sport in Mexico in 1968 and in Los Angeles in 1984. From Barcelona 1992 to Sydney 2000, tennis has firmly established itself as one of the permanent and most attractive events in the Olympic programme.

The cooperation of the ITF and IOC together with the organizing Olympic Committees at all Olympic

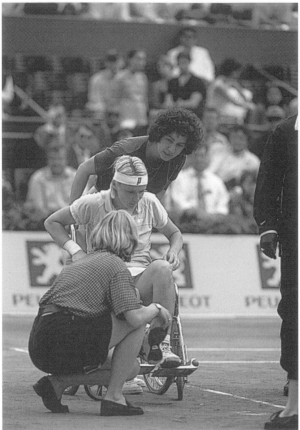

Fig. 23.1 Jana Novotna being wheeled off court at the 1999 French Open. Photo © S. Wake.

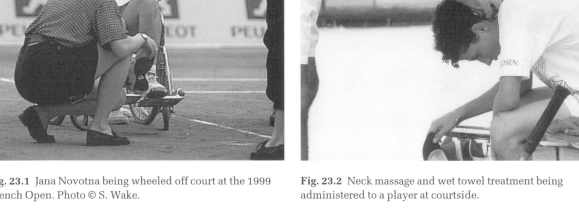

Fig. 23.2 Neck massage and wet towel treatment being administered to a player at courtside.

venues has been instrumental for the successful management of the tennis-related medical issues at each Olympic Games.

Grand Slams

The Grand Slams are the four official International Championships of Australia, France, United Kingdom and the United States. Each Grand Slam is held in accordance with the Grand Slam Rules that have been developed by the Grand Slam Committee.

As per medical issues, these rules specify minimum rest periods between matches and the procedures to be followed during an injury time-out. They further state the need for a medical doctor to be on site at all Grand Slams (Figs 23.1 and 23.2).

Men's tennis and Davis Cup

The Davis Cup is the largest annual team competition in sport and celebrated its centenary in 1999. This most prestigious international team event gives players the chance to represent their country and in doing so, demands unique qualities from its competitors.

Rule 5 of the ITF Davis Cup Regulations for the Competition provide medical control guidelines for the arrangement of the competition. These guidelines state that National Associations entering the Davis Cup and those players nominated to compete on their behalf agree to, as a condition of entry, abide by the ITF Anti-Doping Policy. These regulations also include a waiver of claims.

An appendix is included in the rules with the procedure for anti-doping testing control at Davis Cup ties.

The Davis Cup code of conduct includes an injury/toilet break rule. This rule defines the procedures to follow when a player sustains an accidental injury during the warm-up and match. It also provides examples of accidental injuries and outlines some possible treatments. It states the conditions in which the player may receive consultation, medical supplies and treatment from a medical trainer or tournament doctor, if available, during the injury time-out applied. Guidelines pertaining to the toilet break are also included.

The Davis Cup regulations also include minimum standards for the organization of World Group Davis Cup ties. These standards state that the home nation shall be responsible for the formulation, administration and implementation of a comprehensive safety system that ensures, as far as reasonably practicable, the security, health and safety of all members and officials of both teams and of ITF officials.

In the regulations for ITF Satellite Series Tournaments, it is stated that each tournament must provide at its sole expense a Tournament doctor to be available at all times. Furthermore, to provide sufficient recovery for players and minimize the prospect of excessive fatigue and/or overuse injuries, players may not enter or compete in more than one tournament or circuit per week.

Futures tournaments and satellite circuits are open to all male tennis players based on merit and without discrimination provided, however, that minors under the age of 14 are not eligible for entry. For the purposes of this rule, the player's age as of the first day of the tournament shall be used.

Women's tennis and the Federation Cup

The Federation Cup is the world's premier Women's Tennis Team Event. Like the Davis Cup in the men's game, it gives players the opportunity to represent their country at the highest level. This competition has been attracting the world's best female players for decades.

An important medical issue in the female game is that of age eligibility. The rules governing the issue are applicable to the Federation Cup competition as well as all other professional tournaments worldwide offering prize money of more than US$10 000.

Junior tennis

Through the ITF's member nations, tournaments for players 18 and under are staged throughout the year. More than 150 events, in almost 100 countries comprise the ITF Junior Calendar. The ITF also publishes the official 18 and under junior world ranking for singles and doubles. This ranking includes more than 4500 competitors from all over the world. Other significant junior competitions run by the ITF include the ITF Sunshine Cup and the ITF Conolly Continental Cup as well as the World Junior Tennis Championships.

The importance of addressing medical issues in junior tennis cannot be understated given the delicate balance between growth and development during these early years. Some of the coaching literature published by the ITF includes recommendations pertaining to the appropriate training principles to be followed when working with junior players. These principles include the recommended number of matches per player each year and various training guidelines: correct training intensities, volumes, frequencies and work/rest ratios. All of these principles and guidelines will help players, coaches, parents and officials to ensure a safe tennis practice, which will avoid overtraining and burnout, especially at the junior level (Fig. 23.3).

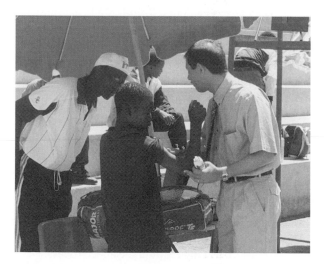

Fig. 23.3 A junior player being attended by a medical doctor at courtside.

An anti-doping education project for junior players is also under study. It is believed that this project is necessary in order to tackle the possible implications of drug abuse at young ages.

Wheelchair tennis

Medical issues are a key aspect of wheelchair tennis. The ITF Rules of Tennis include the rules for wheelchair tennis. These rules outline the medical criteria and provide examples of permanent disabilities that the wheelchair tennis player must satisfy to be eligible to compete. Quadriplegic players are also considered within these rules. The ITF, in the *Wheelchair Tennis Handbook*, provides the regulations for a medical condition (injury or illness) suffered during the match or warm-up. In addition, Appendix 3 of the Rules of Tennis includes the wheelchair tennis player challenges and procedures for a player's eligibility. The appendix details the parties that have the right to question a player's eligibility as well as the procedures of the eligibility subcommittee regarding the medical evidence submitted by the player.

The injury rule for wheelchair tennis provides clarification for treatable and non-treatable medical conditions. It also regulates the conditions treatable on a change-over and the time-out procedure during a match and during the warm-up. This wheelchair injury rule also provides the guidelines for the medical suspension of play.

The ITF has a Wheelchair Tennis Medical Commission, which is comprised of world-renowned medical experts in the field. This commission deals with all medical issues related to wheelchair tennis.

ITF wheelchair tennis coach education publications such as the *ITF Wheelchair Tennis Manual*, and the *ITF Take Two* magazine include specific information on medicine and sports science for wheelchair tennis coaches.

Cooperation with other organizations

As aforementioned the cooperation between the ITF and the IOC in tennis-related medical issues is of great importance. The collaboration between the ITF, ATP and WTA to facilitate the effectiveness of the anti-doping programme has been similarly emphasized.

The ITF is also assisting organizations such as The Society of Tennis Medicine and Science in the spreading of medical and scientific knowledge through the *Medicine and Science Newsletter*. By endorsing several sports medicine tennis congresses worldwide the ITF is also doing its utmost to increase the accessibility of this information.

Additionally, among ITF internet initiatives is the cooperation with the ISBS (International Society of Sports Biomechanics) to establish links between websites in order to better distribute scientific and medical information to all those interested in tennis.

Technology

Nothing has contributed more to establishing tennis as one of the world's major sports than science and technology. The ITF, through their Technical Commission, protects the nature of the game by monitoring developments in racket and ball technology, and the facilities necessary to enjoy the sport at all levels. As custodians of the Rules of Tennis, the ITF decides if innovations bring a genuine benefit to the game, or if they constitute a threat. In 1997, the ITF expanded its technical programme and set up an internal testing laboratory to monitor such innovations.

The ITF has also taken a proactive role in development of rackets, strings, balls and court surfaces. One of the most important ITF initiatives in this regard has been the recognition and use of the bigger ball. Medical implications of this type of ball, as per injuries and load on the player's arm, are currently under study. Preliminary findings seem to suggest that the 6% increase in ball size does not have any adverse effects on the player.

Research and resources on medicine and sports science

It is the aim of the ITF to support research and the publication of resources in the sports sciences. In order to do so, the ITF is fostering tennis-specific research in the areas of: sports biomechanics, exercise physiology, motor learning, sports nutrition, sports psychology and sports medicine.

The ITF Research Grants Programme supports research and the publication of resources specific to tennis, conducted by individuals who are independently, or in conjunction with academic institutions, exploring information related to the teaching or playing of tennis. The results of this research are then distributed to coaches, parents and players around the world. The ITF's aim is to help players be the best they can be; it is hoped that this research programme will help to pave the way.

Expectations are that more substantive and well-supported research will lead to more effective approaches and programmes for developing young talent, as well as for satisfying the concerns of recreational participants.

Coach education

One of the main areas of responsibility of the ITF Tennis Development Department is coach education. Education of coaches on matters pertaining to sports science has been revealed as one of the key factors to increase not only the quality of players worldwide but also the number of people playing the game.

The ITF has produced a syllabus of contents that is delivered in coaching courses. These contents include comprehensive information on all of the sports science disciplines used by coaches such as biomechanics, teaching methodology, exercise physiology, nutrition and sports medicine.

Within the coaching courses, the ITF places considerable emphasis on the idea that the coach, the doctor and the physiotherapist need to understand each other's role in the prevention, treatment and rehabilitation of injuries. All three should be seen by the players to be working together.

The courses further emphasize that coaches should make effective use of sports medicine by having a clear understanding of the mechanisms behind the most common tennis injuries to thus appreciate how they can be prevented. A similar understanding of their role in emergency first response and when dealing with the injured player or assisting with the recuperation, is also of importance.

ITF coach education publications such as the *ITF Level I Manual*, *ITF Advanced Coaches Manual* and the *ITF Coaching Sport Science Review* include specific information on medicine and sports science for tennis coaches.

Conclusion

As illustrated within this chapter, the ITF has an important involvement in medicine and sports science. However, this involvement can be further improved by increasing the direct application of medical and sport science knowledge to the world of tennis.

Successful tennis practice and organization will be enormously benefited by more research in medicine and sports science. Similarly an improvement in the communication between all parties involved will help to achieve a full application of these findings in the practical context.

Medicine, science and technology are impacting on every aspect of the game. The ITF is acting as a catalyst for different tennis initiatives and is eager to increase the tennis specific scientific and medical knowledge of all tennis persons to provide for the further advancement of our sport.

Recommended reading

Crespo, M., Pluim, B. & Reid, M. (eds) (2001) *Tennis Medicine for Tennis Coaches*. ITF Ltd, London.
Grand Slam Committee (2000) *Official Grand Slam Men's Rule Book*.
ITF Ltd (1998) *Advanced Coaches Manual*.
ITF Ltd (1999) *ITF Approved Tennis Balls*.
ITF Ltd (2000) *ITF Junior Circuit Regulations*.
ITF Ltd (2000) *ITF Men's Circuit Rule Book*.
ITF Ltd (2000) *ITF Regulations for the 2000 Competition: Davis Cup 2000*.
ITF Ltd (2000) *ITF Regulations for the 2000 Competition: Federation Cup 2000*.
ITF Ltd (2000) *ITF Rules of Tennis 2000*.
ITF Ltd (2000) *ITF Wheelchair Tennis Handbook 2000*.

Chapter 24

Medical services

in men's and women's

professional tennis

Introduction

The ATP and the Sanex WTA Tour together serve over 1500 professional tennis players worldwide. These players are from over 60 different countries, speak more than 20 different languages and range in age from 14 to 42. The year-long professional tennis season begins in January and continues through November with only a 6-week 'off-season'. There are 75 tournaments played in 21 different countries. The average player travels 80 000 km (50 000 miles) each year on the professional tennis circuit. Matches are played on several different surfaces including clay, hard and grass courts, and can last for more than 5 h. Weather conditions can vary from climate-controlled indoor events to outdoor matches with temperatures over 37°C and humidity over 90%.

Professional tennis is one of the truly major international sports. It is a very physically, mentally and emotionally demanding sport. The players are hard-training and dedicated professionals. These top-level athletes therefore require medical services of the highest quality. It is the goal of the sports medicine team to ensure that the players can perform at safe and optimal levels on court.

With this in mind, the organizational bodies of the ATP and the Sanex WTA Tour have developed high-quality medical services for professional tennis tournaments around the world. The challenges are many. Injury prevention, treatment of musculoskeletal injuries and other medical problems, rehabilitation and player education are all important aspects of the medical services provided on a daily basis at these tournaments.

The medical services of the Sanex WTA Tour

The medical service team on the Sanex WTA Tour is comprised of several members who contribute to the care of the players at tournament sites. The team is headed by a sports medicine trained physician and a Director of the Sport Sciences and Medicine Department.

In addition, there are highly specialized members of the team who have attained formal university degrees in both physical therapy and athletic training (PT, ATC) which we designate as primary health care providers (PHCPs). These PHCPs are the first health care providers that the players see. They evaluate and treat players on court when injuries occur and prepare the players for their matches with various soft tissue techniques, taping skills and warm-up procedures. The care they provide ranges from minor first aid for blisters and abrasions, to emergency care for heat-related illness. They also assist players with therapeutic exercise programmes for rehabilitation of injuries, modalities for pain relief (including ultrasound, electrical stimulation and biofeedback) and manual therapy techniques for joint and soft-tissue injuries (Fig. 24.1).

The PHCPs are supported on-site by a Tournament Physician. This is a sports medicine trained physician who is responsible for all aspects of the medical care of the players on-site.

The massage therapists on the Sanex WTA Tour are trained in providing a wide variety of massage techniques, including neuromuscular, deep tissue, shiatsu, myofascial and neural tension release. Players typically schedule massage after their match or

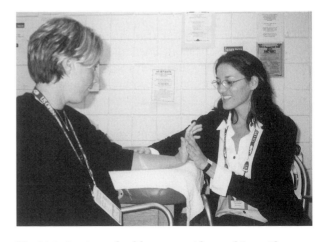

Fig. 24.1 A primary health care provider working with a Sanex WTA Tour player on wrist mobilization techniques.

practice session to promote increased circulation, and relieve muscle tension and mental stress.

The medical services of the ATP

The task of providing medical services to this group of elite athletes is the responsibility of the ATP Medical Services Committee. The committee is headed by an American and a European Medical Director, both of whom are practising sports medicine orthopaedic surgeons. European trained registered physiotherapists (RPTs) and American trained certified athletic trainers (ATCs) comprise the ATP's 'sports medicine trainers' (SMTs). The role of the SMTs is very similar in scope to the PHCPs on the Sanex WTA Tour. A Traveling Sports Medicine Fellow and an Administrative Coordinator are the other members of the Medical Services Committee. In addition to the responsibility of providing medical care to the players, the Medical Services Committee is also involved in player education and tennis-specific sports medicine research.

A worldwide network of tournament physicians has been developed to ensure the availability of high-quality medical care to the players at all tournaments.

Pre-participation medical screening

All players who become eligible for the main ATP tournaments (Division I players) are required to attend the ATP University in Ponte Vedra Beach, Florida, or Monte Carlo, Monaco, where a comprehensive medical evaluation is performed as a requirement for participation on the circuit. This ensures the general health of the player and identifies any special medical needs he may have. The players are instructed about the rules governing medical time-outs and interventions during the course of a match. Educational information about nutrition, hydration, conditioning, injury prevention and rehabilitation is provided.

The Sanex WTA Tour conducts medical screening physicals throughout the year at the tournaments to ensure the health of their players and address any medical concerns the players may have. Healthcare plans and sport-specific therapeutic exercise programmes are given to the players following their physical examination. Educational materials are provided to players throughout the year.

Tournament medical services

Personnel

On-site medical services for the players is overseen by the Tournament Physician who is sports medicine trained and English speaking. The Tournament Physician, who often practises locally, is responsible for coordinating all aspects of medical coverage for the event. A network of specialists including, but not limited to, internal medicine, cardiology, radiology, ENT, dermatology and dentistry should be available for off-site consultation. Availability of an orthotist to fabricate custom orthotics is helpful as biomechanical foot problems are not uncommon.

Between one and three SMTs/PHCPs, depending on the event, are present at every tournament. They travel during the professional tennis season with the ATP or Sanex WTA Tour and serve as the primary medical providers for the players. They are responsible for evaluating, treating and recording injuries during the event and for communicating with the appropriate medical personnel at upcoming events so that continuity of care is assured. Additionally, they provide a written evaluation of the medical services at the completion of each tournament to ensure that the highest level of care is maintained and that any problems are addressed.

Qualified sports-trained massage therapists are required at all tournaments. Their services are utilized at the request of the players or by referral from the SMT/PHCP or Tournament Physician.

A properly staffed first aid station and an emergency medical unit (EMS) are generally present at all tournaments for the care of the spectators. Occasionally, use of the EMS for transportation of a player to the hospital is necessary. The Tournament Physician and SMTs/PHCPs are not responsible for the medical care of the spectators.

An organizational meeting between the Tournament Physician and the SMT/PHCP is held prior to the start of the tournament. Information regarding physician coverage and local hospital and pharmacy accessibility is confirmed along with availability of diagnostic modalities such as radiography, magnetic resonance imaging (MRI) and ultrasound. A tour of the medical facilities concludes the pretournament meeting.

The Tournament Physician or another qualified sports medicine trained physician and the SMT/PHCP are on-site 1 h before play begins until play is completed each day. Communication is maintained between the physician and the SMT/PHCP as well as the tournament referee and the tournament supervisor at all times. All ATP tournament physicians providing on-site medical coverage have reviewed the *ATP Tournament Physician's Handbook* prior to tournament play. This handbook outlines the responsibilities of tournament physicians and provides guidelines for management of all issues related to the medical care of the athletes at the tournament. Similar guidelines are provided by the WTA for their tournament physicians.

Medical facilities and equipment

The medical facility at the tournament site is designated the 'Player Treatment Area' which includes a training room, a separate physician's examination room and a massage area. It should be located adjacent to the players' locker room. There should be easy access to all courts in order to facilitate on-court player treatment.

The training room should be climate controlled to prevent exposure of the players to large variations in temperature. For a 32-player draw, at least one hydraulic treatment table and a separate massage table is needed. More treatment and massage tables are necessary at tournaments with larger draws. Ample shelf and storage space is necessary.

A dedicated television monitor in the training room is helpful so that the players and the SMTs/PHCPs can monitor matches in progress to help in the timing of player preparation for the upcoming matches. A walkie-talkie system is used to maintain communication among the medical staff.

Proper medical equipment and supplies for the evaluation and treatment of player injuries and illnesses are required. The SMT's/PHCP's equipment includes a fully stocked and well-organized training kit, ultrasound and electrical stimulation units, a hydroculator and supplies for athletic taping. Therapeutic exercise equipment such as Swiss balls and elastic resistance bands are also available.

The Tournament Physician's equipment should include a stethoscope, otoscope, ophthalmoscope, blood pressure cuff, oral or otic thermometer and reflex hammer. Intravenous fluids with their accompanying delivery system are on-site. Medications should be stored in a locked cabinet in the physician's room.

A continuously stocked supply of ice and oral fluids including water and sports drinks, both refrigerated and unrefrigerated, is maintained in the Player Treatment Area.

Player treatment

Prematch treatment

In preparation for a match, players often require the attention of the SMT/PHCP directed at either the ongoing treatment of a specific injury or injury prevention in general. Dynamic passive and active stretching of major muscle groups in the upper and lower extremities as well as the spine may be helpful in preventing muscle–tendon injuries and enhancing performance. It is carried out in systematic fashion on the treatment table (Fig. 24.2). Moist heat, warming creams, electrical stimulation and ultrasound may be utilized to manage problems of soreness and stiffness. Heat has the ability to improve tissue elasticity, which may improve muscle function.

Taping of joints is performed to add support to injured areas. Twenty per cent of all treatments include taping. This is most commonly done on the ankle, wrist, knee and finger. Taping may be combined with bracing for ankle sprains and chronic ankle instability.

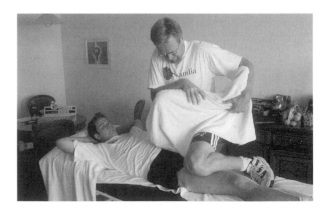

Fig. 24.2 Sports medicine trainer performing prematch stretching on an ATP player.

Strapping of muscles with elastic wraps and tape is utilized to provide compression and support for injured muscles. This technique is most often used for quadriceps and hamstring injuries.

Sports braces are made available to the players. These are most commonly used for the ankle and the knee to add stability. Neoprene sleeves may be helpful by generating heat. They are typically useful for thigh strains and for chronic knee and elbow discomfort.

Protective padding is used to treat pressure areas generally on the feet and hands. The high shear forces and constant pressure on the skin from the shoe and racket grip may result in blistering and callus formation. Tape and antifriction pads are used in the treatment of blisters. Calluses may be carefully shaved when thick and mature. Proper attention to these seemingly minor problems is important as they can be a source of significant discomfort and interfere with player performance.

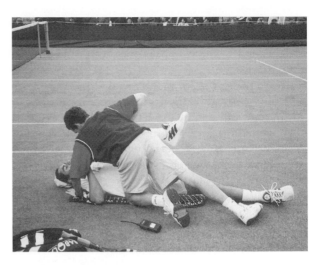

Fig. 24.3 Sports medicine trainer treating an ATP player during a 'court call'. Photo © Dr D. Vilmos.

On-court treatment

Precise rules of the ATP and Sanex WTA Tour at their respective sanctioned events and the ITF at the Grand Slams govern the treatment of players on court during a match. It is the SMTs'/PHCPs' responsibility to be ready and available to respond to any on-court medical problem during a match.

Players are entitled to ask the chair umpire for on-court assistance from the SMT/PHCP at any point in the match. He or she is contacted by walkie-talkie for a 'court call' and arrives on court as quickly as possible to assist the player and avoid any unnecessary delay in the match. They carry to the court a fully stocked trainer's kit, prepared to treat a variety of medical problems that may occur during the course of a match. These most commonly include sprains, strains, blisters, cramping and heat-related problems. More serious conditions such as fractures, dislocations, acute disc herniations, heat stroke and cardiac problems are fortunately much less common. The SMT/PHCP may request the assistance of the Tournament Physician in difficult cases.

The medical time-out begins with the SMT's/PHCP's assessment of the problem. The SMT/PHCP discusses their medical evaluation with the player, after which the player can choose to receive treatment or retire from the match. In making this decision, it is

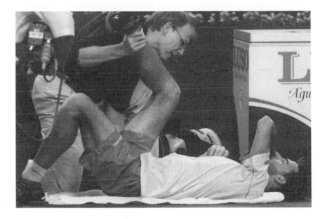

Fig. 24.4 Sports medicine trainer treating an ATP player during a 'court call'.

imperative that the player understands the possible impact of continued play on his or her condition. If he or she chooses to receive treatment, a 3-min time-out is allotted by the chair umpire during which the SMT/PHCP proceeds with on-court medical treatment (Figs 24.3 and 24.4).

Each player is allowed only one medical time-out for treatment of a particular condition. However, the player is entitled to receive further treatment for this same condition by the SMT/PHCP during the 90-s change-overs between games. He or she may also be granted additional time-outs for treatment of other conditions, which may occur during the course of the match.

Postmatch treatment

Following completion of a match, players will often require medical attention. Ice is often utilized to reduce pain and inflammation associated with musculoskeletal injuries following play. Electrical stimulation may also be beneficial in the treatment of inflammation and swelling. Dynamic, passive and active stretching can help prevent the development of activity-related muscle tightness. Any new problems that may have developed during the match as well as all ongoing conditions are fully assessed by the SMT/PHCP and, if necessary, referred to the Tournament Physician for further evaluation.

Many professional tennis players utilize the services of massage therapists. The sports massage can be a general body massage or directed specifically at a problematic area. The therapeutic benefits of massage may include increased local tissue circulation and a feeling of general well being.

Evaluation of injury

The SMTs/PHCPs are the primary health-care providers for the players. An SMT/PHCP is present at every tournament, which is extremely important in establishing and maintaining a sound relationship between the players and the medical team. Although a 'Team Physician' does not travel with the players as in many other professional sports, the tournament physicians, who are generally the same from year to year, together with the SMTs/PHCPs provide the players with the necessary medical team framework. Since 1999, the ATP has also employed a Travelling Sports Medicine Fellow to provide additional medical assistance at selected tournaments to improve continuity of care.

A thorough history is necessary in evaluating injuries and illnesses in these players. Travel-related factors including fatigue, climate variations, dietary changes and sleeping conditions may be important. Performance-related stress may also play a significant role in these athletes. A player who has not been winning may focus more on minor musculoskeletal or general medical symptoms than when he or she is winning matches consistently.

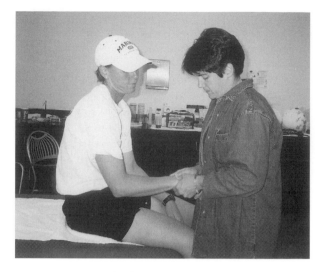

Fig. 24.5 A primary health care provider evaluating a player injury in the training room.

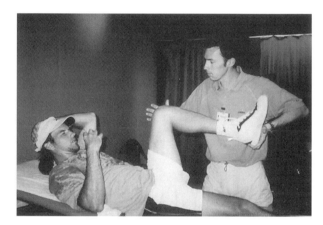

Fig. 24.6 A sports medicine trainer evaluating a player injury in the training room.

A problem-based physical examination follows the history. When evaluating an injury (Figs 24.5 and 24.6), care should be taken to avoid focusing on the injury as an isolated problem, as it may very well be related to an imbalance or other problem elsewhere in the body. For example, elbow pain may be the presenting symptom in a player with a primary shoulder problem. Due to compensatory mechanisms related to the shoulder, the elbow may experience increased stresses resulting in secondary elbow injury. Similarly, lower extremity malalignments may present as knee, hip or back pain.

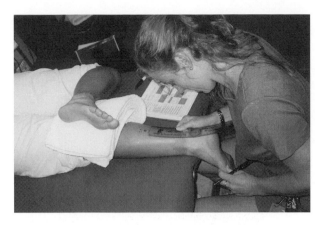

Fig. 24.7 A primary health care provider evaluating alignment in the locker room.

Changes in grip, stroke technique such as more lift on the forehand or more kick on the serve or changes in shoes, racket, strings or string tension, may be an inciting factor in player injuries (Fig. 24.7). Often, a sudden change in the player's fitness and conditioning programme will lead to injury. If a player changes to a new coach, it could mean a change in all these parameters at the same time. Another important risk factor is the playing surface. The stresses on the body vary from surface to surface, related to factors such as friction and shock absorption, and therefore changes in surface during the season may be an additional risk factor. Therefore, it is important for the player, SMT/PHCP, physician and coach to communicate and work together closely.

Following the initial history and physical examination, a provisional diagnosis is usually possible. When indicated, the player may be referred to the Tournament Physician for further evaluation. If further diagnostic testing such as radiographs or MRI scanning is necessary, this is arranged expeditiously, usually at a local facility. The diagnosis is discussed between the Tournament Physician, the SMT/PHCP and the player. The player is educated about his or her condition and alternatives of treatment. Recommendations regarding treatment and return to competition are made. A treatment plan is then outlined and initiated. If the injury precludes the player from continuing to compete in the tournament, the Tournament Supervisor and Tournament Director are notified. Following recovery from an injury, players must be evaluated

and cleared by a tournament physician prior to returning to competition at a subsequent event.

Player injury and confidentiality

All injuries and illnesses that require medical attention are documented. This information becomes part of the player's medical record. Continuous communication among the SMTs/PHCPs and physicians assures the continuity of care necessary to effectively evaluate and treat the athletes. As in any medical practice, however, patient confidentiality is always a priority. Information regarding player injuries must be discussed and signed off with the player prior to its release to the media. All examination and test results are confidential and are used for internal purposes only. The goal is to disseminate accurate information without compromising confidentiality. The Tournament Physician, Tournament Director, Communications Manager and Tournament Supervisor need to be involved when an injury attracts the interest of the media. The Communications Manager will relay information to the media after discussion with the above group. When a press conference is necessary for a player injury, the player may be accompanied by the SMT/PHCP and/or Tournament Physician to discuss the medical aspects of the condition.

Support function of the medical team

Psychologically, the presence of full-time SMTs/PHCPs at all the tournaments is very important. Trust and confidence are established between the players and the SMTs/PHCPs. They play an important role in helping the players deal with the physical and emotional tress of their lives as professional athletes.

When injury or illness does occur, the players rely on the SMTs/PHCPs to coordinate their care. They educate the players about their medical conditions, communicate with treating physicians and assist the players in a safe return to competition.

The future

Providing the highest level of medical care to this unique group of athletes is an ongoing challenge. Efforts continue towards improving medical record keeping and communication among the SMTs/PHCPs, tournament physicians and the players' private physicians through injury-tracking software programs. This will allow for the most effective medical management of injury and illness in the players.

Additionally, it will provide important information that can be utilized for tennis-specific sports medicine research. This, in turn, will result in better insight into injury prevention and treatment in the professional tennis player.

Index